W0050169

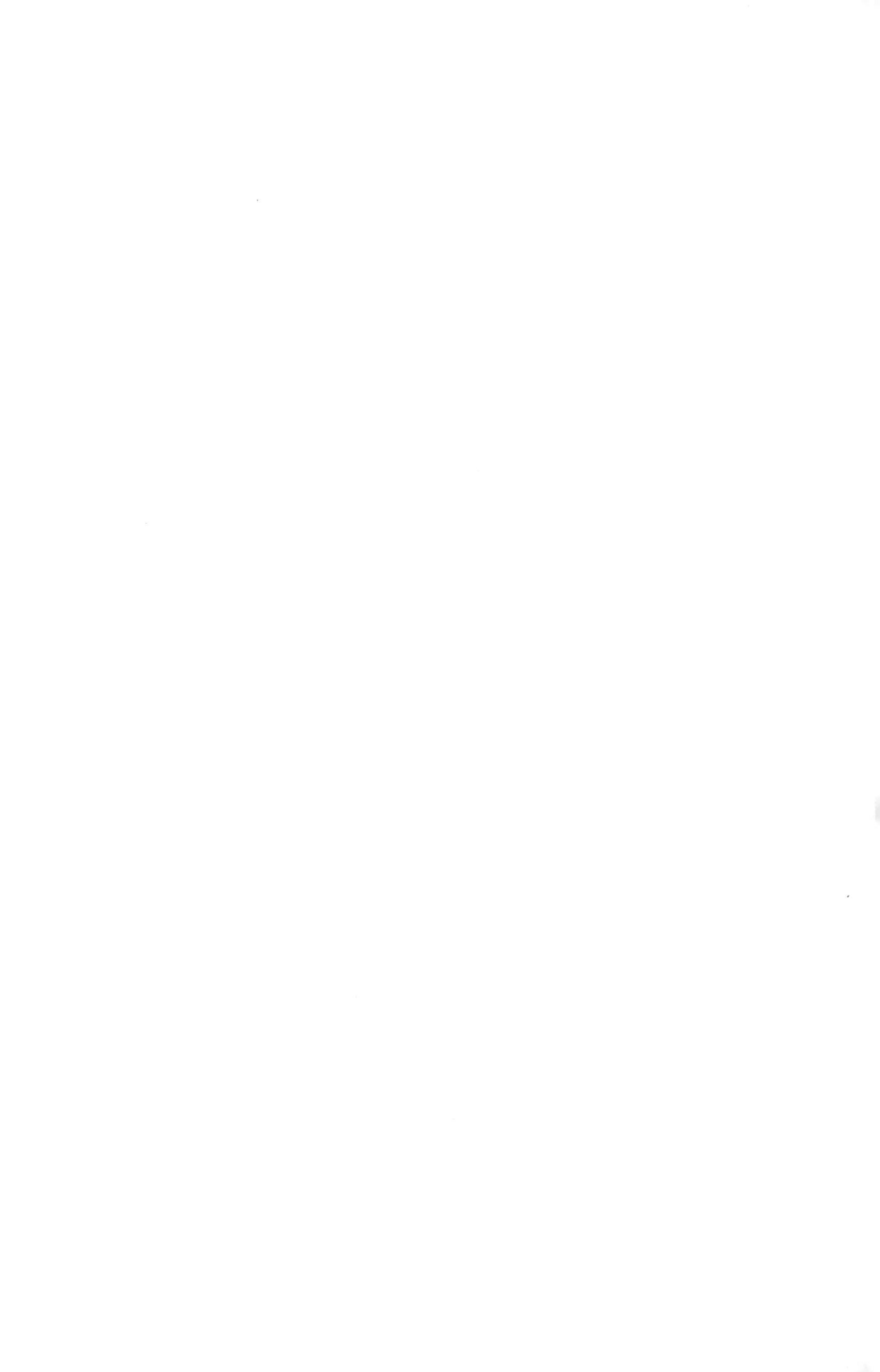

Immunobiology of the
Head and Neck

CONTRIBUTORS

Robert C. Bone, MD
Scripps Clinic and Research Foundation
La Jolla, California

Dennis E. Chenoweth, MD, PhD
Veterans Administration Medical Center
San Diego, California

Sherman Fong, PhD
Scripps Clinic and Research Foundation
La Jolla, California

Michael G. Goodman, MD
Scripps Clinic and Research Foundation
La Jolla, California

Jeffrey P. Harris, MD, PhD
University of California
San Diego Medical Center
San Diego, California

Arnold E. Katz, MD, MS, FACS
Tufts-New England Medical Center
Boston, Massachusetts

Wim Kuijpers, PhD
University of Nijmegen
Nijmegen, The Netherlands

David A. Mathison, MD
Scripps Clinic and Research Foundation
La Jolla, California

Diana Marquardt, MD
University of California
San Diego Medical Center
San Diego, California

Mario S. Nemirovsky, MD
Universite de Sherbrooke
Sherbrooke, Quebec

Marek Rola-Pleszczynski, MD, FRCP(C)
Universite de Sherbrooke
Sherbrooke, Quebec

Bram Rose, MD, PhD, FRSC
McGill University
Montreal, Quebec

Allen F. Ryan, PhD
University of California at San Diego
La Jolla, California

Mary Ann South, MD
NINCDS-Infectious Disease Branch
Bethesda, Maryland

Philip M. Sprinkle, MD
West Virginia University Medical Center
Morgantown, West Virginia

Jan E. Veldman, MD, PhD
University of Utrecht
Utrecht, The Netherlands

Robert W. Veltri, PhD
Cooper Biomedical, Inc.
Malvern, Pennsylvania

Sharyn M. Walker, PhD
Children's Hospital of Los Angeles
Los Angeles, California

Stephen I. Wasserman, MD
University of California
La Jolla, California

Immunobiology of the Head and Neck

Edited by
Jacques F. Poliquin
Allen F. Ryan
Jeffrey P. Harris

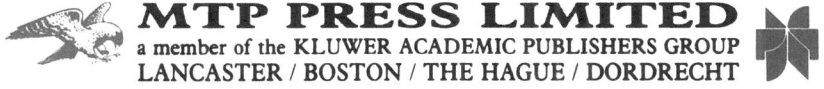
MTP PRESS LIMITED
a member of the KLUWER ACADEMIC PUBLISHERS GROUP
LANCASTER / BOSTON / THE HAGUE / DORDRECHT

MTP Press Limited
a member of Kluwer Academic Publishers Group
Lancaster/Boston/The Hague/Dordrecht

British Library Cataloguing in Publication Data

Immunobiology of the head and neck.

    1. Immunology
    I. Poliquin, Jacques F.   II. Ryan, Allen F.   III. Harris, Jeffrey P.
    616.07'9   QR181

ISBN-13: 978-94-010-8960-9   e-ISBN-13: 978-94-009-5582-0
DOI: 978-94-009-5582-0

College-Hill Press, Inc.
4284 41st Street
San Diego, California 92105

Library of Congress Cataloging in Publication Data
Main entry under title:

Immunobiology of the head and neck.

    Bibliography: p.
    Includes index.
    1. Otolaryngology. 2. Immunologic diseases. 3. Immunology. I. Poliquin, Jacques F., 1941.
II. Ryan, Allen, F., 1945. III. Harris, Jeffrey, P. (Jeffrey Paul), 1949.
RF46.5.I46   1984   617'.51079   83-26312

TABLE OF CONTENTS

PREFACE

This work reviews the basic concepts of immunology and introduces the reader to the latest findings on immunological aspects of diseases of the head and neck. In the past two decades, there has been an explosion of new knowledge in immunology. The contributors to this volume, all of whom have been active in clinical and basic research, describe how recent discoveries in immunology play an increasingly vital role in the understanding and care of patients with head and neck diseases.

An important teaching tool for the resident in training and a valuable reference work for physicians in practice, this book will be of special interest to otolaryngologist-head and neck surgeons, surgical oncologists, pediatricians, allergists, rheumatologists and educators desiring an advanced text in the field.

Jacques F. Poliquin, MD
Allen F. Ryan, PhD
Jeffrey P. Harris, MD, PhD

INTRODUCTION

Immunology has been traced back at least to 1000 AD, when the Chinese discovered that the inhalation of smallpox crusts had some value in prevention of the disease. However, immunology as a science has developed almost entirely within the last 100 years.

Immunity was the primary concept from which this specialty developed, due to clinical preoccupation with host defense against infection. The discovery by Edward Jenner, then a medical student, that inoculation with cowpox crusts protected man from smallpox, assured the future of immunobiology. With the work of Louis Pasteur at the end of the 19th century on fowl cholera organisms and rabies, active rather than passive immunization became the procedure of choice in the prevention of many infectious diseases. Robert Koch, around the same time, discovered delayed hypersensitivity to tuberculosis which unwittingly opened the field of cell-mediated immunity. The last 20 years of the past century were rich in discoveries, primary among them the work of Roux and Yersin on the exotoxin of the diphtheria bacillus. Their work led to that of von Behring on the production of antitoxin and opened the way to immunotherapy. The discovery by Pfeiffer and Border of complement, a substance in the serum distinct from antibody, led to the use of the agglutination reaction in the diagnosis of typhoid fever (Widal test).

At the turn of the 20th century, two different concepts emerged from which modern immunology has developed. Paul Ehrlich proposed the humoral theory of antibody formation, and Elie Metchnikoff developed a competing, cellular theory of immunity. Both were correct and it is now recognized that cellular and humoral aspects of immunity are both interrelated and interdependent. At about the same time, von Pirquet coined the term *allergy* to mean *altered reactivity* of the host.

Immunology has since moved toward defining the mechanisms involved in immunity and in subdividing these responses into specific and nonspecific. It became evident that immunologic responses served three functions—defense, homeostasis, and surveillance. Defense is involved in resistance to infection, homeostasis in removal of worn-out *self* components, and surveillance refers to the detection and destruction of mutant cells. Major discoveries in immunology accumulated slowly over the first half of the 20th century, marked by the work of Landsteiner on the major human blood groups with the ABO system, the work of Prausnitz and Kustner with the PK test, and the description of reagin or IgE. Wiener and Landsteiner in 1940 teamed for the discovery of the Rh antigen system and Witebsky established the criteria which proved the existence of autoimmune diseases. Haurovitz and Burnet are credited with the development of modern theories of antibody formation leading to the concepts of template theory and clonal selection theory.

Since about 1960, a virtual explosion in knowledge about immunobiology has occurred, first in humoral immunity, and more recently in cell-mediated immunity. The knowledge upon which the first section of this volume is based represents the fruits of this period of rapid growth in immunology as a science.

The development of immunobiology has not gone unnoticed by those working in head and neck medicine. Application of the science of immunology to problems in otolaryngology has begun. For example, nasal allergy, asthma, nasal polyps, intolerance to aspirin, and chronic inflammation of the tonsils and adenoids are common clinical conditions facing the otolaryngologist. To some degree, all involve immune responses.

Cancer of the head and neck has been shown to have specific epidemiological factors which predispose to its development, a fact which makes it unique when compared to many cancers that develop in other sites of the body. The roles of cell-mediated reactions, soluble immune complexes, and local reactivity need to be defined with regard to these factors and may give rise to more elegant diagnostic procedures and eventually to more precise modalities of treatment.

The mechanical theory of eustachian tube obstruction is probably of prime importance in serous otitis media with effusion. However, the role of inflammation and the intervention of nonspecific and specific immune responses may significantly hinder the restoration of a normally functioning middle ear. Immune mechanisms involving delayed hypersensitivity may also manifest themselves by chronic infection and/or inflammation in the middle ear. The mucosa of the middle ear is now recognized as a target organ in otitis media with microscopic and biochemical factors that reflect immunologic injury. Greater recognition of these factors in the pathogenesis of ear disease demands a better comprehension of immunology from otolaryngologists. Additionally, a growing knowledge of the pathophysiology of chronic otitis media will probably come in part from the study of protease inhibitors, the subpopulations of lymphocytes in middle ear effusions, and the role and classes of immunoglobulins in the secretions. For example, Yust et al., have shown that impaired cellular immunity of patients with malignant external otitis may be a predisposing factor in the development of their illness. Animal experiments on the immune response of the inner ear will most probably open new horizons in the study of the function of the endolymphatic sac and its role in endolymphatic hydrops.

A better understanding of the immunology of transplantation may possibly lead to improved methods of middle ear reconstruction.

The last half of this volume addresses these and other otolaryngologic problems closely related to immunology. A broad background in immunology is now necessary for clinicians who deal with cancer patients, treat allergies, or are interested in transplantation surgery.

DEFINITION OF TERMS

The term *immunity* was used initially to define the host's resistance to infection. Today, the term refers to the sum of reactions involved in eliminating foreign substances. A broader sense of the term now designates all humoral and cellular factors, specific and nonspecific, protecting the organism against infectious processes or malignant diseases. Sometimes the immune reaction is not favorable to the host and is marked by hypersensitivity reactions (eg, autoimmune diseases, anaphylaxis).

Antigens are customarily defined as any substance that causes the production of antibodies and reacts specifically with those antibodies to produce an immune reaction. By convention, the antigen is schematically represented in this text by a triangle.

In general, there are four characteristics of an antigen: (1) It must be recognized as a foreign substance by the host; (2) It evokes the most vigorous host response when introduced parenterally; (3) It has a high molecular weight; (4) It is proteineic in nature.

Immunogenicity is defined as the capacity to generate an immune reaction, and the degree of immunogenicity is related to the structural and chemical characteristics of the antigenic molecule. There are certain antigenic sites or determinants on the antigen molecule that combine with specific antibodies or sensitized lymphocytes. These may represent only a relatively small portion of the entire molecule. Chapter 2 elaborates on the nature, role, and constituents of antigens.

Haptens are molecules of less than 5,000 molecular weight which alone cannot elicit an antibody response; however, when they are conjugated with larger molecules, they can provide antigenic specificity.

Adjuvants are substances which enhance the immune reaction against an antigen. Adjuvants usually do not modify the specific antigenicity of a substance; however, certain adjuvants may generate different immune responses to the same antigen from the responses generally expected. Adjuvants can be classified as simple (mineral oil) or bacterial (Freund's adjuvant; see chapter 2).

Antibodies are globulins (immunoglobulins, Ig) elaborated by the organism in response to antigenic stimulation. There are five distinct Ig classes which have differing structures and functions (IgA, IgD, IgE, IgG, IgM). These molecules combine with antigens in a "lock and key" fashion and may form an immune complex.

The *complement* system is a series of serum proteins which serves primarily to amplify the effects of an interaction between a specific antigen and its corresponding antibody.

The complement cascade consists of 9 functional entities or 11 discrete proteins which when activated follow two recognized pathways: (1) the classical pathway and (2) the alternative pathway. These are discussed in chapter 3.

Humoral and Cellular Immunity

The immune system may be divided functionally into two main categories, representing two types of effector mechanisms mediating specific immune responses: (1) The humoral immune system mediated by antibody-forming plasma cells (B cells); (2) The cellular immune system mediated by specifically sensitized lymphocytes (T cells).

Various cellular elements and mediators are involved in both the humoral and cellular responses. They are discussed in detail in chapters 1–4.

Lymphocytes

The lymphoid cells (lymphocytes, plasma cells, lymphoblasts) of the immune system react specifically with antigen. The lymphocytes and their products are the means by which antigen is recognized, and thus are responsible for the specificity of host defense. There are two major categories of mature lymphocytes, T cells and B cells, which although morphologically similar, are quite distinct in function (see chapters 1 and 3).

Afferent and efferent limbs. The immune response is further temporally and functionally divided into afferent and efferent limbs. In the afferent limb, the immunogen is processed by macrophages, presented to lymphocytes through macrophage-lymphocyte interaction, and subsequently results in the activation of lymphocytes. In the efferent limb these specifically activated lymphocytes proliferate and differentiate to become engaged in specific humoral and cell-mediated immune responses.

Classification of Gell and Coombs. Gell and Coombs have classified the tissue-damaging allergic hypersensitivity reactions into four reaction types based on animal models. The first three types are antibody mediated and the fourth is cell mediated.

Type I reactions are caused by the secretion of mediators such as histamine and slow-reacting substance of anaphylaxis (SRS-A) from mast cells and/or other cells. Allergic rhinitis is an example of type I mediated reaction.

Type II reactions are mostly cytolytic in nature and usually initiated by antigen-antibody reactions. The mechanisms of cell injury also involve complement-mediated cytolysis. Intravascular hemolytic reactions are the most dramatic expression of the type II.

In the type III reactions, both antigen and antibody are free and react forming complexes which may be soluble and precipitate, or soluble and deposit elsewhere in tissues. Arthus reaction is the best example of type III.

In type IV reactions, various mediators are involved such as chemotactic factors, transfer factor, and migration inhibition factor. Rejection of grafts or tumors best illustrates this last type. This classification is an oversimplification and, in general, the four reactions may be intermingled.

Chapter 1

Cells and Tissues of Immunity

Allen F. Ryan

OUTLINE

INTRODUCTION

LEUKOCYTES
  Hematopoiesis
  Lymphocytes
    T lymphocytes
    B lymphocytes
    Natural killer cells
  The Reticuloendothelial System
    Polymorphonuclear leukocytes
      Neutrophils
      Eosinophils
      Basophils
    Mononuclear phagocytes
  The Mast Cell

LYMPHOID TISSUES
  The Structure of Lymphoid Organs
  Bone Marrow
  Thymus
  Lymph Nodes
  Spleen
  GALT
  Mucosae
  Lymphocyte Circulation
  Response of Lymphoid Tissue to Antigen

* The electron micrographs of human cells in this chapter were provided by Mary Ann Phillips of the Clinical Electron Microscopic Laboratory, UCSD Medical Center, and by Jerry R. Vandeberg, PhD, of the Core EM Facility, San Diego Veterans Administration Medical Center. Supported by grants NS00176 and NS14389 from the NIH/NINCDS.

INTRODUCTION

The cells responsible for the many aspects of immune response are leukocytes, which originate in hematopoiesis. The effector cells of immunity are members of the lymphoid, myeloid, and mononuclear systems. The lymphoid system consists of the lymphocytes, the cells most centrally involved in the expression of immunity. The myeloid group contains the polymorphonuclear granulocytes, while the mononuclear system consists of the monocytes and tissue macrophages. The myeloid and mononuclear systems are frequently referred to collectively as the reticuloendothelial system (RES), classically defined as consisting of those cells that exhibit phagocytic behavior. An understanding of the origins and characteristics of the cells of the lymphoid system and RES is essential to understanding immune responses.

The tissues that play a major role in immunity contain large quantities of lymphocytes, macrophages and plasma cells, and are called lymphoid tissues or organs. Lymphoid tissue is normally present in the organs of the *central* lymphoid system, the bone marrow, thymus, and gastrointestinal-associated lymphoid tissue (GALT), and in the *peripheral* lymphoid organs, the lymph nodes and spleen. Other tissues can also take part in immune responses, when local inflammation leads to accumulation of lymphoid cells. This is especially true of mucosae, some of which appear to have associated with them discrete populations of lymphocytes which are specific to that mucosa. These local populations can generate a local immune response which is independent of systemic immunity.

LEUKOCYTES

Hematopoiesis

The cells of the immune system are formed in the bone marrow. Here they attain at least partial maturity, and it is from the marrow that they are dispersed. The stem cell for all leukocytes is the reticulum cell, which differentiates into a precursor cell for each cell line. Each of the recognized leukocytic cell types originates from a series of intermediate cells. About 75% of the nucleated cells in bone marrow are dedicated to the production of leukocytes. The proportion of leukocytes to erythrocytes in peripheral blood is small because of the relatively short circulation life of most leukocytes. For example, the lifespan of a circulating polymorphonuclear neutrophil is only about ten hours, compared to 120 days for the erythrocyte (Bainton, 1980). After release from the bone marrow some leukocytes, most notably the lymphocytes, undergo further differentiation and maturation. The processes of leukocytic origin, differentiation, and maturation are represented schematically in Fig 1-1.

FIG 1-1. Schematic representation of the processes of hematopoiesis and lymphocyte differentiation. These processes give rise to the mature population of leukocytes which are the effector cells of immunity.

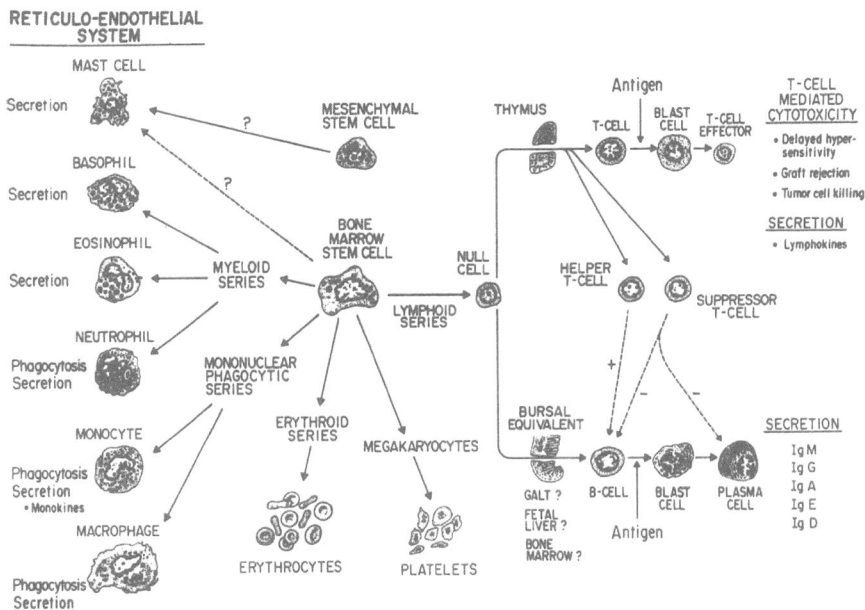

Lymphocytes

The cell which is central to all forms of immune response is the lymphocyte. This small (7 to 8 μm), round leukocyte is found in peripheral blood, lymph nodes, spleen, thymus, tonsils, the appendix, and scattered throughout many other tissues. The typical lymphocyte has relatively little cytoplasm, being composed almost entirely of a circular nucleus with prominent nuclear chromatin, as illustrated in Figs 1-2 and 1-7. The surrounding rim of cytoplasm is almost devoid of cytoplasmic organelles. Lymphocytes in their many recognized forms are the effector cells responsible for recognition of antigen, production of antibodies, cell-mediated immune cytotoxicity, and immunologic *memory*.

FIG 1-2. Lymphocyte from normal human blood. The relatively small amount of cytoplasm, with abundant free ribosomes but few organelles and little endoplasmic reticulum, are typical of the mature lymphocyte (24,000 ×).

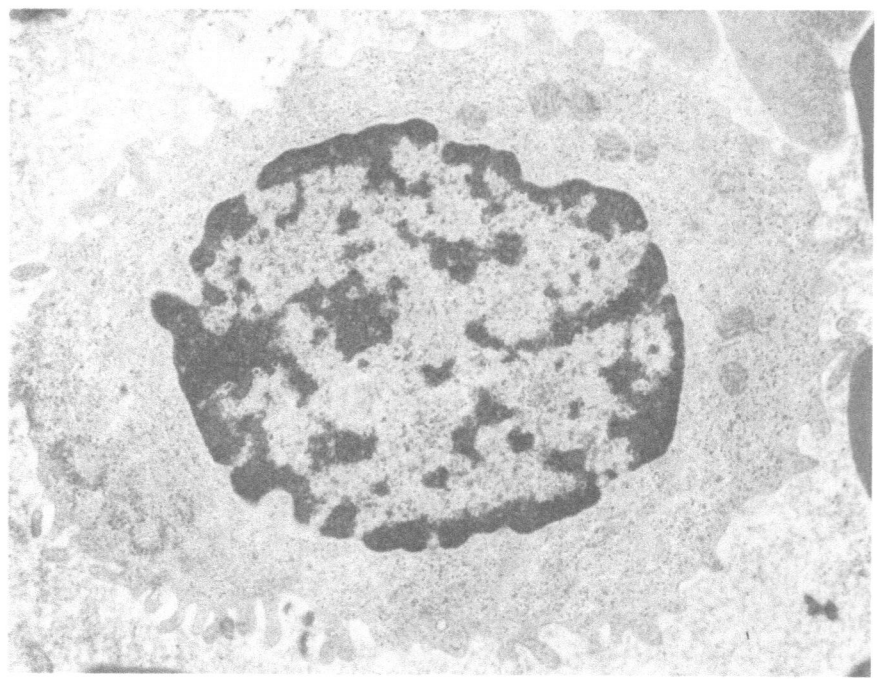

They are often long lived, with their tenure in blood and tissue lasting for months or even years. The secretion products of lymphocytes, both antibodies and lymphokines, regulate a number of other cells and biochemical pathways involved in inflammation.

Lymphocytes also originate in the hematopoietic system, from stem cells in the bone marrow. They differentiate into lymphoblasts at this site. These maturing lymphocytes are then released into the circulation as null cells; that is, they bear none of the cell surface markers which are normally used to identify the two major classes of mature lymphocytes, T cells and B cells. These cellular characteristics are acquired after the lymphocytes leave the bone marrow. The most important events in the terminal maturation of lymphocytes occur in the thymus, and at sites which have not been positively identified in mammals. Recent research has established that there are other classes of mature lymphocytes within the null cell population, such as the natural killer cell.

T lymphocytes

The term T cell is applied to lymphocytes which are derived from the thymus. They enter the circulation from their origin in the bone marrow as precursor lymphoblasts (pre-T cells), and subsequently enter the thymus where they are transformed into T lymphocytes. It is not possible to distinguish T cells from other small lymphocytes on morphological grounds (Dantchev & Belpomme, 1977). However, the surface membranes of T cells are quite distinct from those of B cells (Dwyer, 1976). Several techniques which take advantage of these differences in membrane markers have been used to differentiate between lymphocyte populations. For example, T cells adhere to sheep erythrocytes, while B cells do not. If T cells and sheep erythrocytes are incubated in the proper proportions, they will form rosettes with a T cell in the center of a surrounding layer of erythrocytes. There are also surface markers on T cells to which an antibody can be formed. An antibody to this *T antigen* will not react to B cells. These markers have been used to demonstrate that about 80% of lymphocytes in peripheral blood are T cells.

The process of initial T-cell sensitization is not completely understood. However, when a T cell which has been sensitized to antigen encounters that antigen again, it undergoes a period of growth and cell division known as lymphocyte transformation or blast transformation. The lymphocyte transforms into a blast cell, which then divides to form a large population of T cells which are all sensitized to the original antigen.

Several functional subpopulations of T lymphocytes have been identified. *Helper T cells* assist B cells in the production of antibodies to what are called T-cell–dependent antigens. These antigens are more complex than those to which B cells can respond directly. *Suppressor T cells* retard or even completely suppress the production of antibody by B cells. *Killer T cells* act directly to eliminate tumors or transplanted tissues. Other T cells are responsible for the development and expression of delayed hypersensitivity.

Many of the functions of T cells appear to be mediated by soluble factors which are distinct from the immunoglobulins. This diverse family of lymphocyte mediators are known as lymphokines. Via the lymphokines, T lymphocytes can regulate the antibody production of B cells, inhibit the spread of viruses, and kill foreign or neoplastic cells. The lymphocyte mediators are discussed in detail in chapter 3.

B lymphocytes

The term B cell is used to describe those small lymphocytes which are the precursors of antibody-producing cells. In birds, B-cell maturation occurs in an organ known as the bursa of Fabricus, and B lymphocyte is shorthand for bursal lymphocyte. Mammals lack this organ, and their bursal equivalent has not been identified with any certainty. While the GALT has been the leading candidate, recent evidence suggests that fetal liver, spleen or even the bone marrow itself may be more likely sites of B-cell determination.

B lymphocytes are similar to T cells in their morphological appearance. A number of differences in surface membrane characteristics exist, as discussed above. However, the most important surface marker by which B lymphocytes can be distinguished from T cells is the presence of large quantities of immunoglobulin on the B cell membrane

(Dwyer, 1976). In the case of the B lymphocyte, it is this surface antibody which serves as the cell receptor for antigen.

When a B lymphocyte encounters an antigen to which it is sensitized, it undergoes blast transformation similar to that of the T cell. The blast cell then produces a large number of progeny which are all of the same clone; that is, they all produce antibodies directed against the same antigen. The plasma cell, which is specialized for the production of large quantities of specific antibody, is the terminal stage of this replication.

There are at least five recognized classes of B lymphocytes, which correspond to the five classes of immunoglobulin: IgM, IgG, IgA, IgD, and IgE. At any one time, each B cell or antibody-produced cell manufactures only one class of antibody, directed toward one antigenic determinant. However, B cells may switch from one antibody class to another. It has recently been demonstrated that virtually all B cells synthesize IgM in the very early stages of their development, and most then switch to another antibody class during their development into active antibody-forming cells (Hammerling, 1981).

While lymphokine production is usually associated with T cells, it has recently been demonstrated that B cells can, under certain circumstances, also produce lymphocyte mediators (Rocklin, Bendtzen, & Greineder, 1980).

Plasma cells are the final stage of B-cell blast transformation. The plasma cell is a small oval or round cell characterized by an eccentric nucleus, and abundant cytoplasm which consists primarily of laminated rough endoplasmic reticulum, is illustrated in Fig 1-3. The nucleus of the plasma cell often has a "cartwheel" appearance due to the condensation of chromatin along the nuclear membrane with filaments extending toward the nuclear center. Plasma cells are a prominent feature of lymph nodes, the spleen, and sites of chronic inflammation. They increase in numbers in draining lymphoid organs approximately 1 week following an antigenic challenge.

Natural killer cells

A new nonclassical subpopulation of lymphocytes, designated natural killer cells, has recently been described (Herberman, Nunn, & Lavrin, 1975; Kiessling, Klein, & Wigzell, 1975). While these cells have not yet been fully characterized, it is clear that they are an important surveillance mechanism against certain tumors and allografts, which operates independently of the T-cell cytotoxic system. While the cytotoxicity of killer T cells is dependent upon antibody, that of the natural killer cells occurs in unimmunized hosts, and appears to be completely independent of antibody or sensitization to the target cell. The recognition of the target cell by the natural killer cell is under genetic control, and surface glycoproteins on the target cell membrane are important for recognition (Roder, Karre, & Kiessling, 1981). The recognition receptor has not been identified. It has recently been reported that natural killer cells bear a unique glycolipid marker, asialo-GMI (Kasai et al., 1980), which should aid greatly in the investigation of this lymphocyte type. Natural killer cells represent about 1% to 2% of the total circulating lymphocyte pool (Roder & Kiessling, 1978). The independence of natural killer cell cytotoxicity from sensitization suggests that this system may be the initial defense against neoplasms.

FIG 1-3. Human plasma cell. The most characteristic feature of the plasma cell at the electron microscopic level is the laminated rough endoplasmic reticulum which occupies virtually all of the extranuclear space. The chromatin of the plasma cell nucleus occurs in large clumps along the nuclear membrane, with occasional bridges into the center of the nucleus. The electron-dense bodies in the cytoplasm of this cell (arrows) may be lysosomes or Russell bodies, suggesting an early stage of cell degeneration (20,000 ×).

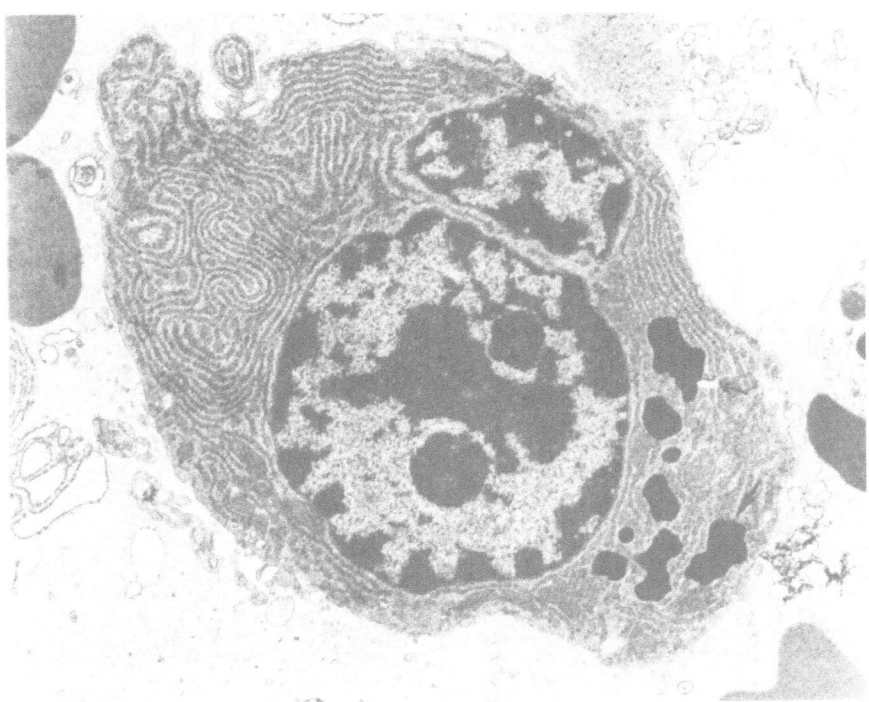

The Reticuloendothelial System

Polymorphonuclear leukocytes

Polymorphonuclear leukocytes are phagocytic cells characterized by their relatively small size (9 to 12 μm) compared to other phagocytic cells, by a multilobate nucleus, and by prominent cytoplasmic granules. This system is usually subdivided into three cell types, based upon the staining characteristics of their granules: neutrophils, basophils, and eosinophils.

FIG 1-4. Human polymorphonuclear neutrophil. The nucleus of the neutrophis is lobed, with the divisions connected by chromatin bridges. The larger azurophilic granules (ag) are rich in lysosomal enzymes and peroxidase, and thus are well equipped for a role of killing and digesting bacteria. The smaller neutrophilic granules (ng) contain lysozyme, collagenase, and lactoferrin. Their function is not known (20,000 ×).

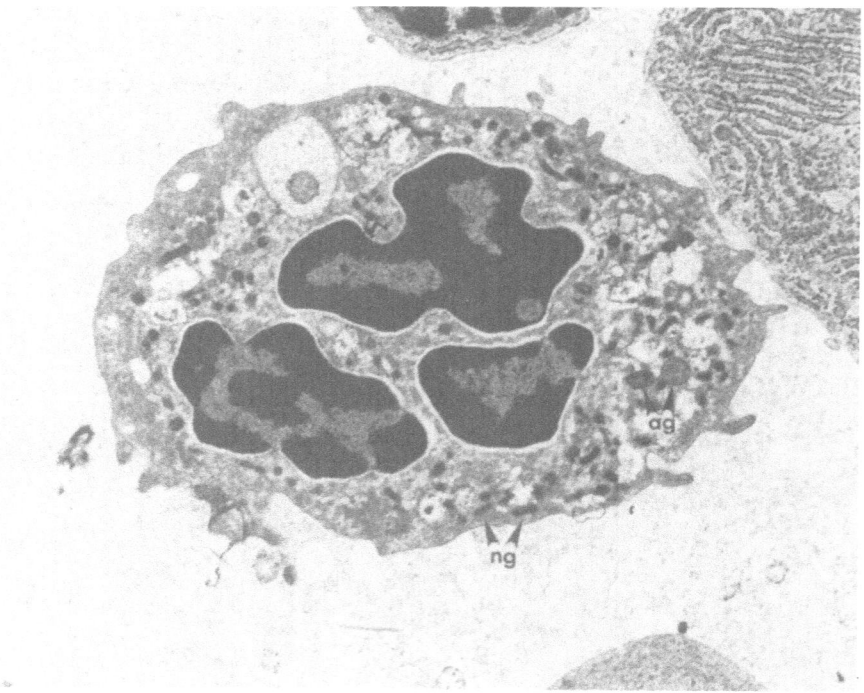

Neutrophils. Neutrophils are those polymorphonuclear leukocytes which do not take on strong acidophilic (red) or basophilic (blue) staining with the dyes normally used for staining blood smears. As illustrated in Figs 1-4 and 1-7, the abundant cytoplasmic granules which characterize the neutrophil are small and their contents are amorphous in appearance. There are two morphologically distinct types of granules. Azurophilic granules contain microbicidal elements such as peroxidase and lysozyme as well as a variety of digestive enzymes. The smaller neutrophilic granules have not been as well characterized, but while they contain lysozyme and collagenase, they have neither peroxidase nor acid hydrolases, and thus cannot be considered true lysosomes (Baggiolini, 1981). The multilobed nucleus is surrounded by a prominent perinuclear space. Neutrophils are the most common leukocyte in peripheral blood, making up from 50% to 70% of the total

FIG 1-5. Human eosinophil. The large cytoplasmic granules of the eosinophil are relatively uniform in size. Each contains a dense crystalline core of one or more cationic proteins. The configuration of the core crystals is characteristic for a given species, apparently determined by the types of proportions of cationic proteins which make up the core. The remaining, amorphous portion of the granule is rich in peroxidase and other lytic enzymes (20,000 ×).

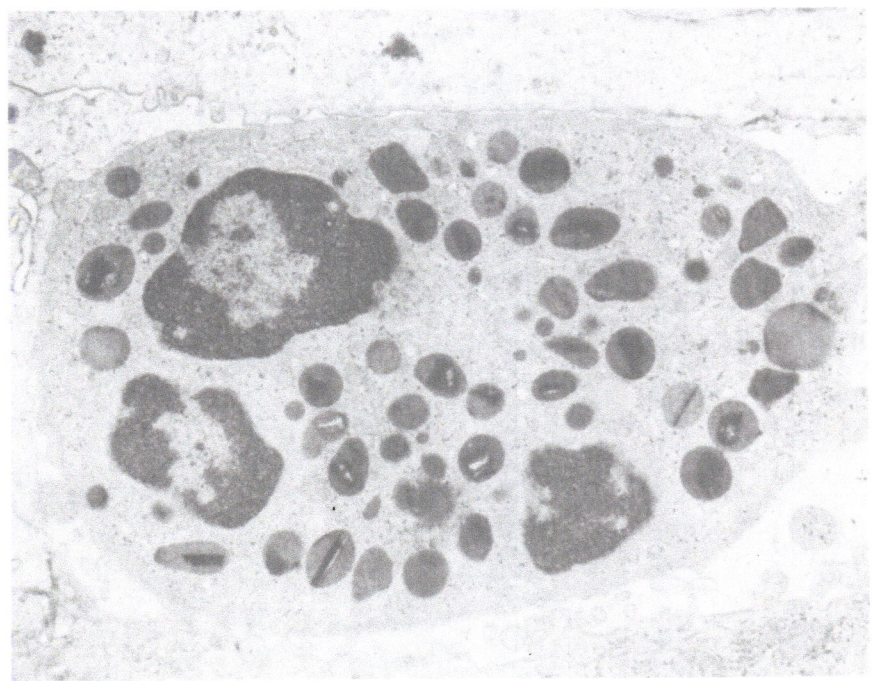

white blood cell population. They are rapidly migrating, highly phagocytic, cells which are frequently the first cells to appear in areas of inflammation.

Eosinophils. The large cytoplasmic granules of eosinophils stain a bright red with standard stains. This cell type constitutes only 1% to 3% of the leukocytes in peripheral blood. As can be seen in Figs 1-5 and 1-7, under electron microscopy the granules of the eosinophil consist of a crystalline core, composed of cationic protein of unknown function, and a noncrytalline component rich in peroxidase, lysosomal enzymes, and histaminase (Smith & Goetzl, 1981). Eosinophils respond to specific chemotactic factors which are released during the activation of the complement pathways, during mast cell degranulation, and during arachidonic acid metabolism. They thus are drawn to the sites of several types of immune reaction. They can be the predominant leukocyte in certain allergic responses, such as allergic rhinitis. The function of eosinophils is poorly

FIG 1-6. Human basophil. Only a small portion of the nucleus (n) of the cell is visible in this section. The granules of the basophil are approximately the same size as those of the eosinophil, but they are uniformly amorphous. Basophil granules are similar in some respects to mast cell granules, although with lower levels of histamine (43,000 ×).

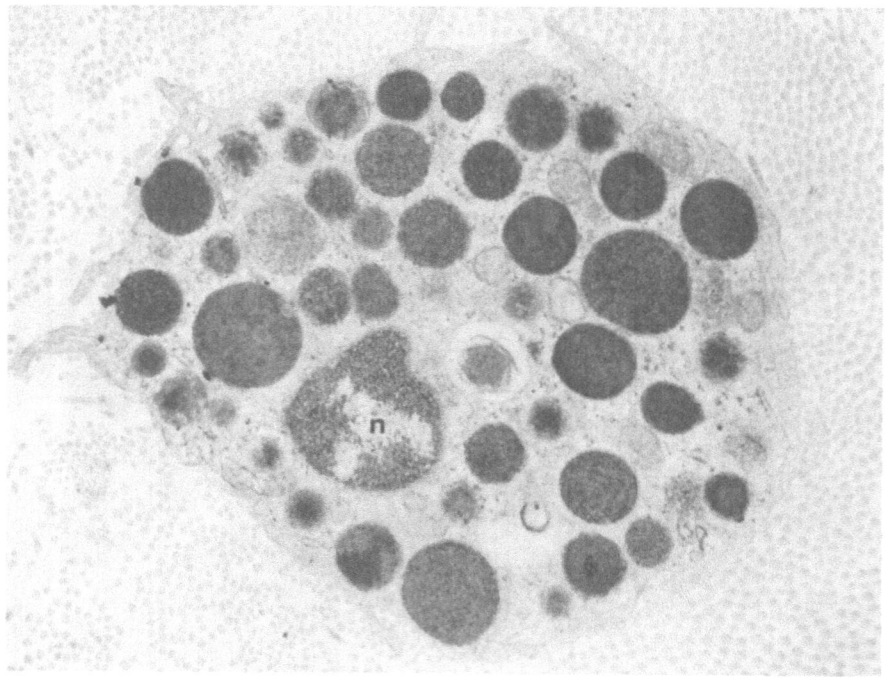

understood, but they appear to subserve several distinct roles. While eosinophils exhibit typical polymorphonuclear traits such as phagocytosis and are at least weakly microbicidal, they also mediate antibody-dependent destruction of nonphagocytosable parasites. They also appear to modulate mast cell reactions via the inactivation of mast-cell–derived mediators (Wasserman, 1976). The eosinophil may thus be both an effector cell and a regulator cell.

Basophils. Basophil cytoplasmic granules, like those of the eosinophil, are large. However, they stain blue with standard blood smear stains and, as shown in Figs 1-6 and 1-7, they appear uniformly amorphous in electron micrographs. Basophils constitute only 0.5% of the leukocytes in peripheral blood, and depend upon chemotaxis to be drawn into tissues. While basophils originate from a different cell line, they are in many ways analogous to mast cells, with somewhat similar granule contents and physiological responses. The granules of basophils contain histamine, although in much smaller

FIG 1-7. **Leukocytic infiltration of the guinea pig middle ear mucosa during a secondary immune response. Three days after antigenic challenge of the middle ear cavity of an immunized guinea pig, both the eipthelium and submucosa are heavily populated by neutrophils (PMN), eosinophils (Eo), basophils (Ba), and lymphocytes (Ly) (2,500 ×). From Ryan and Catanzaro, 1983.**

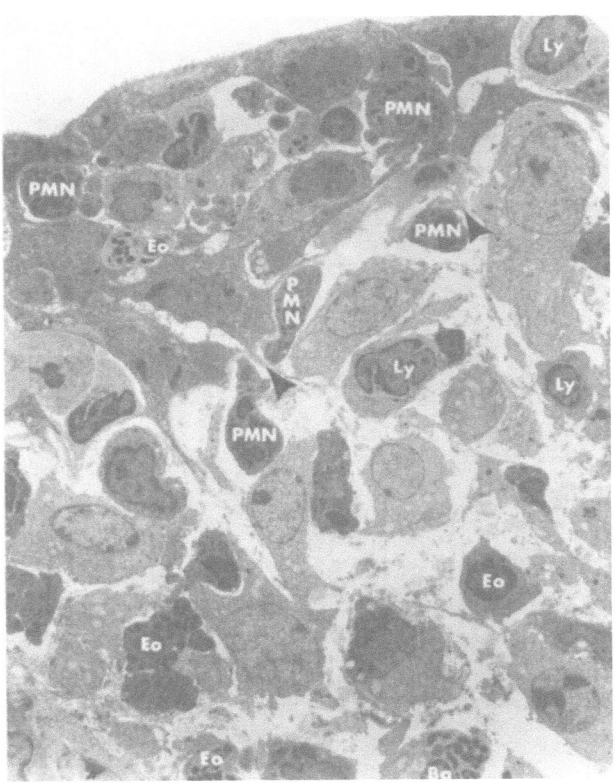

quantities than found in mast cell granules, and they degranulate in response to IgE interaction with antigen (Lagunoff & Chi, 1980). The normal function of basophils is unknown. However, their participation in certain types of inflammatory responses, such as delayed cutaneous hypersensitivity, is well documented.

Mononuclear phagocytes

The other major cell group in the reticuloendothelial system is the mononuclear phagocytes, consisting of the monocyte and the tissue macrophage. The structure of a typical macrophage is illustrated in Fig 1-8. The monocyte or blood macrophage, at 12 to 15 μm, is the largest cell in peripheral blood. The tissue macrophage or histocyte differs

FIG 1-8. Human tissue macrophage. Macrophages are specialized for phagocytes and locomotion. Their cytoplasm is rich in primary lysosomes (ly) containing hydrolytic enzymes. Vacuoles (v) or phagosomes containing phagocytosed material merge with lysosomes to form secondary lysosomes (sly). The numerous pseudopodia (ps) suggest that this cell is a wandering rather than a fixed, state (20,000 ×).

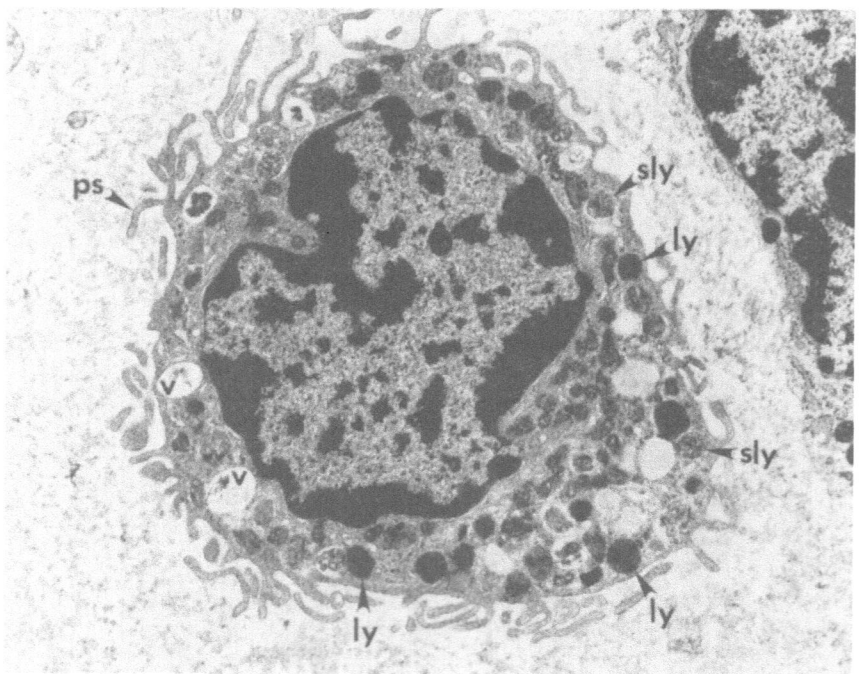

from the monocyte primarily in its greater number of cytoplasmic vacuoles. The major function of the macrophage is phagocytosis. Ingested material is encapsulated in phagosomes, which merge with the primary lysosomes which are abundant in the cytoplasm of macrophages. The hydrolytic enzymes of the lysosomal granule digest the particles within the membrane-bound compartment, called a secondary lysosome, formed by phagosome-lysosome fusion.

The uptake of antigens by macrophages is an important step in the process leading to production of circulating antibody. Through a process which is still incompletely understood, antigen is not completely degraded by hydrolysis, but becomes bound to macrophage RNA or membranes. This macrophage processing somehow enhances the ability of lymphocyte to recognize the antigen.

In addition to their phagocytic function, macrophages also secrete a family of mediators known as monokines (Rocklin et al., 1980). These regulatory proteins include factors which stimulate the differentiation of both T and B cells, T-cell maturation, leukocyte colony formation in bone marrow, and the production and release of prostaglandin, collagenase, and various proteinases by monocytic cells. Macrophages also have been shown to synthesize and secrete a pyrogenic factor and complement components C2, C4, and factor B.

Macrophages play an important role in the late phases of inflammation, replacing the neutrophil which dominates the early phase. The movement of macrophages into a site of inflammation is controlled in part by the release of chemotactic factors from lymphocytes, which can also regulate their phagocytic and digestive behavior.

The Mast Cell

The mast cell represents a special case in the leukocytic series. The structure of the human mast cell is illustrated in Fig 1-9. These cells are characterized by an unlobed nucleus, numerous metachromatically staining cytoplasmic granules, and a villous or ruffled cell membrane. In many ways mast cells resemble basophils, and for some time they were regarded as tissue basophils. However, it has now become clear that there are many differences between these two cell types. The mast cell appears to originate, in some if not all cases, from stem cells outside of the bone marrow, perhaps a mesenchymal stem cell. Their life span is much greater than that of the basophil. More important, the granule contents of mast cells are distinct from those of basophils, implying differences in function. In man, the mast cell granule is morphologically quite distinct from that of the basophil, as is obvious from a comparison of Figs 1-6 and 1-8. The mast cell is an important mediator of immediate hypersensitivity and inflammation, and is discussed in detail in chapters 3 and 8.

LYMPHOID TISSUES

Lymphoid tissues are characterized by accumulations of lymphocytes, plasma cells, and macrophages. They are the sites at which many of the important events in immune responses, such as antigen recognition and antibody production, are most likely to occur. There are a number of lymphoid tissues and/or organs which are present in the normal organism. The spleen and the GALT are often referred to as the central lymphoid organs, because of their role in lymphocyte development. Many authors also classify bone marrow as a lymphoid organ, and if so it certainly falls within the central category. The peripheral lymphoid organs, the lymph nodes, and spleen, are more concerned with postmaturational lymphocyte function. During inflammation, other tissues may acquire accumulations of lymphoid cells and briefly qualify for the designation of lymphoid tissue.

FIG 1-9. Mast cell from human lung. The large granules of the mast cell contain high levels of histamine and other mediators. In the human, mast cell granules are characterized by a scroll-like internal arrangement, as is apparent in this cell (27,000×).

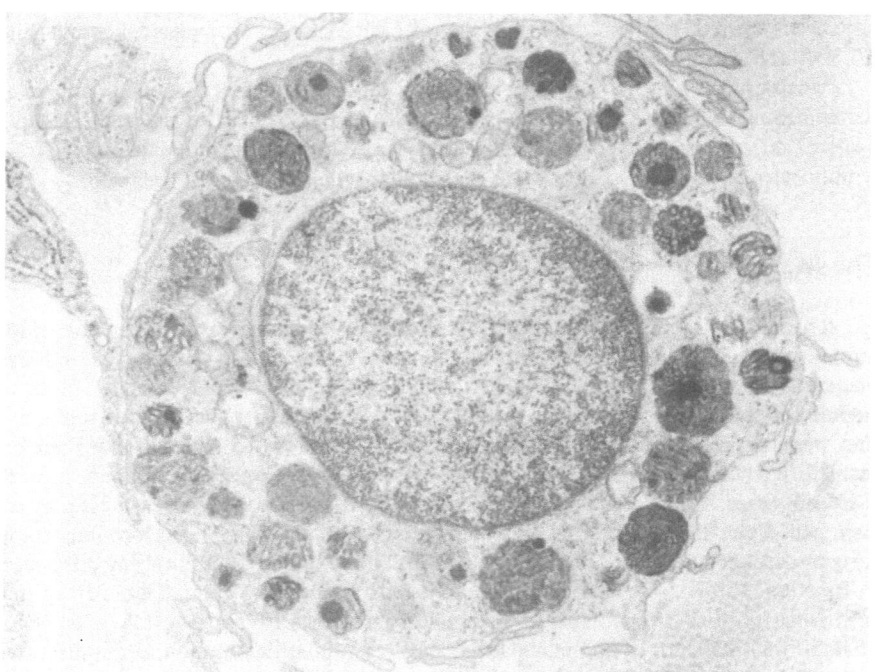

The Structure of Lymphoid Organs

All permanent lymphoid organs, with the exception of the bone marrow, have similarities in structure. They are encapsulated in a layer of collagenous connective tissue. The arterial and venous supply to the organ enters through an indentation in the capsule known as the hilus. The parenchymal tissue which makes up the organ is divided into lobules by connective tissue strands known as trabeculae. The parenchyma is divided into two areas, the cortex and the medulla, which differ markedly in their composition. The cortex lies between the organ capsule and the medullary tissue. It contains tightly packed lymphoid cells and is the area of B-cell and/or T-cell proliferation. The medulla occupies the center of the organ and contains fewer lymphocytes. It consists primarily of a supporting framework of reticular phagocytic cells, and may contain plasma cells. Most lymphoid organs are supplied by efferent and/or afferent lymphatics. This general model varies considerably among the several lymphoid organs, as described below.

Bone Marrow

The bone marrow, as the site of origin of the cells of immunity rather than an organ of immune expression, differs markedly in structure from other lymphoid organs. Encased in bone, the marrow has no need of a connective tissue capsule. The stem cells of hematopoiesis are organized into islands of cells located in the fatty tissue of the marrow. The cell types are admixed so that the precursors of all of the hematic elements are quite closely spaced. While all stem cells are virtually identical in appearance, they are surrounded by their progeny in various states of maturation. Bone marrow lacks lymphatic supply, and mature blood cells exit the marrow via the venous drainage.

While the bone marrow is the site of origin of most of the cells involved in immune responses, it is not usually involved in response to antigen. Plasma cells represent less than 1% of bone marrow cellular elements in normal organisms. Given this lack of effector function, it is interesting to note that in humans myelomas appear to originate exclusively within the bone marrow. Of the mature lymphocytes which are found in the bone marrow, the majority are B cells.

Thymus

As shown in Figure 1-10, the thymus has a typical fibrous capsule, a cortical area of tightly packed lymphoid cells, lobular organization with trabeculae dividing the lobules, and a medulla of reticular cells. However, the thymus differs from other lymphoid organs in that its cortex entirely lacks follicles or germinal centers. Also, in the medulla there are small, concentric rings of epithelial cells of uncertain function known as Hassall's corpuscles. The thymus has efferent but no afferent lymphatics, with drainage probably occurring through the veins.

The thymus is necessary neonatally for the normal development of T lymphocytes, and thus for immune resistance of the cellular type as well as other T-cell functions. The cortex of the thymus consists of packed small T lymphocytes and many proliferating cells in the T lymphocyte series. Very few B lymphocytes can be identified in the thymus.

Lymph Nodes

Lymph nodes are located in areas of lymphatic drainage and serve as filters for the tissue fluid in lymphatic vessels. As such, they remove foreign material that has entered the lymph via tissue, and are often the site of antigenic recognition by the lymphocytes accumulated within each lymph node. The structure of the typical lymph node is illustrated in Fig 1-11. Lymph nodes are similar to the thymus in structure, as described above. However, the cortex of the lymph nodes contains tightly packed nodules of lymphocytes called primary follicles, and more loosely packed nodules with a rim of tightly packed cells called germinal centers or secondary follicles. The follicles contain mostly B cells, and function primarily in the production of plasma cells. The remainder of the cortex,

FIG 1-10. A schematic representation of the structure of the thymus. The cortical tissue of the thymus contains no germinal centers, but consists entirely of tightly packed T cells. The medullary tissue contains numerous Hassall's, or thymic, corpuscles. The function of these concentric rings of eipthelial cells is not known. Adapted from Weiss (1972).

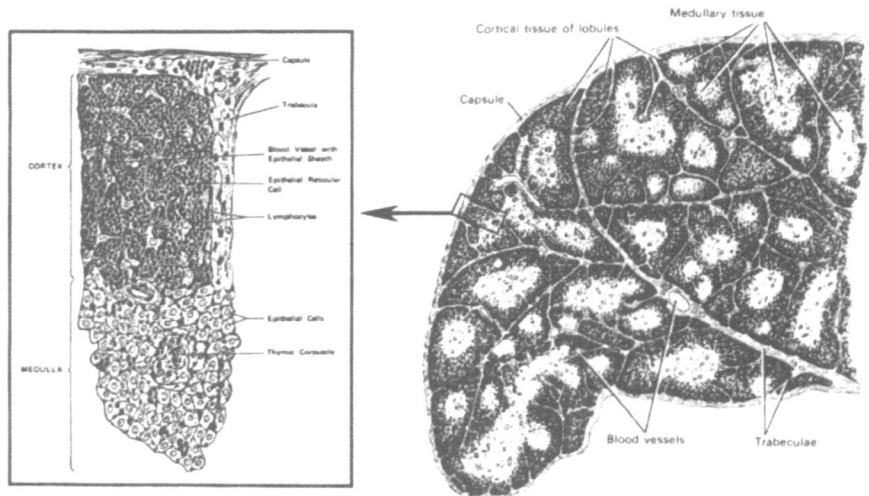

the paracortical area, is called the thymus-dependent portion because it does not develop in neonatally thymectomized animals. It is the focus of T lymphocyte production. The medulla of the lymph node consists of a network of draining sinusoids formed by the reticular phagocytic cells. The lymph node receives afferent lymphatics which drain through the fibrous capsule into a subcapsular sinus. Lymph sinusoids drain through the cortex into the medullary sinusoids, which empty into the efferent lymphatics, which exit the node at the hilus. The structure of the lymph node reflects its functions: filtration of the lymph, with ingestion of foreign material by reticular phagocytes, and presentation of lymphocytes for recognition and response. The lymph node is the primary site of generation of circulating IgG and of peripheral blood IgG-producing B cells.

Spleen

The structure of the spleen is analogous to that of the lymph node, but the arrangement of the elements is different. There is a fibrous capsule and trabeculae which divide the spleen into lobules. However, there is no cortex as such. The spleen is composed of a network of sinusoids, which are filled primarily with red blood cells. This network

FIG 1-11. Schematic representation of a typical lymph node. The lymphoid tissues of the node are segregated by lymphocyte type. The cortex consists of B-cell generating germinal centers surrounded by T-cell containing paracortical tissue. Plasma cells and macrophages (insert) occupy the medullary cords. The cords line the medullary sinuses, which are drained by efferent lymphatics.

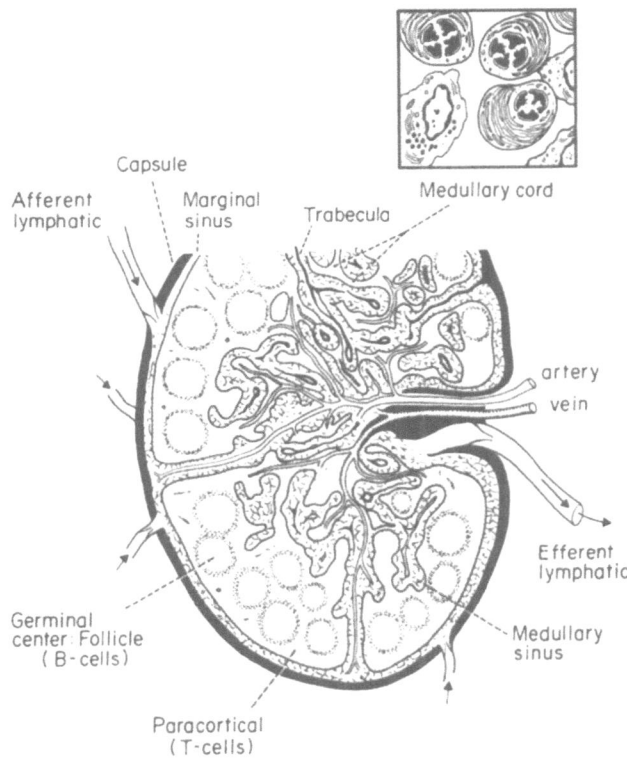

forms the red pulp of the spleen. The lymphoid tissue of the spleen forms lumpy, cylindrical sheaths which surround the splenic arterioles prior to the point at which they supply the sinuses of the red pulp. Within the lymphoid tissue, called the white pulp of the spleen, the thymus-dependent area is a relatively small region of densely packed lymphocytes, immediately adjacent to the arteriole. The remainder of the lymphoid tissue sheath consists of primary and secondary follicles containing B cells. The spleen contains several types of phagocytic cells within and lining the sinusoids, and reticular cells around and sometimes within the lymphoid tissue. The spleen has neither afferent or efferent lymphatic supply. The arterioles around which the lymphoid tissue is located double back to supply it with capillaries. The circulation through the lymphoid tissue drains into a marginal sinus, which surrounds it and separates the lymphoid tissue from the red pulp. Lymphocytes enter the lymphoid tissue by traversing the marginal sinus.

A major function of the spleen is the removal of aged and damaged erythrocytes from the circulation. However, the spleen also performs many of the same functions of lymph nodes: filtration by phagocytosis, antigen entrapment, and the production of antibodies and replication of lymphocytes. The spleen operates on the circulatory system, while the lymph nodes serve the lymphatics.

GALT

Local collections of lymphoid tissue are found under the submucosa of many areas of the gastrointestinal tract. Some of these are large and specialized enough to be identified as individual lymphoid tissues or organs: the tonsils, appendix, and Peyer's patches. It has long been suggested that the GALT in mammals plays the role of the bursa of Fabricius in birds, mediating the development of B lymphocytes, although more recent evidence implicates other structures (Waksman & Ozer, 1976). Whether or not it serves as the site of B-cell maturation the GALT is an important source of B cells and IgA, and plays an important role in immunization via oral administration of antigens. It has been estimated that the production of IgA by GALT equals that of IgG by the rest of the body. The relatively low proportion of IgA in serum (12% v 80% for IgG) is due in part to the more rapid catabolism of IgA, which has a half life in serum of only six days as compared to 22 days for most IgG (Tomasi & Shorter, 1978). Production of secretory component and secretion of IgA into the lumen of the gastrointestinal tract are also important functions of GALT.

The tonsils and Peyer's patches, described in detail in chapter 5, are only briefly discussed here. The tonsils are overlain by an epithelium appropriate to their site, overlying a cap of lymphocytes and plasma cells which invade the epithelium. Beneath the cap, a cortical region contains typical germinal centers and surrounding paracortical tissue, and reticular tissue analogous to a medulla lies beneath the cortex. The cortex and the epithelial layers of the tonsils are highly convoluted, forming deep surface crypts, which appear to fulfill the function of afferent lymphatics, which the tonsils lack. The tonsils are drained by efferent lymphatics. Unlike other elements in GALT, the B cells of the tonsils are primarily IgG-containing, which had led some authors to suggest that they should perhaps be classified with bronchial-associated lymphoid tissue (BALT). The Peyer's patches are focal collections of lymphoid tissue rich in germinal centers, found mainly in the submucosa of the distal ileum. They are supplied by afferent lymphatics which drain the intestinal villi above the germinal centers, while efferent lymphatics drain into the thoracic duct. The function of the Peyer's patches is not entirely clear. While rich in both B and T lymphocytes, they are almost devoid of antibody-producing cells, and stimulation with a variety of antigens has failed to demonstrate specific antibody production in a Peyer's patch.

Appendix

The appendix is the most readily studied element of the GALT, and its function has been extensively documented. The B-cell elements of the appendix consist of tightly packed follicles, each with an overlying coronal region of small lymphocytes, and above the corona a dome of large lymphocytes and lymphoblasts, but few plasma cells. The dome is adjacent to the lumen of the appendix and is covered by a simple epithelium. Wedged between the adjacent B-cell regions, at the level of the corona and upper end of the follicle, are small thymus-dependent areas rich in T cells. As with the Peyer's patches, the lymphocytes of the appendix do not appear to produce antibody in response to in vivo antigenic stimulation, although they can be induced to do so in culture. It appears that both structures are sites of priming of memory B cells which are dispersed to the lamina propria of the gut and, upon reexposure to antigen, differentiate into IgA-producing plasma cells (Waksman & Ozer, 1976).

Mucosae

Mucosae make up a major part of the epithelial capsule which protects the body from potentially harmful agents in the environment. As a major site of antigen contact, they are often involved in immune responses. While normal mucosa cannot be defined as a lymphoid tissue or organ, there is frequently lymphoid tissue associated with mucosae. In the gastrointestinal tract, some of this tissue has been formalized as GALT, and lymphoid tissue in the bronchi has been termed BALT. In most instances, however, patches of lymphoid tissue and individual lymphoid cells are scattered through mucosal tissue in relative isolation. Mucosal lymphoid tissue is sometimes involved in a local immune response, limited to that particular mucosa and site, and independent of systemic immunity. Mucosal epithelia produce secretory component, and can also store and secrete at the luminal surface antibodies produced at a distant site (Virella, Montgomery, & Lemaitre-Coelho, 1977), presumably via immunoglobulin complexing with secretory component and concurrent secretion. Mucosal immune responses are discussed in detail in chapter 5.

Lymphocyte Circulation

Lymphocyte populations in lymphoid tissues are by no means static. Lymphocytes which mature at a particular location often leave that site and circulate through the blood stream. They then may enter the same or another lymphoid organ. While the proportion of fixed to circulating lymphocytes is not known, it is assumed that a large fraction do circulate. One purpose of circulation is undoubtedly to maximize the exposure of lymphocytes to various antigens. The degree of effectiveness of this exposure may be observed during antigenic stimulation. Introduction of an antigen into an organism produces a marked decrease in the circulating population of lymphocytes sensitized to that antigen, at least for a short period of time, as the cells become localized to the site of the foreign material.

The circulation of lymphocytes between lymphoid organs is not a random phenomenon. Lymphocytes which originated from GALT have a tendency to lodge in the lamina propria of various mucosae, a phenomenon known as "homing." The degree of specificity of homing is not known. However, it has been demonstrated that both B and T lymphocytes from GALT demonstrate this behavior.

The T cells which circulate tend to be long lived, with life spans of up to ten years. About 80% to 90% of thoracic duct cells are such long-lived T cells.

Response of Lymphoid Tissue to Antigen

What has been described as the normal structure of lymphoid organs is in fact dependent upon the organism's history of antigen contact. In animals raised under germ-free conditions, in which relatively little antigenic contact would have occurred, the lymphoid organs contain few primary or secondary follicles and markedly attenuated paracortical areas. The sinusoids of the medullary area contain relatively few mononuclear phagocytes. The lymphocyte population of the mucosae is also less than 10% of that seen normally. If antigen is then introduced, the lymphoid organs assume a much more "normal" appearance, and the lymphocytic population of the mucosae increases dramatically. This provides an extreme example of the response of lymphoid tissue to antigen.

In normal animals, induction of a relatively pure B-lymphocyte response results in an increase in germinal centers of the cortex of lymphoid organs. After several days, plasma cells migrate from the germinal centers to the medullary cords, where they secrete antibody into the medullary sinusoids. If a relatively pure T lymphocyte response is elicited, as in delayed hypersensitivity, antigenic challenge is followed by proliferation of paracortical areas.

REFERENCES

Baggiolini M: The neutrophil, in Weissman G (ed): *The Cell Biology of Inflammation*. New York, Elsevier, 1980, pp 163–188.
Bainton DF: The cells of inflammation: a general view, in Weissman G (ed): *The Cell Biology of Inflammation*. New York, Elsevier, 1980, pp 1–26.
Dantchev D, Belpomme, D: *Biomedicine* 1977; 27: 202.
Dwyer JM: *Prog Allergy* 1976; 21: 178.
Hammerling U: Differentiation of B lymphocytes in lineage development and in the immune response. *Prog Allergy* 1981; 28: 40.
Herberman RB, Nunn ME, Lavrin DH: Natural cytotoxic reactivity of mouse lymphoid cells against syngeneic and allogeneic tumors. I. Distribution of reactivity and specificity. *Int J Cancer* 1975; 16: 216.

Kasai M, Iwamori M, Nagai Y, Okumura K, Tada T: A glycolipid on the surface of mouse natural killer cells. *Eur J Immunol* 1980; 10: 175.

Kiessling R, Klein E, Wigzell H: Natural killer cells in the mouse. I. Cytotoxic cells with specificity for mouse Moloney leukemia cells. Specificity and distribution according to genotype. *Eur J Immunol* 1975; 5: 112.

Lagunoff D, Chi EY: Cell biology of mast cells and basophils, in Weissman G (ed): *The Cell Biology of Inflammation*. New York, Elsevier 1980, pp 217–266.

Rocklin RE, Bendtzen K, Greineder D: Mediators of immunity: Lymphokines and monokines. *Adv Immunol* 1980; 29: 55.

Roder JC, Karre K, Kiessling R: Natural killer cells. *Prog Allergy* 1981; 28: 66.

Roder JC, Kiessling R: Target-effector interaction in the natural killer cell system. I. Co-variance and genetic control of cytolytic and target-cell-binding subpopulations in the mouse. *Scand J Immunol* 1978; 8: 135.

Ryan AF, Catanzaro A: Passive transfer of immune-mediated middle ear inflammation and effusion. *Acta Otolaryngol* 1983; 95: 123.

Smith JA, Goetzl EJ: Cellular properties of eosinophils: Regulatory, protective and potentially pathogenic roles in inflammatory states, in Weissman G (ed): *The Cell Biology of Inflammation*. New York, Elsevier, 1980, pp 189–216.

Tomasi TB, Shorter RG: Immunology of the gastrointestinal tract and inflammatory bowel disease, in *Samter M (ed): Immunological Diseases*. New York, Little, Brown, 1978, pp 1478–1501.

Virella G, Montgomery PC, Lemaitre-Coelho IM: Transport of oligomeric IgA of systemic origin into external secretions. *Adv Exp Med Biol* 1977; 107: 241.

Waksman BH, Ozer H: Specialized amplification elements in the immune system. *Prog Allergy* 1976; 21: 1.

Wasserman, SI: The mast cell: Its diversity of chemical mediators. *Int J Dermatol* 1980; 19: 7.

Weiss, L: *The Cells and Tissues of the Immune System*. Englewood Cliffs, NJ, Prentice-Hall, 1972.

Chapter 2

Immunochemistry

Sherman Fong

OUTLINE

ANTIGENS
Physical and Chemical Requirements for Immunogenicity
Antigenic Determinants
Haptens
Immunopotency
Immunodominance
Antigenic Determinants of Complex Antigens
Size of Antigenic Determinants
Antigenic Determinants and Cell Collaboration
Immunogenic Determinants for T Lymphocytes
T-Independent Antigens
Adjuvants

IMMUNOGLOBULINS
Structure of Immunoglobulins
Heterogeneity
Light chain types
Heavy chain classes
Heavy chain subclasses
Variable Regions
V region subgroups
Hypervariable regions
Antibody diversity
Idiotypes
J Chain
Secretory Component
Genetic Markers on Immunoglobulins
Carbohydrate Moieties of Immunoglobulins

Biological Activities of Immunoglobulins
Placental and gut transfer
Complement activation
Cytophilic antibodies
Cell membrane immunoglobulins

ANTIGEN-ANTIBODY REACTIONS
Forces That Participate in Antigen–Antibody Reactions
Precipitation Reactions
Agglutination Reactions
Conformational Changes in the Antibody Molecules upon
        Interaction with Antigen
Hapten-Antibody Interactions.

ANTIGENS

Physical and Chemical Requirements for Immunogenicity

Substances which provoke humoral and/or cellular immune responses when introduced into animals are antigens or immunogens. A variety of substances, including macromolecular proteins, synthetic polypeptides, lipoproteins, polysaccharides, glycoproteins, lipopolysaccharides, nucleic acids, and nucleoproteins can be antigens (Kabat, 1956; Race & Sanger, 1975; Rapport & Graf, 1969; Stollar, 1973). The feature of the antigen molecule which influences its immune capabilities is its antigenicity (Sela, 1969). Whether antigenic substances become immunogenic depends on the type of animal being immunized, the dose of antigen used, the conditions under which it is introduced, and the sensitivity of the methods used to detect the immune response (Borek, 1972).

Early studies empirically established that proteins from plants and animal body fluids were strongly immunogenic when injected into animals across species lines. This gave rise to the general thought that foreignness to the host was a basic requirement for immunogenicity. However, many substances not foreign to the host are antigenic and can induce autoimmune responses. Tissue extracts from brain, kidney, testis, and crystalline lens of the eye are immunogenic when injected into animals syngeneic to the species from which they originated. The discrimination between self and nonself must be redefined in terms of recognizable foreignness to the immune system and to the circulation.

Molecular size has been important in establishing the antigenic potential of a substance. The most potent antigens are macromolecular proteins with molecular weights greater than 100,000. Small molecules such as amino acids or monosaccharides are not antigenic. Substances such as insulin with molecular weights of 6,000 may be antigenic, but as a general rule molecules smaller than 10,000 mol. wt. are only weakly antigenic if at all (DeWeck, 1974).

A molecule must also possess a certain degree of chemical complexity to be antigenic. Antigenicity increases with structural complexity. For example, homopolymers composed of a single amino acid are poorly immunogenic in most species tested; copolymers of two or three amino acids may be immunogenic, regardless of size. The presence of aromatic amino acids in proteins and polypeptides contributes more to antigenicity than the presence of nonaromatic residues. Polypeptides containing tyrosine are better antigens than those without. Gelatin when conjugated with as little as 2% peptide chains of tyrosine becomes immunogenic in animals. It is not exclusively tyrosine that is found as an enhancer of antigenicity. The presence of other amino acids such as phenylalanine, tryptophan, glutamic acid, lysine, and cystine, in their natural L-forms in protein, also have the same effect.

Polymers containing high electric charge are poor antigens, despite the fact that most natural antigens are charged. Even the addition of tyrosine to highly charged polymers will not enhance their antigenicity. Polypeptides bearing no net charge can be antigenic also, showing that the presence of electric charge on the antigen is not a requirement for its antigenicity.

The genetic constitution of an animal greatly influences whether a particular substance, when introduced into the animal, will result in an immune response. In one experiment strain 2 guinea pigs responded readily to poly-L-lysine, whereas strain 13 guinea pigs did not. The ability of the animals to respond was shown to be inherited as an autosomal dominant trait (Benacerraf & McDevitt, 1972). In other words, antigenic substances are nonimmunogenic in genetically nonresponsive animals. Polymers composed of two different amino acids are immunogenic in rabbits and guinea pigs, but not in man and mouse. Linear and branched synthetic polymers composed of three of four different amino acids are highly immunogenic in most species tested. Polysaccharides are immunogenic in the mouse and human, but not in the guinea pig.

Physical forms of the antigen influence antigenicity. The immunogenic potential of poorly antigenic proteins, such as ribonuclease and human gonadotropin, can be increased by chemically cross-linking the proteins. The aggregation of poor antigens with macromolecules of opposite charge has also greatly enhanced antigenicity. In general, insoluble aggregated molecules are more antigenic than unaggregated molecules.

Antigenic Determinants

Injection of a protein antigen, even if uniform and chemically pure, always leads to the production of different antibodies, each of them directed against one of the various groups on the surface of the protein molecule. The groups determine the immunological specificity of the antigen and are called antigenic determinants.

Much of the information on the composition, structure, and size of antigenic determinants has been derived from studies with three general approaches. The first examined patterns of cross-reactivity of an antibody with antigens other than the one which induced its formation. The second involved the degradation of complex macromolecular antigens into fragments bearing intact antigenic determinants in order that the structure might be elucidated. The third approach, and the most productive, has been the study of natural or synthetic homopolymers of a single amino acid or sugar, synthetic polypeptides of defined structure, or synthetic antigens coupled to macromolecular carriers such as proteins (Sela, 1966).

Haptens

Karl Landsteiner (1945) described, at the turn of the 20th century, small, chemically defined compounds which were not immunogenic unless coupled to a carrier protein, in which case antibodies of the appropriate specificity were formed against both the protein and the attached chemical group. The attached groups were called haptens, from the Greek word *haptein*, "to fasten."

Although most haptens are small molecules, macromolecules may also function as haptens. The definition is bound not by size, but by immunogencity. Types of haptens studied include aromatic compounds, sugars, steroids, peptides, purines, pyrimidines, drugs such as penicillin, fluorescent compounds such as fluorescein and rhodamines, and electrondense material such as the ion-containing protein, ferritin.

The successful coupling of haptenic groups to carrier proteins and the ability of the conjugate to induce the formation of antihapten-specific antibodies have made possible the analysis of antigen structure and immune specificity.

Landsteiner's studies showed that antibody could distinguish between structurally similar haptens thereby demonstrating antibody specificity. Antibodies raised to three different isomeric *m-*, *o-*, and *p*-aminophenylsulfonic acids could be differentiated from each other serologically. Antibodies to *p*-aminophenylsulfonic acids could be differentiated from each other serologically. Antibodies to *p*-azophenylsulfonate-conjugated proteins reacted best with other proteins containing this chemical group. They reacted weakly with proteins containing the *m-* and *o-* isomeric derivatives of azophenylsulfonate. Similarly, antibodies against the *m*-azophenylsulfonate reacted best with the *m*-form of the derivative, weakly with azoproteins containing *o-* or *p-* derivatives. In contrast to the azoproteins, protein-free azodyes are not immunogenic.

Studies further showed that antibodies against *d*-isomers were different from those formed against *l*-isomers, and that *cis* and *trans* isomers could be differentiated. These experiments show clearly that antibodies react with definite chemical groups of the antigen and not with the entire antigenic molecule. The goodness of fit of antigen and antibody determine the immune specificity of the reaction.

Immunopotency

The most exposed portion of an antigen molecule would likely be the most immunogenic. Strong evidence for this was provided by Sela and his collaborators (Sela, 1966, 1969) who prepared antibodies to a synthetic polypeptide with the general structure of a backbone of poly-L-lysine, its ε-amino side chain residues linked to oligopolymers of poly-D, L-alanine. A polypeptide chain consisting of poly (tyrosine, glutamic acid) was attached to poly-D, L-alanine. Antibodies to the intact polypeptide were inhibited by the addition of free random copolymer poly (tyrosine, glutamic acid) but not by poly-L-lysine, nor by poly-L-alanine. The terminally exposed copolymer poly (tyrosine, glutamic acid) proved the most highly immunogenic portion of the polypeptide.

Sela termed the antigenic determinant provoking formation of a high concentration of specific antibody "immunopotent." Other determinants not inducing antibody production were termed "immunosilent." These latter only became immunopotent following chemical modification or fragmentation.

Important conditions for immunopotency of an antigenic determinant are accessibility and conformation. These points are illustrated in the antigenic structural studies by Atassi of sperm whale myoglobin (Atassi, 1975) and hen egg white lysozyme (Atassi, 1978). Since precise three-dimensional structures of these two proteins have been delineated by x-ray crystallography, and their amino acid sequences have been defined, their antigenic determinants have been located and described. All determinants are on the surface of the molecule, easily accessible for interaction with antibody. The determinants generally are comprised of six or seven amino acids.

The importance of conformation was born out by studies showing that, at low concentrations, the larger peptides of a myoglobin antigenic determinant region were better able to inhibit the same fraction of anti-myoglobin antibody than smaller peptides. The larger peptides showed greater inhibiting capacity because of their more favorable conformation.

Antibodies to another site of myoglobin, the C-terminal antigenic determinant, were shown to be inhibited by either the hexapeptide or heptapeptide of the region. Inhibition was found to be sometimes greater by one or the other peptide in different animals. It was suggested by these studies, that individual animals might not recognize exactly the same sequence of amino acid residues, and thus that the myoglobin molecule might have antigenic regions, rather than determinants. The recognition pattern of individual animals might involve different portions of the same antigenic region.

The immunopotent antigenic determinants of hen egg white lysozyme are also dependent upon conformation. Studies with antibodies to different animal lysozymes have shown that a high level of cross-reactivity tended to correlate closely with the presence of similar amino acid sequences occurring at the surface of the lysozyme molecule. Moreover, antibody activity to the determinants in the region of residues 60 to 83 bearing disulfide bonds, termed the "loop" region, is destroyed by change in conformation brought about by breakage of the disulfide bonds.

Immunodominance

The attachment of an antigenic determinant to an antibody combining site involves the regions of antigen and antibody which contribute the highest proportion of binding energy. On the antigenic determinant, these regions are termed immunodominant. They define the specificity of, or the degree of, reactivity with antibodies. Many factors which influence the immunopotency, or quantitative expression of the strength of an antigenic determinant, also play a role in determining immunodominance. Accessibility of the determinant and structural conformation of the antigen are two such factors.

Terminal sequences of polypeptide chains and polysaccharides are often exposed portions of these molecules. The terminal sequences are frequently antigenic determinants. The terminal amino acid peptides exert a dominant effect on the specificity of antigen interaction with antibody. The terminal nonreducing sugar residues of polysaccharides are often the immunodominant sugars in their reaction with antibody. These terminal residues were demonstrated by Landsteiner to contribute a large proportion of the binding energy in the interaction between the antigenic determinant and specific antibody. A gradient of binding energy was demonstrated to decrease from the most exposed portion of the molecule inward.

Antigenic Determinants of Complex Antigens

The major attribute of all antigenic determinants is their specificity, or selective reaction with antibody. For protein antigens, antibodies are directed against antigenic determinants. The salient properties of protein determinants will be dependent of: primary structure (the sequential arrangement of amino acids in the polypeptide chain), secondary structure (dictated by the backbone of polypeptide, such as the α-helix and β-structure), tertiary structure (conferred by the interaction between various reactive groups on the polypeptide chain and expressed by the folding of the chain), or quaternary structure such as the combination between α and β chains of the hemoglobin molecule (Benjamini, Michaeli, & Young, 1972; Crumpton, 1974; Reichlin, 1975).

Sequence-dependent antigenic determinants have been demonstrated for many polypeptides and proteins. Antibodies to ACTH, to gastrin, and to angiotensin have been shown to react with determinants which depend upon their amino acid sequence rather than the more complex architectural features of the peptide.

On the other hand, antibodies to bradykinin can be demonstrated to bear specificity to those secondary structural aspects which are governed by the polypeptide backbone. Antibodies to several collagens and gelatins and the polymer $(pro\text{-}gly\text{-}pro)_n$ will cross-react with one another. All these antigens form, in solution, triple-stranded helixes, indicating secondary structure-dependent determinants. Studies with myoglobin also show that secondary structure-dependent determinants in the form of tryptic peptides occupy several corners in the configuration.

A great proportion of antibodies induced by immunization with protein antigens are directed against specific determinants resulting from the tertiary structure of the protein. Antibodies can distinguish between oxy- and deoxy- forms of hemoglobin and myoglobin, forms which differ from each other only in their conformation. The antigenicity of myoglobin with metalloporphyrins other than heme can be differentiated. Reduced and carboxymethylated lysozyme do not cross-react with native lysozyme; performic acid-oxidized RNAase poorly cross-reacts with RNAase. All of these examples show a reduction in reactivity with antibodies parallel to conformational alterations.

Immunochemical studies with protein antigens composed of more than one polypeptide chain or subunit indicate that some of the antibodies elicited in response to immunization with native protein are directed against architectural aspects present only in the intact molecule. Studies with hemoglobin show that antibodies reactive to native A_1 hemoglobin ($\alpha_2\beta_2$) contain populations which react specifically with determinants formed from the interaction between α and β chains. Some antibodies against the isolated α chains of hemoglobin recognize determinants expressed when the α chains are either in free state or complexed with β chains in the normal $\alpha_2\beta_2$ tetramer, but not expressed when the α chains are complexed with γ chains to form $\alpha_2\gamma_2$ (fetal hemoglobin).

Quaternary structure-dependent determinants may consist of areas formed by the juxtapostion of two or more interacting subunits. They may also consist of structures on a given subunit which are induced by interaction with other subunits.

The simple sugars and oligosaccharides are not immunogenic, but can be converted into antigens by coupling to proteins. Isolated bacterial capsular polysaccharides are immunogenic in man and mouse, but not in horse or rabbit unless they are injected conjugated to protein carriers. Heidelberger and co-workers demonstrated that synthetic polyglucans are precipitated by antibodies to the pneumococcal polysaccharides and concluded that the determinant groups of these polysaccharides contained glucose residues.

Antigenic determinants on nucleic acids have been analyzed, although purified nucleic acids are poorly immunogenic (Stollar, 1973). Antibodies to DNA can be found in rabbits immunized with lysates of T_2, T_4, and T_6 bacteriophages. Such antibodies were specific for glucosylated hydroxymethylcytosine residues exposed to denatured single-stranded phage DNA. Antibodies to RNA have been induced by immunization with ribosomes. Antibodies to single-stranded DNA have been readily induced by immunization of animals with denatured DNA complexed with methylated bovine serum albumin plus adjuvant. Attempts to induce antibodies to native double-stranded DNA with similar complexes have not been successful.

Antibodies with specificity to antigenic determinants present in both native and denatured DNA have been isolated from human subjects with lupus erythematosus and from strains of mice and dogs with similar diseases. Antibodies to double-stranded RNA, histones, and nucleoproteins have also been identified. The mechanism by which these antibodies are induced is not clear.

Fatty acids, triglycerides, and other pure lipids do not have antigenic properties. To obtain antibodies to these substances, they must be complexed to protein carriers or other complex molecules. The specificity of antibodies to glycolipids is directed against the carbohydrate portion and little against the lipid (Rapport, 1969). The specificity of antibodies to cytolipin H, from human epidermoid carcinoma, and the antibodies to globoside from human red blood cells are both directed predominantly against the sugar moiety of their respective antigens, and some to the lipid. Similarly, antibodies to endotoxic lipopolysaccharides of gram-negative bacteria may also be directed against the core polysaccharide.

Size of Antigenic Determinants

The estimation of the size of an antigenic determinant was first accomplished by Kabat in 1966. Using the inhibitory activity of a series of oligosaccharides of increasing size on the precipitation reaction between dextran and human antidextran, he showed that with six different sera the hexasaccharide was the best inhibitor. In its most extended form, the dimensions of isomaltohexose are $34 \times 12 \times 7$ Å. This was taken to be the maximum size of the antigenic determinant of dextran. On the other end of the scale, he found that the determinant groups of dextrans must consist of more than a single glucosyl residue. The determinants of other polysaccharides contain only one or two monosaccharide units. Similarly, the glycolipid red blood cell A, B, Le, and H blood group substances owe their serological specificity to their carbohydrate portion, of which the determinant groups are not much larger than a single monosaccharide residue (Kabat, 1956; Race & Sanger, 1975).

Analysis of the size of determinant of a protein antigen has resulted in an estimate of comparable size. The optimal size of the capsular polypeptide antigen of *Bacillus anthracis*, poly-γ-D-glutamic acid, was concluded to be equivalent to a hexapeptide, with the dimensions of $36 \times 10 \times 6$ Å.

Antigenic Determinants and Cell Collaboration

Immunogenic molecules will induce both humoral and cellular immune responses when introduced into immune responsive animals. Immunization with hapten-carrier conjugates will elicit antibodies directed against the haptenic determinant and the carrier molecule, whereas the cellular immune response is generally directed against the carrier molecule only. Studies with well-defined protein antigens have clarified the difference between humoral and cellular immune specificities (Bullock, 1978; Goodman et al., 1978; Hashim, 1978). Investigations of the structure of the hormone bovine glucagon and its tryptic peptides have distinguished between the antigenic determinants involved in humoral, and in cellular immunity (Senyk et al., 1971). Immunized guinea pigs produced antibodies primarily directed against the amino-terminal heptadecapeptide, whereas cellular immunity was predominantly directed against the carboxyl-terminal undecapeptide.

This dichotomy of the immune response can be understood on the basis of cellular collaboration in the generation of antibody responses. Many studies have clearly demonstrated that the thymus-derived T lymphocytes, which do not secrete antibody, must interact with the bone-marrow-derived cells, the B lymphocytes, for induction of B lymphocyte antibody secretion. Both cell types are functionally distinct and antigen specific. It is therefore believed that an immunogen generally requires at least two determinants in order to form an "antigen bridge" between the two cells and thereby stimulate antibody formation. The spatial arrangements between haptenic and carrier determinants have been found to be important in the induction of antibody formation

(Fong et al., 1978). Effective interaction between T and B cells was estimated to lie between 69 and 97 Å. Antigens requiring this collaboration between B lymphocytes and T lymphocytes are termed T-dependent antigens.

Immunogenic Determinants for T Lymphocytes

Several functional subpopulations of thymus-derived, or T lymphocytes have been described. Two of these are important in the regulation of antibody synthesis. Those T lymphocytes which aid in the induction of antibody formation are called helper T cells. Those that suppress antibody production are called suppressor T cells. Recently different antigenic determinants specific for such T-cell functions have been identified on protein molecules such as β-galactosidase from *E. coli* (Sercarz et al., 1979). A specific determinant on a cyanogen bromide cleavage peptide termed CB-2 was demonstrated to induce suppression of the antibody response to any determinant on the β-galactosidase molecule. Two other cyanogen bromide cleavage products, CB-M and CB-C, were shown to induce helper T-cell function. Studies of this protein molecule have led to the identification of distant determinants responsible for immune regulatory functions. Moreover, they suggest that the repertoire of β-galactosidase specific determinants for suppressor T cells is more limited than, and different from, those determinants responsible for the initiation of T-cell helper function.

T-Independent Antigens

Some molecules are immunogenic because they are able to trigger B lymphocytes to secrete antibodies without the collaboration of the T lymphocytes. Although the principal feature of these molecules is repeating units, not all molecules with repeating units can be T-independent antigens. Bacterial polysaccharides and polymerized proteins such as bacterial flagellin can trigger antibody responses independent of any T-cell involvement. The antibodies produced are almost exclusively of the IgM class. The mechanism by which this class of antigen induces antibody production is not understood.

Adjuvants

Agents which nonspecifically enhance immune responses by increasing the intensity of the response, increasing the rate of development, prolongation, or induction of responses to immunologic or weakly immunogenic substances, are termed adjuvants (Jolles & Paraf, 1973; Munoz, 1964). Such agents can be subdivided into two major categories: those that potentiate both cellular and humoral immunity to antigens and those that enhance specific responses to certain antigens only. A wide variety of substances can act as general potentiators of immune responses.

Freund's complete adjuvant (Freund, 1951), a water and oil emulsion, is thought to function by releasing antigen slowly, and by enhancing the inflammatory responses. This mixture contains mineral oil, lanolin, and killed mycobacteria. The cell wall lipids, mucopolysaccharides, and mycobacteria RNA are the potent components. The same mixture, minus the mycobacteria, is termed Freund's incomplete adjuvant.

Inorganic compounds such as alum (potassium aluminum sulfate), aluminum hydroxide, and calcium phosphate also act to potentiate antibody responses. All of these substances act nonspecifically.

Synthetic polyribonucleotides in double- and single-stranded form act to enhance immunoresponsiveness. The homoribopolymer poly adenylate and poly uridylate (poly AU) can potentiate helper T cell, cytotoxic T cell, and delayed hypersensitivity responses as well as antibody production.

Other nonspecific immunostimulatory agents such as BCG, the methanol-extracted residue (MER) of BCG, *Corynebacterium parvum*, and the antihelmintic drug levamisole have been used in clinical trials of cancer therapy. The value of these agents as immunopotentiators in clinical use must await further trials.

Two experimental immunopotentiators that have been shown to endow specific immunoresponsiveness are immunogenic RNAs and transfer factor. It has been reported that RNA isolated from murine peritoneal lymphocytes and macrophages can transfer to recipient animals the ability to respond to an antigen, even in the absence of that antigen. The precise nature and role of the RNA as an immunopotentiator is unknown. It is thought that the RNA may couple to fragments of the antigen and yield an immunogenic "super antigen." A dialyzable, DNAase-resistant human peripheral blood extract was demonstrated to transfer specific skin test sensitivity to PPD from an immune donor to a recipient in the absence of antigen. The substance was termed transfer factor by Lawrence (1969).

IMMUNOGLOBULINS

In 1931, Felton observed that antipneumococcal antibodies in horse serum were water-insoluble proteins, or euglobulins. Tiselius and Kabat, in 1938, demonstrated that antibodies were proteins which migrate in the γ mobility region of an electrophoretic pattern. Antibodies were in the γ-globulin fraction of serum. Today, antibodies are classified as a group of related serum proteins termed immunoglobulins. They are glycoproteins composed of 82% to 96% protein and 4% to 18% carbohydrate. Based on such chemical properties as size, amino acid sequence, carbohydrate content, and electrophoretic mobility, they are subdivided into five major classes in the human. The accepted World Health Organization designations are IgG, IgM, IgA, IgD, and IgE.

Antibody molecules are structurally similar and yet show enormous diversity with respect to antigen binding and biological function. Antibodies of any specificity can be found in any class. Our present understanding of their structure is based on enzymic degradation of immunoglobulins into characteristic fragments (Edelman et al., 1969; Porter, 1973). This approach, and the realization that homogenous myeloma proteins are related to normal immunoglobulin, have been two major factors instrumental in enabling their structure to be analyzed in detail. Tabulation of the physical and chemical properties of the human immunoglobulins is shown in Table 2-1 (Gergely & Medgyesi, 1975; Nisonoff, Hopper, & Spring, 1975).

Structure of Immunoglobulins

All normal immunoglobulins are composed of a basic unit made of four polypeptide chains, or multiple of this unit. The basic four chain units consist of two identical heavy chains and two identical light chains differing in molecular weight. A bilaterally symmetric polypeptide structure is held together by covalent interchain disulfide bridges and by noncovalent forces. Dissociation of light and heavy chains can be accomplished by reduction and alkylation of the disulfide bonds.

The five classes of immunoglobulins are defined by antigenic differences on their heavy chains. The light chains are divided into kappa (x) or lambda (λ). Their distinction is one of serology which is based on primary structural differences. Both the heavy and light chains bear variations in amino acid sequences in the NH_2 terminals; therefore these portions of the chains are designated the variable regions (V regions to distinguish them from the relatively constant region (C region) on the remainder of the molecule. The chains exist as linear polypeptides with discrete regions of globular loops formed by the intrachain disulfide bonds termed domains. The light chain is composed of the V_L region domains of constant size (100 to 110 amino acid residues), which are designated V_x and V_λ depending on the light chain type, and the C_x or C_λ region domains. The heavy chain is composed of the V_H domain and three C region domains termed C_H1, C_H2, and C_H3.

The antibodies can be split by proteolytic enzymes without losing their specificity. IgG was the first immunoglobulin to be split by papain, an enzyme from papaya, into three pieces. Papain cleaved the IgG molecules at the hinge region between the C_H1 and C_H2 domains. Two separate antigen-combining fragments with electrophoretic mobilities similar to the parent antibody molecule, termed Fab fragments, and a third crystallizable piece, termed Fc fragment, were obtained.

The enzyme pepsin cleaves the immunoglobulin molecule on the COOH terminal side of the inter-heavy chain disulfide bonds, yielding a fragment termed $F(ab')_2$ a molecule composed of two Fab units and the hinge region. The Fc fragment is extensively degraded by pepsin treatment. See Fig 2-1 for a simplified and stylized diagram of the human IgG molecule.

TABLE 2-1. Physical Properties of Human Immunoglobulins

Properties	WHO Designations				
	IgG (γG)	IgA (γA)	IgM (γM)	IgD (γD)	IgE (γE)
Heavy chain class	γ	α	μ	δ	ε
Heavy chain subclass	γ1,γ2,γ3,γ4	α1,α2	μ1,μ2	Ja,La	—
Light chain types	κ and λ	κ and λ	κ and λ	κ and λ	κ and λ
Molecular weight	150,000	160,000 (monomer) 400,000 (secretory)	900,000	180,000	190,000
Sedimentation coefficient	7S	7S, 9S, 11S (secretory)	19S	7S	8S
Molecular formula	$\gamma_2\kappa_2, \gamma_2\lambda_2$	$\alpha_2\kappa_2, \alpha_2\lambda_2$ $(\alpha_2\kappa_2)_2 SJ,$ $(\alpha_2\lambda_2)_2 SJ$	$(\mu_2\kappa_2)5$ $(\mu_2\lambda_2)5$	$\delta_2\kappa_2, \delta_2\lambda_2$	$\epsilon_2\kappa_2, \epsilon_2\lambda_2$
Antigen binding valency	2	2	5 or 10	?	2
Concentration in serum—mg/ml	8-16	1.4-4.0	0.5-2.0	0-0.4	17-450 ng/ml
% of Total immunoglobulin	80	13	6	1	0.002
Electrophoretic mobility	γ	Fast γ to β	Fast γ to β	Fast γ	Fast γ
% Carbohydrate content	3	8	12	13	12

FIG 2-1. Structure of human immunoglobulin G. Diagram shows the enzyme-mediated cleavage sites for papain and pepsin, the cleavage products, and the variable and constant region domains.

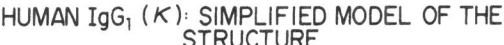

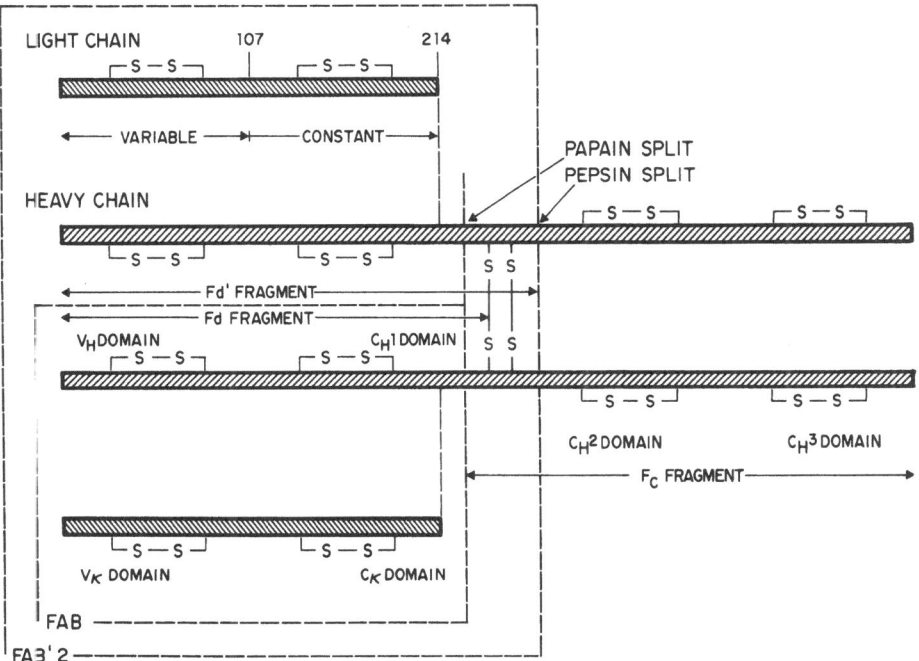

Heterogeneity

Light chain types

Light chains have a molecular weight of approximately 23,000 and are classified into two types, x and λ, based on multiple amino acid sequence differences in the constant region of the polypeptide chain. The proportion of x to λ chains in humans is approximately 2:1. A given immunoglobulin will bear identical chain types, never a mixture of the two.

The x chains do not exhibit C region subclasses. However, four distinct λ chains have been detected in humans and are termed subtypes.

Heavy chain classes

There are five classes of heavy chains based on structural differences in the constant region of the polypeptide chain. The class of heavy chain, γ, α, μ, δ, or ϵ determines the class of immunoglobulin: IgG, IgA, IgM, IgD, or IgE, respectively. The IgG molecule is composed of two γ chains and two light chains. The subunit IgM molecules are composed similarly of two v and two light chains (Metzger, 1970). IgM as a macromolecule is composed of five basic four-chain units.

Monomeric IgA is structurally composed of two α heavy chains and two light chains (Tomasi & Grey, 1972). However, it can be found as a mixture of varying proportions of monomers, dimers, and tetramers.

IgD (Möller, 1977) and IgE (Bennich & Bohr-Lindström, 1974), similarly to IgG, each consist of a single four-chain unit. The heavy chain classes vary in the number of constant region domains. The μ and ϵ chains possess four C-domains rather than three as in γ and α chains. The δ chain has three C-domains, but has an extended hinge region, the area between the first and second C region domains (C_H1 and C_H2) of the heavy chain.

Heavy chain subclasses

The heavy chains have been further divided into subclasses based upon physiochemical differences in the constant regions. There are four subclasses of the human γ chains, γ_2, γ_1, γ_3, and γ_4. The IgG_1 and IgG_4 subclasses have four, whereas the IgG_3 subclass may have as many as seven.

There are two subclasses of the α chain, α_1 and α_2, in IgA_1 and IgA_2 molecules, respectively. The IgA_2 molecule is unique among immunoglobulins because the light chains are bonded to the α_2 chain by noncovalent forces instead of disulfide bonds.

The subclasses of μ chains of IgM have been identified and are termed μ_1, and μ_2. Similarly antigenic heterogeneity has been reported for the δ chain of IgD-two subclasses, Ja and La, have been identified. No subclasses for the ϵ chain of IgE have been reported.

Variable Regions

V region subgroups

The V region comprises the NH_2 terminal end of both the light and heavy chains. The region has been divided into three main groups, V_H group (for H groups), $V_\varkappa$ group for $\varkappa$ light chains, and the V_λ group for λ light chain. The V region has been divided into subgroups based on length and position of invariant amino acid sequences. These subdivisions exist for $\varkappa$ and λ light chain types as well as for heavy chains. The V_L region subgroups are designated $V_\varkappa I$-$V_\varkappa IV$ and $V_\varkappa I$-$V_\varkappa VI$. The V_H region subgroups are classified $V_H I$-$V_H IV$.

Hypervariable regions

The chemical differences responsible for the specificity of the antibody molecule are embodied in the amino acid sequences of the variable region. The alignment of the

FIG 2-2. Variability at different amino acid positions for human *x*, human λ, and mouse *x* light chain populations. GAP designates the amino acid positions in which insertions or deletions have been found. Three hypervariable regions for these light chains have been detected. (From Wu TT, Kabat EA. *J Exp Med* 1970; 132: 211).

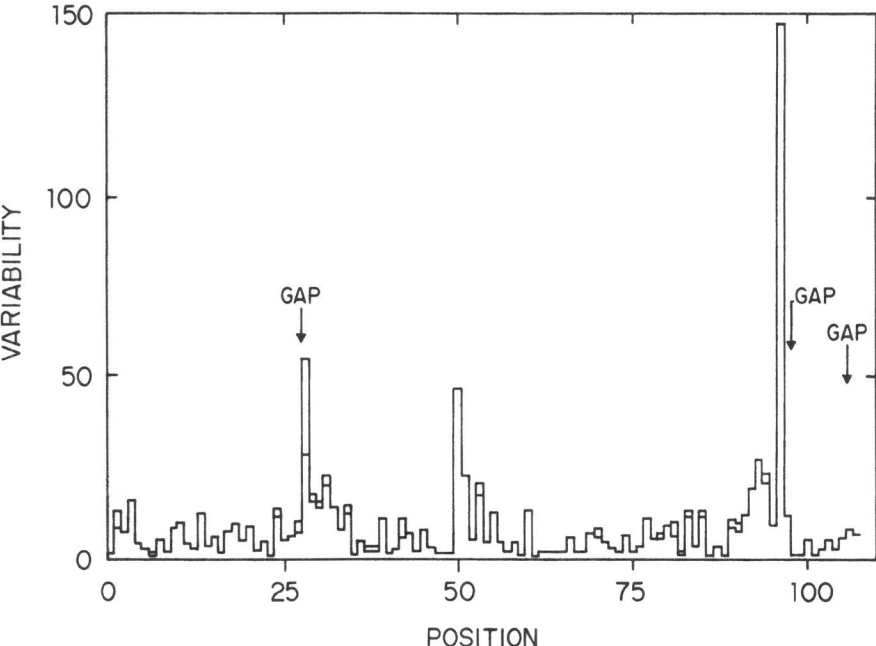

light and heavy chain variable regions create a specific combining site to which antigenic determinants attach. Within the variable domains of both light and heavy chain several hypervariable regions have been found (Wu & Kabat, 1970). These regions show increased frequency of heterogeneity in amino acid sequence and have been termed "hot spots." The light chain appears to have three hypervariable regions, and the heavy chain, four, as illustrated in Figs 2-2 and 2-3. These regions are intimately associated with the formation of the antigen binding site of the antibody molecule (Cebra, Koo, & Ray, 1974) and thus are known as the complementarity-determining regions.

Antibody diversity

Extensive sequence analysis of many immunoglobulins suggested that they are encoded by distinct variable and constant region genes in germ-line cells (Dreyer & Bennett, 1965). Two opposing hypotheses have been proposed to explain such antibody diversity that may be composed of as many as 10^6 to 10^8 (Sigal & Klinman, 1978). According to the germ-line gene theory, each variable region is encoded by a separate variable gene

FIG 2-3. Variability at different amino acid positions for human heavy chain hypervariable regions. Four hypervariable regions for the heavy chains have been detected. (From Kabat EA. Structural concepts in immunology and immunochemistry, p. 295. New York, Holt, Rinehart & Winston, 1976).

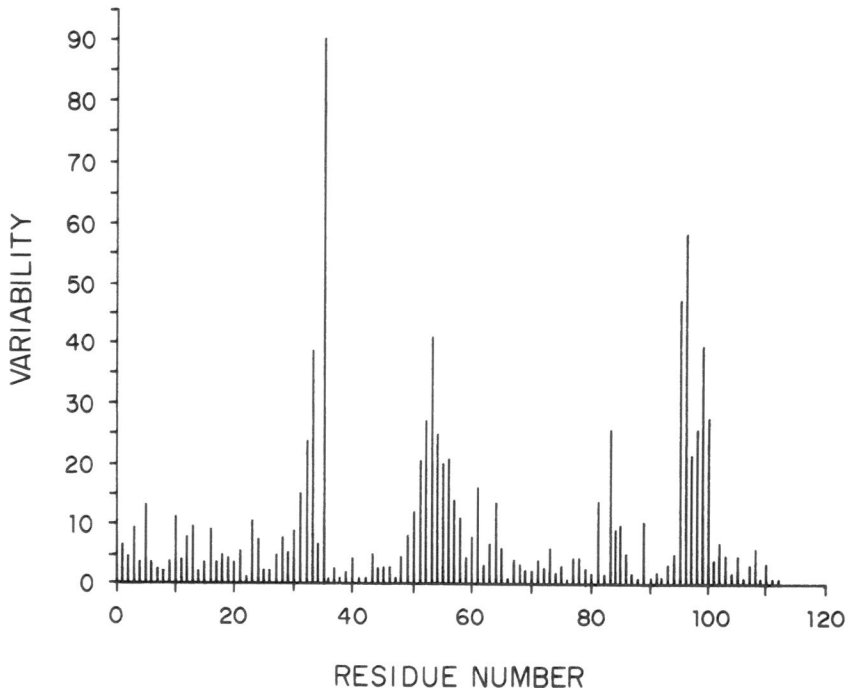

(Hood & Talmage, 1970). The somatic diversification theory postulated that there are only a few inherited genes, which undergo extensive somatic mutation to generate thousands of genes (Weigert et al., 1970). Recent restriction enzymes and recombinant DNA technology have resolved that the immunoglobulin peptide chains are encoded in multiple gene segments scattered along a chromosome of the germ-line genome. The gene segments must be brought together to form a complete immunoglobulin gene active in B lymphocytes. In addition, mutations are introduced somatically into immunoglobulin genes at a high rate. Both the recombination and mutation result in diversification of the genetic information carried in the germ-line genome.

The variable regions of λ and x light chains are encoded by two gene segments termed variable (V_L) and joining (J_L). The joining gene segment encodes a peptide region between the variable and constant region. The V_L and J_L gene segments contribute to the third hypervariable region. The variable regions of the heavy chains are specified by third gene segments called variable (V_H), diversity (D), and joining (J_H) regions. The D segment encodes the major portion of the third hypervariable region. The assembly of the variable gene from several gene segments is thought to enable creation of antibody diversity (Tonegawa, 1983).

Idiotypes

Unique V region amino acid sequences have been identified by immunization of genetically similar animals with specific antibodies. The only antigenic differences between the immunoglobulin donor and recipient were unique V region sequences. The antibody response was restricted to these unique antigenic determinants. The term idiotype was used to denote these unique V region determinants which are recognized by anti-idiotypic antibodies (Natvig & Kunkel, 1973; Sakato & Eisen, 1975). Many studies have shown that idiotypic determinants are located close to or within the antigen binding site of the antibody molecule. Idiotypic determinants have been regarded as immunologic markers for the antibody combining site and thus are associated with the hypervariable region. Whether this dictates antibody specificity is not clear, since similar idiotypic determinants have been detected on antibodies of different specificities.

Early experimental work in the 1950s suggested the presence of individual specific determinants in human myeloma proteins and Waldenström macroglobulins. Subsequent work showed that myeloma proteins and macroglobulins possessed determinants not present in any other myeloma or macroglobulin tested. Similarly, human Bence Jones proteins (L chains) of x and λ types were also shown to possess unique antigenic determinants. These determinants were found to be present in the V regions of the light and heavy chains. Such idiotypic determinants in man have been detected even on IgM cold agglutinins in patients with acquired hemolytic anemias.

In addition to unique determinants, cross-idiotypic specificities, or antigenic specificities common to human IgM cold agglutinins but not to Waldenström macroglobulins have been identified. These cross-reacting cold agglutinins were hypothesized to bear a common antigenic determinant in the combining site. Similarly, human IgM antibodies to human IgG from patients with mixed cryoglobulin syndrome have been found to have cross-idiotypic specificities that divide them into two major protein groups. The prototypes are termed Wa and Po.

These two prototypes have been studied extensively. They have been found to bear similar amino acid sequences in all four hypervariable regions on the V_H domain, with only three differences in amino acid sequence out of 41 potential hypervariable positions. The studies on the light chain of the Wa group of proteins have shown that they possess the same V_{xIII} subgroup with similar amino acid sequences exhibited in at least the first hypervariable region. The first hypervariable region of the light chains of cold agglutinins have also been found to be similar.

These studies suggest that the chemical basis for proteins exhibiting cross-idiotypic specificities have the same light chain, heavy chain, or both, belonging to the same V_L or V_H subgroup, and have similar antigenic determinants on the hypervariable regions.

J Chain

Monomeric IgA and IgM are covalently linked by disulfide bonds and by the J or joining chain (Koshland, 1975) to form polymeric IgM and secretory IgA (sIgA) as illustrated in Fig 2-4. The J chain is believed to have the function of initiating or facilitating polymerization of IgM or IgA and is present in the stoichiometric ratio of one J chain per polymer, regardless of size. The J chain is glycopeptide with a molecular weight of 15,000. IgA myeloma molecules have been found which lack the J chain; its presence is not invariably required for polymerization. The J chain is rich in half-cystine groups (7 to 8 residues per molecule). In human IgM, the single J chain is disulfide-bonded to the penultimate half cystine of one, or possibly two, μ chains. The accommodation of the J chain in the IgM pentamer suggests that the molecule may be asymmetric, but this requires further clarification. The J chain is synthesized by the same cells that produce the immunoglobulin to which it is attached . It is linked to IgM or to polymeric IgA before they are secreted from the lymphocyte. Electrophoretic or ion-exchange chromatography purified J chain appears to be homogeneous, although minor polymorphism has not yet been ruled out.

Secretory Component

Secretory IgA is composed of an IgA dimer, a molecule of secretory component, and a molecule of J chain. The secretory, or S component is a single chain polypeptide of about 70,000 mol wt, containing about 9% carbohydrate. It can be found in unbound form in the saliva of persons lacking IgA, in the saliva of the newborn, in the gastrointestinal fluid, and in colostrum and milk. The secretory component is not synthesized by the lymphoid cells but by the mucosal epithelial cells. The biological significance of the component is not known, but it does increase the resistance of sIgA molecule against digestion by trypsin and pepsin.

Genetic Markers on Immunoglobulins

Inherited differences on human immunoglobulins have been detected and are termed allotypes, allotypic markers, or genetic markers. The human IgG heavy chain bear Gm markers. The IgA heavy chains bear Am markers, and the light chains of x bear the Km markers (formerly Inv). Each allotypic marker is restricted to one IgG or IgA subclass.

The human chain allotypic markers have been found only on the C region of the IgG and IgA heavy chains. Each determinant is associated with a specific domain of the heavy chain. Human population studies have demonstrated that different combinations of allotypic markers are inherited as units of haplotypes. The Gm and Am markers are genetically linked to each other, but not the Km markers.

FIG 2-4. Schematic illustration of the structures of IgA, the secretory IgA molecule with J chain secretory component, and IgM with its J chain.

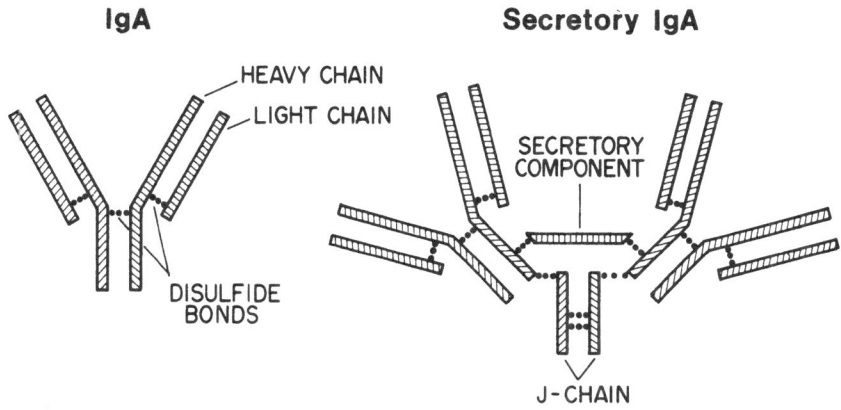

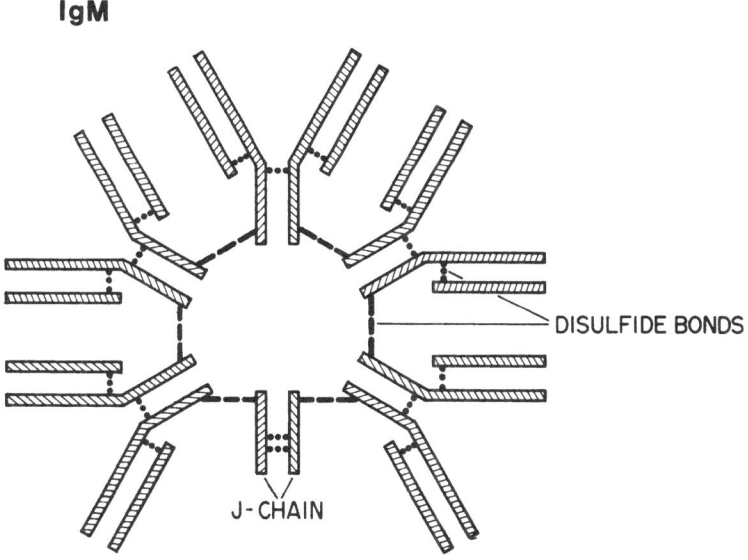

Carbohydrate Moieties of Immunoglobulins

Carbohydrates are found covalently bonded to the polypeptide chains of immunoglobulins. The function of these moieties is poorly understood, but it is proposed that they play a role in the secretion of immunoglobulins by plasma cells, and in biological functions associated with the C region of the heavy chain. The carbohydrate is found associated with the secretory component, the J chain, and the C region of the heavy chain. IgM and IgE have an average of five oligosaccharides each, IgG has one, and IgA two or three. The attachment in most cases is by means of N-glycosidic linkage between N-acetylglucosamine residues of the carbohydrate side chain and an asparagine residue of the polypeptide chain.

Biological Activities of Immunoglobulins

Immunoglobulins exhibit many different biological activities (Spiegelberg, 1974) as shown in Table 2-2. Some of these functions follow the interaction between antigen and antibody, others do not. The structure that governs biological activity other than interaction with antigen is localized in the constant region of the heavy chain, particularly the Fc fragment. For instance, the concentration and distribution of immunoglobulins in body fluids are regulated in part by the constant region of the heavy chain. The rate of immunoglobulin synthesis per plasma cell is similar for all classes. Therefore the number of plasma cells and the rate of catabolism also influence serum concentration of immunoglobulins. IgG_1 and IgG_2 are the two most abundant immunoglobulins in serum. The normal synthetic rate of IgG is also the greatest, and its half-life is the longest. The turnover rate of intact immunoglobulins is similar to the rate of Fc fragments. The Fc fragments of IgG are catabolized relatively slowly as compared to Fab fragments and light chains, both of which are rapidly eliminated from the circulation.

IgG immunoglobulins are predominantly located in the extravascular spaces, as are IgA immunoglobulins. IgM and IgD immunoglobulins are predominantly located in the intravascular spaces. The rate of exchange of an immunoglobulin between intra- and extravascular space depends primarily on its diffusion coefficient. There is an inverse relationship between the diffusion coefficient of a particular immunoglobulin, and the ratio expressed as its concentration in serum compared to that in extravascular fluid. IgG has a high diffusion coefficient, IgM has a low one.

Placental and gut transfer

Maternal immunoglobulins can be transferred to offspring prenatally, postnatally, or both ways. The Fc fragment plays an important role in the transfer, since isolated Fc fragments are passed across the placenta but Fab fragments are not. In man, prenatal transfer of immunoglobulin to the fetus is the major route—all IgG subclasses can pass the placental barrier.

Transfer of immunoglobulins through the gut does not appear to be important in man.

TABLE 2-2. Biological Properties of Human Immunoglobulins

Properties	IgG	IgA	IgM	IgD	IgE
Total body pool intravascular spaces (%)	45	42	76	75	51
Intravascular pool catabolized per day (%)	6.7	25	18	37	89
Cerebrospinal fluid (μg/ml)	2.5-7.5	—	—	—	—
Normal synthetic rate mg/Kg/day	33	24	6.7	0.4	0.02
$T_{1/2}$ (half-life in serum in days)	23	5.8	5.1	2.8	2.3
Complement fixation classical pathway	yes	no	yes	no	no
alternate pathway	no	yes	no	weakly	weakly
Crosses placenta	yes	no	no	no	no
Cytophilic for mast cells and basophils	no	no	no	no	yes
Antibacterial activity	yes	yes	yes	?	?
Antiviral activity	yes	yes	yes	?	?

Complement activation

Immunoglobulins can activate complement by two different pathways, the classic pathway involving complement components C_1 to C_9 or the alternate pathway involving factors C_3, and C_5 through C_9. IgG_1, IgG_2, IgG_3, and IgM can activate the classic pathway. IgA_1 and IgA_2 can activate the alternate pathway. Aggregated IgA, IgD, and IgE proteins do not fix classic components of complement, but Fc fragments of aggregated IgD and IgE can fix late complement components.

The C_H2 domain of IgG (the NH_2 terminal half of the Fc fragment) is associated with complement fixation. Fab or $F(ab')_2$ fragments do not fix complement.

Cytophilic antibodies

Leukocytes have surface receptors specific for immunoglobulins. Cytophilic antibodies are bound to the cell receptors by the Fc portion of their molecules. The Fc receptors are distributed evenly on the cell surface. The binding of immunoglobulins to cells is highly specific. In man, monocytes and macrophages have receptors for IgG_1 and IgG_3. These cytophilic antibodies aid opsonization of foreign particles. The human B lymphocytes bear Fc receptors for IgG. Similarly, the human T lymphocytes bear Fc receptors. The helper T lymphocytes bear receptors for IgM and the suppressor T lymphocytes bear Fc receptors for IgG. Neutrophils bear receptors for IgG and IgA immunoglobulins. Platelets bear receptors only for IgG. The functions of these receptors are not known.

The IgG molecules are associated with lymphocyte-mediated cytotoxicity. The lysis of ^{51}Cr-labeled chicken erythrocytes coated with anti-erythrocyte antibodies by unsensitized human lymphocytes is inhibited by human IgG_1, IgG_3, or by aggregated IgG_2, but not by IgG_4. The inhibitory activity has been located on the Fc portion of the IgG molecules.

IgE can bind to basophils or mast cells present in the skin and lungs and is termed homocytotropic because it attaches to cells of animals of the same species (Ishizaka & Dayton, 1973). Cell-bound IgE molecules are attached to basophils and mast cells by the Fc fragment. IgE is in this way responsible for passive anaphylaxis in the Prausnitz-Kustner reaction, and reaginic activity in man. The binding of allergens to the cell-bound IgE initiates the release of vasoactive substances such as histamine, and slow-reactive substance of anaphylaxis (SRS-A) from basophils and mast cells. The IgE mediated release of vasoactive substances is thought to require cross-linking of the IgE molecules on the cell surface by specific antigen. Experimentally induced release by cross-linking the IgE molecules with anti-IgE Fc specific antibodies has also been demonstrated.

Cell membrane immunoglobulins

Antigen-specific receptors on the surface of lymphocytes are immunoglobulins (Warner, 1974). IgD and IgM comprise the dominant membrane immunoglobulin classes on the human peripheral blood B cells. IgA- and IgG-bearing cells account for fewer of the peripheral blood lymphocytes in the normal person.

The lymphocytes from the newborn and adults stain for surface IgD. These same cells also stain for IgM surface immunoglobulin. The IgM and IgD molecules form caps independently on the same cell, so indicating that they are not linked. It has been proposed that IgD is the antigen receptor initially present, and is followed by synthesis and expression of IgM only after contact with antigen.

ANTIGEN-ANTIBODY REACTIONS

Forces That Participate in Antigen-Antibody Reactions

The specificity of the antibody reaction with antigen, the forces that participate in their interaction, and the biological consequences of their reactions have been the subject of intensive study. The chemical basis for the combinations of antigens and antibodies are much the same as those found for enzymes and transport proteins. They do not involve covalent bonding. Their interaction can easily be visualized as occurring in two stages. The first stage is the specific combination of the antibodies with the determinant groups of the antigens. This takes place rapidly and is accompanied by energy changes. The second stage is an observable reaction such as precipitation, agglutination, or complement fixation. This reaction may occur very slowly and is accompanied by little energy change.

The combination of antigen and antibody can be explained by their complementariness, but many forces influence the goodness of fit. Involved in the interaction are electrostatic forces such as Coulomb forces. The positively and negatively charged groups, in their appropriate spatial arrangements on antigens and antibodies, can endow strong attraction or repulsion to each other. The force of attraction is inversely proportionate to the square of the distance between the charges. The closer the charges, the stronger the attracting force.

Other forces also play a role in determining the strength of binding. Weaker forces such as dipole-dipole bonds, dipole-ion bonds, Van der Waal's forces, and hydrogen bonds influence intramolecular attraction. Hydrophobic and hydrophilic interactions are also important, since antigen–antibody reactions occur in aqueous environments. The weak and reversible hydrogen bonds can form between hydrophilic groups such as NH_3^+, COO^-, and OH depending upon the closeness of the antigen and antibody bearing these groups. When hydrophobic groups containing nonpolar groups (alanine, valine, leucine, isoleucine, proline, phenylalanine, tryptophan, and methionine) on the surface of the antigen and antibody come into contact, water molecules are excluded between them. The reduction of contact with water means more water molecules are in the H-bonded state and the lower force-energy state of the system influences stronger attraction rather than repulsion. Antibody molecules possess many hydrophobic amino acids in their antigen combining region.

Weak forces such as Van der Waal's forces require close proximity of both antigen and antibody to become an important factor. Their formation depends on the complementary electron-cloud formation between the combining site of the antibody and the surface of the antigenic determinant. The smaller the intermolecular distance, the stronger the force, which is inversely proportional to the seventh power of the distance.

Precipitation Reactions

The precise method of quantitative measurement of soluble antigens and antibodies and their interactions was introduced by Heidelberger and his colleagues in 1929 (Heidelberger, 1949). The classical precipitation reaction was accomplished by titration of solutions of increasing antigen concentration into a constant amount of antibody. The mixtures were incubated for from five to seven days to ensure maximum precipitation of antigen-antibody complexes. The precipitates formed were recovered and quantitatively measured by the micro-Kjeldahl method for protein nitrogen (antibodies contain about 16% nitrogen). Today, a variety of other analytical methods exist, including those which use antigens labeled with a radioisotope, and spectrophotometric measurements. A typical precipitation curve is obtained as shown in Fig 2-5.

The addition of increasing concentrations of antigen to a constant amount of antibody will result in a precipitation curve manifesting three zones or regions. The zone of antibody excess is the portion of the curve showing a steep rise. Precipitation requires that the antigen as well as the antibody have two or more binding sites or valencies. All the antigen is contained in the precipitate. Precipitation will increase until a maximum is reached. A zone of equivalence is detected when neither free antigen nor free antibody are found in the supernatant. All are bound in the large three-dimensional lattice of the immune precipitate. With still further addition of antigen, a zone of antigen excess is finally reached and the curve falls off as the quantity of precipitation between antigen and antibody decreases.

Agglutination Reactions

The interaction of antibodies with particulate antigens such as viruses, bacteria, fungi, cells, or antigen-coated beads results in agglutination. Their reactions have three distinct patterns: antibody excess, antigen-antibody equivalence, and antigen excess, similar to the precipitation reaction. The ability of particulate antigen to be agglutinated by antibodies depends also on the number of antigenic determinants and the antibody valency. IgM antibodies, bearing ten antigen-binding sites, are better agglutinators than IgG antibodies, with two. The net electric charge or Z potential of the particulate antigen greatly influences its reaction with bivalent molecules such as IgG. Some cells bearing net charge groups fail to agglutinate because of repulsion forces. Agglutination will result if the charges are neutralized by buffering protein solutions or by removal of the undesired charged groups by enzymatic cleavage.

FIG 2-5. Schematic diagram of the quantitative precipitin reaction between a soluble antigen and antibody. Top panel illustrates possible patterns of precipitation for divalent antigen and IgG antibody. The bottom panel shows the degree of precipitation expected with increasing antigen concentration in the presence of a constant amount of antibody.

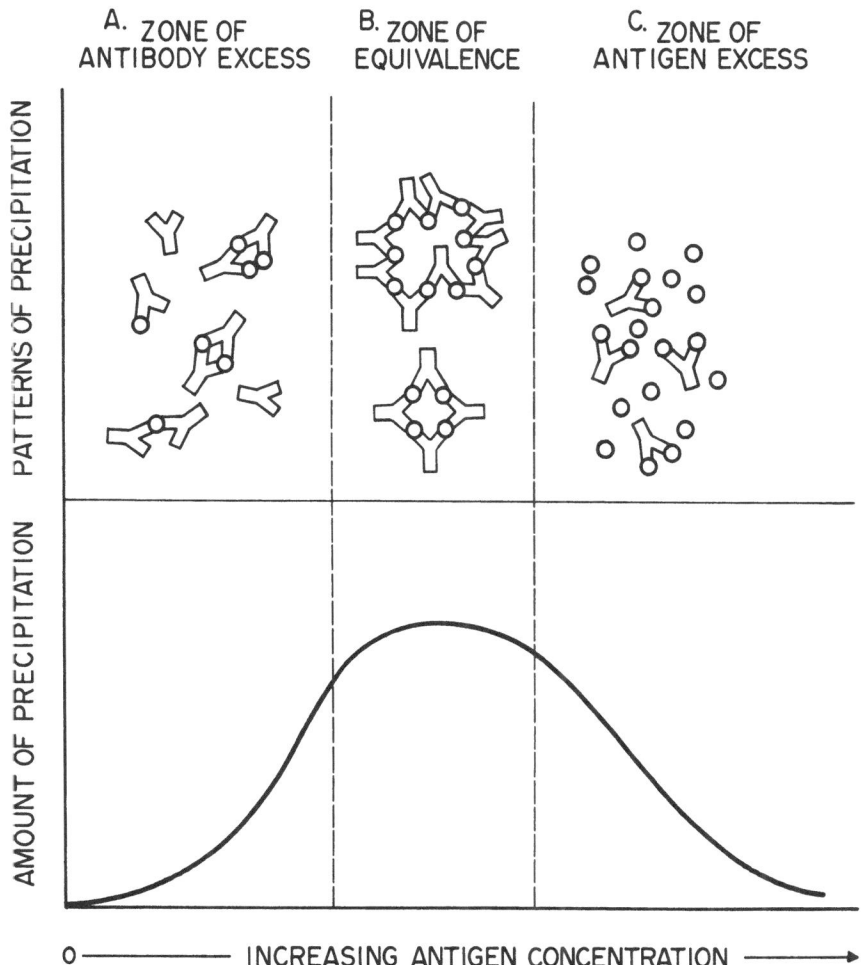

Conformational Changes in the Antibody Molecule Upon Interaction with Antigen

It is attractive to explain certain biological properties of antibodies by conformational changes that may occur within the antibody molecule after interaction with antigen (Metzger, 1974). The fixation of complement to the Fc region of the antibody molecule occurs after reaction of the Fab region with antigen. Moreover, such conformational changes may explain how immune cells bearing immunoglobulin receptors are triggered by antigen.

One piece of evidence that conformational changes can occur in antibodies comes from electron microscopic analysis. IgG antibody molecules attached to two virus particles were observed to be in extended form, or in a "horseshoe" shape, with both combining sites attached to the same particle. This suggests the potential of movement for the two Fab segments in relation to each other. The freedom of rotation can be attributed to the flexibility in the hinge region of the two heavy chains.

Changes in circular dichroic spectra, sedimentation coefficient, and volume contraction, and decrease in radius of gyration of the antibody molecule upon interaction with antigen have been interpreted as indicating conformational changes in the antibody. The mechanism of internal conformational changes upon interaction of the antibody molecule with antigen remains unsettled.

Hapten-Antibody Interactions

The nature of the antibody affinity, or strength of binding to a hapten, can be determined by studying the reaction between antibody and hapten. Studies of the antigen-antibody reaction have shown that frequently a gradual increase in the affinity of circulating antibodies with time occurs after initial immunization (Eisen & Siskind, 1964), with IgG more likely to increase in affinity than IgM. Immunization with a low dose of antigen has been shown to favor the production of high-affinity antibodies. The affinity of a receptor on a B cell has been shown to reflect that of the antibody produced by the cell and its descendents.

A general method for measuring the association constant is equilibrium dialysis (Eisen, 1964). The antibody affinity is determined by dialyzing a solution of antibody in a dialysis membrane sac in a solution of hapten of known concentration. Only the hapten will diffuse through the membrane, which is permeable to small molecular weight molecules, but impermeable to large ones such as antibodies. The external hapten concentration at equilibrium will be equal to the concentration of unbound hapten within the dialysis sac. The combination between antigen and antibody is fully reversible, so the amount of bound hapten will depend on the final concentration of unbound or free hapten in solution. A test of different concentrations of hapten with the same antibody concentration will provide the necessary information for the determination of the average affinity constant (K) of the antigen-antibody reaction.

The method of measuring the affinity of antibodies is to analyze the interaction between antigen and antibody. Their interaction can be formulated by the following equation according to the law of mass action:

$$Ab + H \underset{k_2}{\overset{k_1}{\rightleftharpoons}} AbH \tag{1}$$

Kinetic studies have shown that antigen-antibody reactions have a high forward rate and a low backward rate. Equation (1) can be expressed as follows:

$$\frac{[AbH]}{[Ab][H]} = \frac{k_1}{k_2} = K \tag{2}$$

$[AbH]$ is the concentration of antigen-antibody complexed.
$[Ab]$ is the concentration of free antibody.
$[H]$ is the concentration of free hapten.
K is the average association or affinity constant at equilibrium.

Since

Ab_t (total Ab concentration) $= [Ab] + [AbH]$, then

$$[Ab] = [Ab_t] - [AbH]$$

Therefore

$$K = \frac{[AbH]}{[(Ab_t)-(AbH)][H]}$$

$$K = \frac{[AbH] \, [1+K \, H]}{[H][Ab_t]}$$

$$\frac{[AbH]}{[Ab_t]} = \frac{K[H]}{1+K[H]} = R$$

50   Fong

FIG 2-6. A Scatchard plot of a simple case of an interaction between two identical and independent antibody binding sites with hapten. The slope is − K, the X-intercept is the number of binding sites, and the Y-intercept is nK.

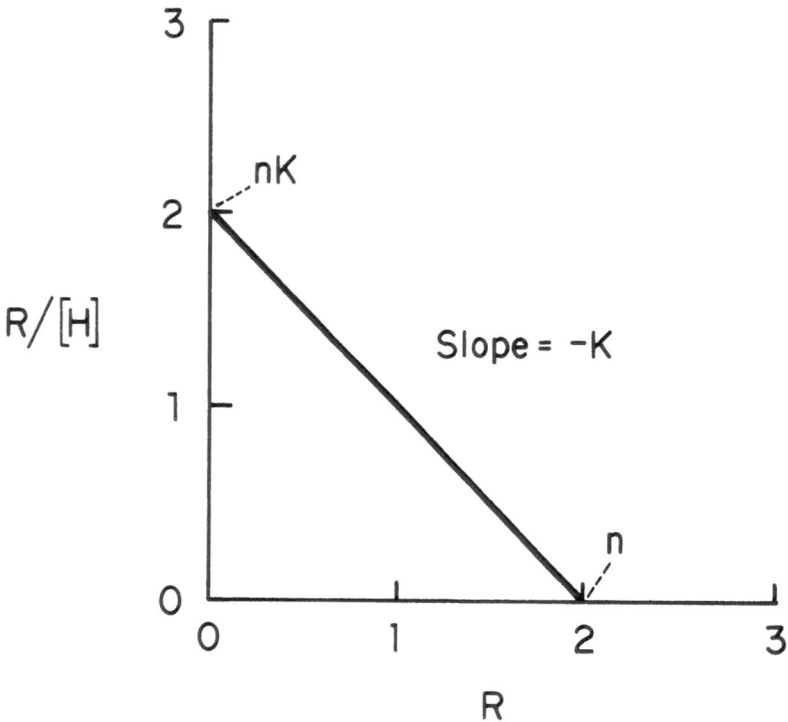

R is the ratio of the moles of bound hapten per mole of antibody. A Scatchard plot $R/[H]$ v R (Scatchard, 1949) graphically represents the data (Fig 2-6). If the antibody-binding sites are identical and independent, a straight line will result with a slope of $− K$. The X-intercept is equal to the number of binding sites, n. The association constant of the antibody is determined from the relationship between free and bound hapten and antibody. The constant can be obtained directly from the binding plots.

Homogeneity of association constants will result in a straight line or linear relationship between $R/[H]R$. Antibody populations with mixed or heterogeneous association constants will show nonlinear or curved line relationships.

Most antibodies have association constants in the range of 10^5 to 10^{12} L/mol. The low-affinity antibodies have association constants near 10^5 L/mol, whereas the high-affinity antibodies have association constants near 10^{12} L/mol.

Through analyses of antigen-antibody reactions, antisera have been found to consist of a heterogeneous population of antibodies with a range of affinity constants, even though these antibodies bear the same specificity. Thus, the term antibody is a collective noun referring to a set of molecules defined by their capacity to bind a given antigen.

REFERENCES

Atassi MZ: Antigenic structure of myoglobin. *Immunochemistry* 1975; 12: 423.

Atassi MZ: Precise determination of the entire antigenic structure of lysozyme. *Immunochemistry* 1978; 15: 909.

Benacerraf B, McDevitt HO: The histocompatibility-linked immune response genes. *Science* 1972; 175: 273.

Benjamini E, Michaeli D, Young JD: Antigenic determinants of proteins of defined sequences. *Current Topics in Microbiology and Immunology* 1972; 58: 85.

Bennich H, Von Bohr-Lindström H: Structure of immunoglobulin E (IgE). *Progress in Immunology, II* 1974; 1: 49.

Borek F (ed): *Immunogenicity*. Amsterdam, North-Holland Publishing, 1972.

Bullock WW: ABA-T determinant regulation of delayed hypersensitivity. *Immunological Reviews* 1978; 39: 3.

Cebra JJ, Koo PH, Ray A: Specificity of antibodies: Primary structural basis of antibody binding. *Science* 1974; 186: 263.

Crumpton MJ: Protein antigens: The molecular bases of antigenicity and immunogenicity, in Sela, M. (ed): *The Antigens, II:* p. 1. New York, Academic Press, 1975.

DeWeck EL: Low molecular weight antigens, in Sela, M. (ed): *The Antigens, II:* 141. New York, Academic Press, 1974.

Dreyer WJ, Bennett JC: The molecular basis of antibody formation: A paradox. *Proc Natl Acad Sci USA* 1965; 54: 864.

Edelman GM, Cunningham BA, Gall WE, Gottlieb PD, Rutishauser U, Waxdal MJ: The covalent structure of an entire γG immunoglobulin molecule. *Proc Natl Acad Sci* 1969; 63: 78.

Eisen HN: Equilibrium dialysis for measurement of antibody-hapten affinities. *Methods in Med Research Yearbook* 1964; 10: 106.

Eisen HN, Siskind GW: Variations in affinity of antibodies during the immune response. *Biochemistry* 1964; 3: 996.

Felton LD: Use of ethyl alcohol as precipitant in concentration of anti-pneumococcus serum. *J Immunol* 1931; 21: 357.

Fong S, Nitecki DE, Cook RM, Goodman, JW: Spatial requirements between haptenic carrier determinants for T-dependent antibody responses. *J of Experimental Med* 1978; 148: 817.

Freund J: The effects of paraffin oil and mycobacteria on antibody formation and sensitization. *Am J of Clin Path* 1951; 21: 645.

Gergely J, Medgyesi GA (eds): *Antibody Structure and Molecular Immunology.* Amsterdam, North-Holland Publishing Co, 1975.

Goodman JW, Fong S, Lewis GK, Kamin R, Nitecki DE, DerBalian G: Antigen structure and lymphocyte activation. *Immunol Review* 1978; 39: 36.

Hashim GA: Myelin basic protein: Structure, function and antigenic determinants. *Immunol Review* 1978; 39: 60.

Heidelberger M: Quantitative absolute methods in the study of antigen-antibody reactions. *Bacteriological Review* 1949; 3: 49.

Hood L, Talmage DW: Mechanisms of antibody diversity: Germ-line basis for variability. *Science* 1970; 168: 325.

Ishizaka K, Dayton DH Jr (eds): *The Biological Role of the Immunoglobulin E System.* US Dept of Health, Education and Welfare, 1973.

Jolles P, Paraf A: *Chemical and Biological Basis of Adjuvants.* New York, Springer-Verlay, 1973.

Kabat EA: *Blood Group Substances—Their Chemistry and Immunochemistry.* New York, Academic Press, 1956.

Kabat EA: The nature of an antigenic determinant. *J Immunol* 1966; 97: 1.

Koshland ME: Structure and function of the J chain. *Adv Immunol* 1975; 20: 41.

Landsteiner K: The specificity of serological reactions. Cambridge, Mass, Harvard University Press, 1945.

Lawrence HS: Transfer factor. *Adv Immunol* 1969; 11: 195.

Metzger H: Structure and function of IgM immunoglobulins. *Adv Immunol* 1970; 12: 57.

Metzger H: Effects of antigen binding on antibody properties. *Adv Immunol* 1974; 18: 169.

Möller G (ed): Immunoglobulin D: Structure, synthesis, membrane representation and the function. *Immunological Review* 1977; 37: 1.

Munoz T: Effect of bacteria and bacterial products on antibody response. *Adv Immunol* 1964; 4: 357.

Natvig JB, Kunkel HG: Immunoglobulins: Classes, subclasses, genetic variants, and idiotypes. *Adv Immunol* 1973; 16: 1.

Nisonoff A, Hopper JE, Spring S: *The Antibody Molecule.* New York, Academic Press, 1975.

Porter RR: Structural studies of immunoglobulins. *Science* 1973; 180: 713.

Race RR, Sanger R: Blood groups in man. Oxford, Blackwells, 1975.

Rapport MM, Graf L: Immunochemical reactions of lipids. *Progress in Allergy* 1969; 13: 273.

Reichlin M: Amino acid substitution and the antigenicity of globular proteins. *Adv Immuno* 1975; 20: 71.

Sakato N, Eisen HN: Antibodies to idiotypes of isologous immunoglobulins. *J of Experimental Med* 1975; 141: 1411.

Scatchard G: The attractions of proteins for small molecules and ions. *Annals of the New York Academy of Sciences* 1949; 51: 660.

Sela M: Immunological studies with synthetic polypeptides. *Adv Immunol* 1966; 5: 29.

Sela M: Antigenicity: Some molecular aspects. *Science* 1969; 66: 1365.

Senyk G, Williams EB, Nitecki DE, Goodman JW: The functional dissection of an antigenic molecule: Specificity of humoral and cellular immune responses to glucagon. *J of Experimental Med* 1971; 133: 1254.

Sercarz EE, Yowell RL, Turkin D, Miller A, Araneo BA, Adorini L: Different functional specificity repertoires for suppressor and helper T cells. *Immunological Reviews* 1978; 39: 108.

Sigal NH, Klinman NR: The B-cell clonotype repertoire. *Adv Immunol* 1978; 26: 255.

Spiegelberg H: Biological activities of immunoglobulins of different classes and subclasses. *Adv Immunol* 1974; 19: 259.

Stollar BD: Nucleic acid antigens, in Sela M (ed): *The Antigens, I.* p. 1. New York, Academic Press, 1973.

Tiselius A, Kabat EA: An electrophoretic study of immune sera and purified antibody preparations. *J Exp Med* 1939; 69: 119.

Tomasi TB, Grey HM: Structure and function of immunoglobulin A. *Progress in Allergy* 1972; 16: 81.

Tonegawa S: Somatic generation of antibody diversity. *Nature (London)* 1983; 302: 575.

Warner NL: Membrane immunoglobulins and antigen receptors on B and T lymphocytes. *Adv Immunol* 1974; 19: 67.

Weigert MG, Cesari IM, Yonkovich SJ, Cohn M: Variability in the lambda light chain sequences of mouse antibody. *Nature (London)* 1970; 228: 1045.

Wu TT, Kabat EA: An analysis of the variable regions of Bence Jones proteins and myeloma light chains and their implications for antibody complementarity. *J Exp Med* 1970; 132: 211.

Chapter 3

Nonspecific Immune Response: The Role of Accessory Systems in the Expression and Regulation of Specific Immunity

Dennis E. Chenoweth
Stephen I. Wasserman
Allen F. Ryan

Dr. Chenoweth is an established investigator of the American Heart Association. Dr. Wasserman is the recipient of Allergic Diseases Academic Award AI 00431 from the NIH/NIAID. Dr. Ryan is the recipient of Research Career Development Award NS 00176 from the NIH/NINCDS. Portions of this work were supported both by a grant-in-aid from the American Heart Association and USPHS/NIH Grants AI 18731 and NS 14389.

OUTLINE

INTRODUCTION

COMPLEMENT
  Overview
  The Classical Pathway
  The Alternative Pathway
  Complement-Derived Inflammatory Mediators
    C3b opsinization
    The anaphylatoxins
    Summary

INTRODUCTION

Each of us is protected from the many potentially dangerous microorganisms in the environment by epithelia which serve as a mechanical barrier. These epithelia, sheets of cells such as those of the skin or mucous membranes, are our first line of defense in combating infection. Mounting a specific immunologic response when an epithelium is breached would be a slow and inefficient initial reaction to injury. The response which does occur is immediate and predictable: inflammation. The acute inflammatory response has three major components: hemodynamic changes, alterations in the permeability of vessels, and changes in the location and concentration of leukocytes. These events are triggered by a variety of chemical mediators derived from many sources. They lead to exudation of fluid and migration of white cells, especially polymorphonuclear leukocytes, into sites of injury. Inflammation thus marshals the attack on an injurious agent. By drawing lymphocytes and macrophages into the site of injury, inflammatory mediators also help to initiate specific immune responses. Since the vascular and cellular events that characterize the acute inflammatory response are basically similar whatever the injurious agent, they can be considered nonspecific responses (Ryan & Majno, 1977).

By contrast, the chronic inflammatory response, which is characterized by the appearance of lymphocytes, plasma cells, and macrophages at the site of injury, is considered to represent a highly specific immune response by specifically informed or programmed cells. However, recent evidence supports the hypothesis that inflammatory mediators may play a role in modulating these conceptually more specific immune responses. Thus, the distinction between nonspecific and specific immune mechanisms, although a useful construct, appears to be blurring as biochemical and biological experimentation attempts to unravel the intricacies of host defense mechanisms.

Immediate inflammation can be triggered by a variety of nonimmunologic events. Tissue injury, with release of cellular constituents and blood proteins, is an important cause. For example, inflammatory mediators are released during coagulation. Also, platelets are an important source of inflammatory mediators, such as the products of arachidonic acid metabolism.

Alternatively, the triggering event for inflammation can be the recognition of antigen. The interaction of antigen with IgG can activate the complement cascade. Antigen interaction with IgE on the surface of mast cells triggers degranulation, releasing a host of mediators. Antigen recognition by lymphocytes can stimulate the release of lymphokines. Thus, inflammation can be an important factor in both immune host defense and in immunopathologic conditions. In this chapter, we consider those inflammatory systems which are released as accessories of specific immune response.

COMPLEMENT

Overview

The human complement system has long been recognized as being responsible for erythrocyte lysis under appropriate circumstances. More recently it has become clear that complement functions most importantly to facilitate killing of bacteria and viruses and to serve as the source of soluble immune mediators (Muller-Eberhard, 1975).

The term complement refers to a group of at least 20 plasma proteins that interact in a concerted fashion to constitute an important portion of the humoral immune system. The various complement proteins may be functionally defined to act as either recognition factors, proteolytic enzymes, positive modulators, or inhibitors. The complement system is conceptually similar to the coagulation system in that an initiating stimulus triggers a cascade-like series of enzymatic reactions. Complement activation may proceed through two different routes, termed the classical or alternative pathways. By-products of the activated complement components constitute the biologically active inflammatory mediators.

The Classical Pathway

As shown in Fig 3-1, a variety of agents may serve to activate complement by classical pathway mechanisms. Binding of the first complement component, C1, takes place on a specific region of the Fc portion of immunoglobulin. Typically, immunoglobulins, either IgM or clustered groups of IgG molecules, initially bind to specific cell-surface antigens. This binding interaction promotes a conformational change in the Fc domain of the molecule that exposes a potential binding site for the recognition protein C1q. Binding of C1q to the immunoglobulin in turn facilitates proteolytic conversion of the inactive proenzyme C1r to its enzymatically active form, $C\overline{1r}$. This protease then acts upon the proenzyme C1s to specifically cleave this molecule to its active form, $C\overline{1s}$. The net result of this series of sequential reactions is the formation of an enzymatically active complex (C1 esterase) on the surface of an antibody-attached foreign surface. This active complex may undergo two fates. It may either be neutralized and inactivated by the regulatory protein C1 esterase inhibitor or it may continue to function as an active enzyme responsible for propagation of the activation signal.

If the activation stimulus is of sufficient intensity, classical pathway activation proceeds in the following way. Active $C\overline{1rs}$ simultaneously cleaves both C2 and C4 to yield the subcomponents C2a and C2b and C4a and C4b, respectively. The C2a portion of C2 possesses marginal proteolytic activity, but when combined with C4b by noncovalent forces, a potent enzyme known as the C3 convertase ($C\overline{4b2a}$) results. This C3 convertase is responsible for cleaving C3 into two components, the low molecular weight C3a anaphylatoxin which is released into the fluid phase and C3b which remains bound to the foreign surface. The surface-bound C4b2a3b constitutes an active enzyme, C5 convertase, that acts to cleave C5 into two components, C5a analphylatoxin and membrane-bound C5b. Deposition of C5b on the surface of cells or particles permits subsequent assembly of the potentially lytic membrane attack complex composed of C6, C7, C8, and C9. In this manner, antibody binding to specific surface antigenic determinants is recognized, amplified, and terminates in potential cellular destruction by complement-mediated lysis. Of equal importance, potent inflammatory mediators such as the anaphylatoxins C3a, C4a, and C5a are generated as a result of these reactions.

The Alternative Pathway

A second means of activating complement, the alternative or properidin pathway, may be initiated by a diverse series of agents (Fig 3-7). Striking analogies between the classical and alternative pathways exist. The initial recognition event consists of the binding of metastable C3, trace amounts of which arise spontaneously following hydrolysis of a critical active site, to suitable activating surfaces. This binding interaction protects C3 from inactivation by β1H globulin and C3b inactivator (C3INH). The signal is then amplified as surface-bound C3b interacts with factors B and D to form the alternative pathway C3 convertase enzyme termed $C3b_nBb$. From this point onward, the alternative and classical pathway converge at the level of C3.

FIG 3-1. Activation of the classical pathway and assembly of the membrane attack complex. Activation of the C1(q,r,s) recognition complex by an appropriate stimulus results in formation of the enzymatically active C1(q, r, s) complex. This enzyme cleaves both C4 and C2 to liberate the fragments C4a and C2b and form an active enzyme, C4b2a. This enzyme in turn specifically hydrolyzes a peptide bond in C3 to release the polypeptide C3a and the larger molecule C3b. The C3b thus formed complexes with C4b2a to form the active C5 convertase, C4b2a3b, which cleaves C5 to liberate C5a and form C5b, the cornerstone of the spontaneously assembled C4a, C3a, and C5a which result from classical pathway activation and are enclosed in dashed lines for emphasis.

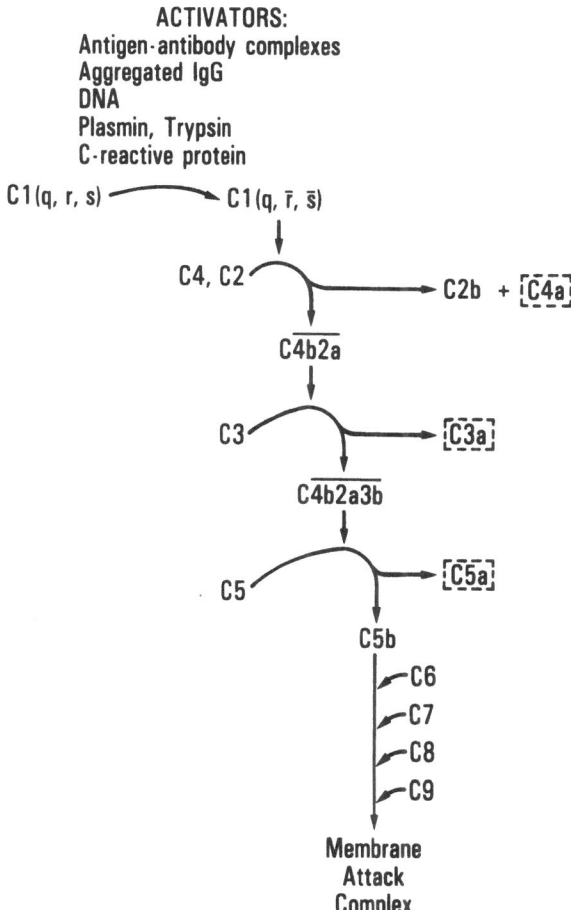

Complement-Derived, Inflammatory Mediators

C3b opsonization

Activation of complement by either alternative or classical pathway routes results in the deposition of surface-bound C3b. This bound C3b, either alone or in conjunction with IgG, serves as a major source of opsonic activity, enhancing the ability of phagocytes to engulf the bound surface (Stossel, 1974). Phagocytes that bear C3b receptors are thus able to recognize and ingest foreign complement-activating agents.

The anaphylatoxins

Low molecular weight cleavage products of the complement proteins C4, C3, and C5, termed C4a, C3a, and C5a anaphylatoxins, respectively, have been implicated as potent inflammatory mediators (Hugli & Muller-Eberhard, 1978, 1981).

Each anaphylatoxin, denoted by dashed squares in Figs 3-1 and 3-2, possesses spasmogenic activity. That is, each induces smooth muscle contraction, increased vascular permeability, and promotes cellular reactions such as the release of histamine from mast cells and basophils. Generally C5a is regarded as a more active spasmogen than C3a, which is in turn considerably more potent than C4a. These observations suggest that the anaphylatoxins, generated by local complement activation, may participate in nonspecific immune responses by altering vascular permeability and local blood flow either through direct action or by stimulating local histamine release (Hugli & Muller-Eberhard, 1981).

Human C5a, but apparently not either human C3a or C4a, appears to play a unique role in acute inflammatory events by promoting a variety of neutrophil-related biological responses (Table 3-1). The anaphylatoxin C5a is the predominant complement-derived neutrophil chemotactic factor (Chenoweth & Hugli, 1980). Additionally, this stimulant causes these cells to demonstrate increased aggregation, release their lysosomal constituents, and generate toxic oxygen species. Thus, a single mediator may account for many of the changes observed in inflamed tissues;   ie, neutrophil margination within vessels, migration of these cells into tissues, and their destruction of foreign agents.

Human C5a exerts its biological effects on the neutrophil after binding to specific cellular receptors (Chenoweth & Hugli, 1978). Quantitative studies indicate that the human neutrophil C5a receptor has an apparent dissociation constant of 2 and 3 nanomolar and there are approximately 200,000 C5a receptors per cell. Once bound to its cell-surface receptor, C5a is rapidly internalized and degraded to biologically inactive peptides and amino acids. Thus, in addition to destroying inflammatory stimuli, the C5a-activated neutrophil is capable of inactivating its own chemotactic stimulus.

Recent investigations have provided support for the hypothesis that C5a not only serves as an acute inflammatory mediator, but may play a critical role in regulating cellular events normally associated with the chronic inflammatory responses. Binding studies have been utilized to demonstrate that macrophages, as well as neutrophils, possess C5a receptors (Chenoweth, Goodman, & Weigle, 1982). Binding of C5a to these receptors not only initiates macrophage chemotaxis but, most interestingly, causes these cells to

FIG 3-2. Activation of the alternative pathway and assembly of the membrane attack complex. Binding of metastable C3 to an appropriate activating surface triggers the activation process by facilitating factor B association. Cleavage of bound factor B by the enzyme factor D creates the active C3 convertase C3bBb. This enzyme amplifies the initial signal by promoting further surface deposition of C3b. When sufficient surface-bound C3bBb is finally formed, an active C5 convertase is produced.

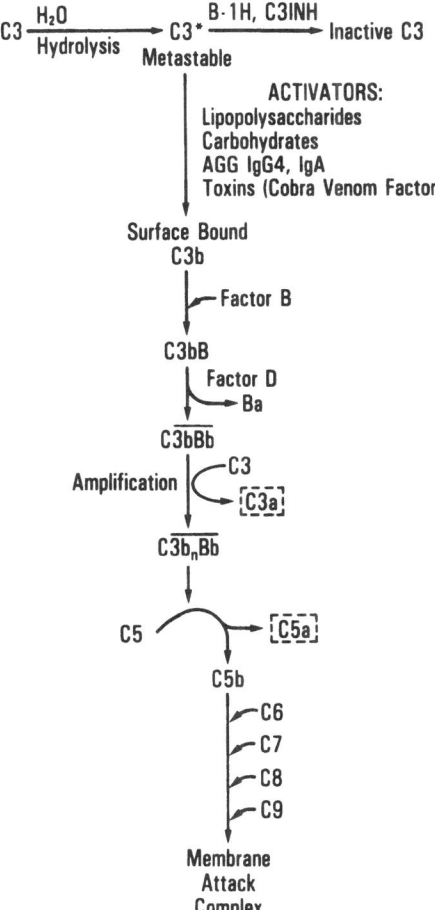

elaborate a soluble factor, identified as interleukin-1, that augments the B lymphocytes's primary humoral immune response to antigens such as sheep red cells. Thus, current evidence suggests that the complement-derived anaphylatoxin C5a may function as an

TABLE 3-1. Biological Activities of C5a Anaphylatoxin

Spasmogenic

    Contraction of smooth muscle
    Increased vascular permeability
    Histamine release from mast cells/basophils

Leukocyte related

    Chemotactic (directed) migration and chemokinesis
      (stimulated random migration)
    Degranulation
    Production of toxic oxygen species
    Aggregation

---

important link between nonspecific or acute inflammatory events and more specific immune responses.

Summary

The human complement system plays a critical role in initiating and modulating nonspecific immune phenomena classically associated with the acute inflammatory response. Certain complement proteins possess the capacity to specifically recognize foreign agents and initiate a cascade-like series of enzymatic reactions that eventuate in the production of potent inflammatory mediators. These by-products of complement activation may facilitate opsonization and alter blood flow and vascular permeability, as well as promoting leukocyte accumulation in inflammatory foci. In addition, certain of these mediators may act on macrophages to cause regulation of immune responses such as antibody production by B lymphocytes. Thus, the complement system ought to be considered as a critical entity that provides interdigitation of both nonspecific and specific immune responses.

THE MAST CELL

Overview

The mast cell, with its specific immunologic receptors, is positioned at portals of entry of potentially toxic or noxious exogenous material. In the lung, mast cells are located free in the bronchial lumen; in the gastrointestinal, nasal, middle ear, and bronchial mucosae they are found in intraepithelial locations, as well as in deeper perivenular collections (Tomita, Patterson, & Susko, 1974; Selye, 1965). In the skin, mast cells are found at the dermal–epidermal junction and in perinvenular locations. As the mast cell's presence at entry of noxious agents frees it from the requirements of mobilization and localization, it may be the sentinel cell for induction of local inflammatory responses. The development of inflammation by the mast cell is consequent to the release of its content of potent biologic mediators as well as by its capacity to generate, de novo, active biologic materials from the local microenvironment. The knowledge that mediators are active in vivo follows from the in vitro definition of their biologic activities which relate to the known pathophysiology of inflammation. The inflammatory processes induced by mast cell mediators are both acute and chronic and are subject to both positive and negative feedback controls inherent in the properties of the mediators themselves. It is the purpose of this review to delineate the mast cell mediators generated upon mast cell activation and the regulation of mast-cell–dependent inflammatory events.

Mast Cells

Mast cells are present in human tissue at concentrations of 1 to 10×10^6 cells/g (Paterson et al., 1976; Mikhail & Miller-Milinska, 1964). Each mast cell possesses several hundred metachromatically straining granules each surrounded by a bilayer membrane. The granules possess a definite subgranular architecture of unknown functional significance. The mast cell membrane is ruffled and possesses 50,000 to 300,000 receptors for the Fc portion of IgE and for C3b, and functionally defined receptors for C3a and C5a. In addition, mast cells may be degranulated by such nonimmunologic stimuli as enzymes, ionophores, polycations, radio-contrast media, and opiates. While it is generally assumed that atopic individuals exhibit their antigen-induced symptomatology as a result of IgE-dependent mast cell activation, the demonstration of non-IgE mediated mechanisms for mast cell mediator release yields additional information on potential mechanisms for recruitment of mediators.

Activation and Degranulation of Mast Cells

The IgE-dependent degranulation of mast cells is initiated by the bridging of pairs of cell-bound IgE molecules by specific antigen, and terminates rapidly. Bridging results in an alteration of the cell membrane, which is associated with increased entry of energy-dependent calcium into the cell, increases in cyclic AMP, and alterations in membrane phospholipid metabolism; it is postulated that it causes cytoskeletal reorganization. Following the ordered completion of these processes, the perigranular membranes fuse with each other and with the cell membrane, and the granules are extruded. Degranulation may be modulated by endogenous or exogenous agents which affect cyclic nucleotide

FIG 3-3. Schematic representation of mast cell–dependent humoral and cellular inflammatory events.

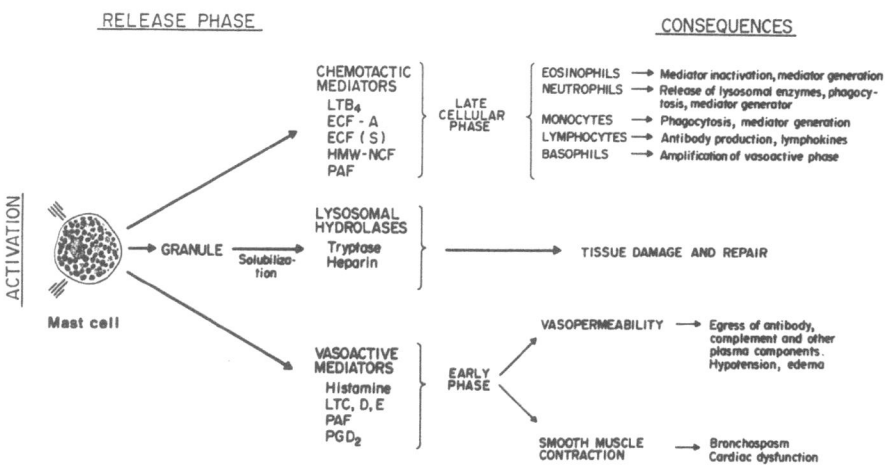

levels in mast cells. Thus, elevations in intracellular levels of cyclic AMP, which may be induced by prostaglandins, histamine, and β-adrenergic agents, inhibit degranulation; whereas α-adrenergic- or prostaglandin-induced falls in cAMP or rises in intracellular cyclic GMP due to cholinergic stimuli may enhance degranulation (Kaliner & Austen, 1973).

Mast Cell–Dependent Mediators

Mast cells possess within their granules a large number of vasoactive/spasmogenic and chemotactic mediators, as well as a variety of active enzymes and structural proteoglycans. Mast cell activation leads to the release of these preformed granular elements as well as to the de novo generation of potent vasoactive/spasmogenic and chemotactic substances. Although this process is best delineated in the rat mast cell, it is likely that the human mast cell will be found to function similarly. The mast cell mediators are listed in Table 3-2, and are described briefly below. A more detailed discussion of the biochemistry and pharmacology of these mediators is given in the Appendix to this chapter.

Vasoactive/bronchospastic mediators which have been identified as originating from the mast cell include histamine, which acts through interaction with two classes of receptors designated H_1 and H_2. Slow-reacting substance of anaphylaxis (SRS-A) is actually a family of leukotrienes, which are products of arachidonic acid metabolism (Fig 3-3). Several of the many other derivatives of arachidonic acid, including the prostaglandins (PGs),

TABLE 3-2. Mast-Cell–Dependent Mediators

Mediator	Mol wt	Function
Histamine	111	Increased vascular permeability, smooth muscle contraction, stimulation of suppressor T cells, prostaglandin generation, H_1 chemotaxis and inactivation of eosinophils, H_2 inhibition of neutrophil chemotaxis and activation, elevation of cAMP (H_1) and cGMP (H_2)
Serotonin	182	Contraction of smooth muscle, increased vascular permeability
PAF	400	Release of platelet amines, platelet aggregation, sequestration of platelets
Arachidonic acid metabolites Cyclooygenase PGD		Increased vascular permeability, contraction of smooth muscle, increase of cAMP, inhibition of platelet aggregation
Lipoxygenase Leukotriene C, D, E (SRS-A)		Contraction of smooth muscle, increased vascular permeability, generation of PGs
Leukotriene B		Chemotaxis of neutrophils
ECF-A	360–390	Eosinophil and neutrophil chemotaxis and deactivation
EDF-oligopeptides	1300–2500	Eosinophil and neutrophil chemotaxis and deactivation
NCF	750,000	Neutrophil chemotaxis and deactivation
Heparin	60,000	Anticoagulation, antithrombin III interaction, inhibition of complement activation
Chondroitin sulfate		Platelet factor IV interaction
Chymase	29,000	Proteolysis with chymotryptic specificity
Tryptase	140,000	Proteolysis with tryptic specificity, cleavage of C3, Hageman factor, and kinin from kininogen
Arylsulfatase A	60,000	Hydrolysis of various sulfate esters
N-acetyl-β-D-glucoseaminidase	158,000	Cleavage of glucosamine residues
β-Glucuronidase	300,000	Cleavage of glucuronide conjugates

thromboxanes, and monohydroxy fatty acids, have been shown to be vasoactive, as has platelet activating factor (PAF). Chemotactic mediators associated with mast cells include eosinophil chemotactic factor of anaphylaxis, intermediate molecular weight eosinophil chemotactic peptide, high molecular weight neutrophil chemotactic factors, and lipid chemotactic factors. Histamine also displays chemotactic properties. Other mast cell mediators include the anticoagulant heparin and the enzymes chymase, tryptase, hexosaminidase, and arylsulfatase.

Determinants of Activity of Mast Cell Mediators

Following activation of mast cells by IgE-dependent or other mechanisms, the variety of mediators generated and released and their many potential interactions provide the substrate for induction of inflammatory events. The putative role of the mast cell and its mediators in both the homeostatic as well as pathophysiologic induction of inflammation is strengthened by the location of the mast cell at host–environmental interfaces. Thus, the interaction of surface mast cells with antigen or noxious agents could, by the action of locally released permeability factors, lead to alterations of the epithelial barrier, thereby permitting access to the large number of more deeply situated mast cells. Of more direct relevance has been the in vivo demonstration that mast-cell–dependent events alone can indeed cause both immediate and more persistent inflammatory processes. A biphasic cutaneous response to IgE-dependent mast cell activation has been defined (Dolovitch et al., 1973; Solley et al., 1976). In the skin a wheal and flare response reflects altered vascular permeability at that site, whereas later local inflammatory events are accompanied by an intense cellular infiltration (Solley et al., 1976). Immunochemical studies have not revealed the participation of immune complexes or complement during this later inflammatory phase (Solley et al., 1976). Elicitation of both phases by purely IgE-dependent mechanisms has been accomplished and this fact indicates that mast cell activation can contribute to subacute and chronic as well as to acute pathobiologic processes. This fact is central to according the mast cell an important role in persistent diseases. Whether continued alteration in the threshold of tissue responses is due to mast cell mediators directly or to cellular infiltration is not established, but mast-cell–derived mediators could be critical by either route alone or in combination.

A possible mechanism by which mast cell mediators might provoke such biphasic inflammatory responses is illustrated in Fig 3-3. The mast-cell–dependent generation of spasmogenic and vasoactive mediators could establish a local vasodilatory or humoral phase of inflammation while the release of chemotactic mediators provokes a cellular phase of inflammation. The humoral phase, apparent within minutes, could lead to egress from the circulation of immunoglobulin and complement components as well as fibrinolytic, procoagulant, and kinin-generating proteins. This response could be expected to be rapidly beneficial to the host by aiding removal of invading microorganisms, by localizing and removing noxious agents, and by facilitating leukocyte migration through venular disconnections. On the other hand, an unregulated humoral phase might be expressed in disease as acute exacerbations of brochospasm, or urticaria, or as upper airway obstruction due to angioedema. The generation and release of chemotactic factors would, in a period of several hours, be expected to call into the local inflammatory focus both eosinophilic and neutrophilic polymorphonuclear leukocytes. These cells could prove beneficial not only by their phagocytic function but also by their ability to inactivate mediators (see below). Conversely, if accumulation of leukocytes were uncontrolled, the pathobiologic consequences of tissue infiltration with leukocytes would ensue. Clinically, such infiltration has been noted in the late phase of the IgE–mast-cell–dependent cutaneous response where eosinophils, neutrophils, basophils, mononuclear leukocytes, and lymphocytes are seen in the skin and may be accompanied by frank necrotizing venulitis. In addition, such infiltration could be detected by the action of leukocytic lysosomal enzymes in the destruction of tissue and the induction of fibrosis. By their capacities to deactivate leukocytes to subsequent chemotactic activation, mast cell chemotactic mediators might also inhibit localization of leukocytes (Center et al., 1979). Such an inhibitory action of chemotactic factors could prove beneficial by blunting exuberant inflammation, but, if prolonged or ill-timed, might be harmful by preventing adequate host response to local insult. The release of mast cell proteases and lysosomal enzymes may itself lead to alterations in ground substances and to activation of such protein inflammatory cascades as complement, fibrinolysis, and coagulation. These processes would amplify inflammatory events and might prove beneficial to the elimination of micro-organisms or toxic agents but might also, if unregulated, lead to tissue destruction, chronic inflammation, and fibrosis.

Regulation of Mast Cell Mediator Release and Activity

The events which lead to the generation and release of mast cell mediators and thereby to the elicitation of mast-cell–dependent inflammatory events are subject to regulation at several critical points. Activation of the mast cell, the secretion of granules, the release of the preformed mediators and generation of unstored mediators, the effect of mediators upon target cells, and finally the persistence in tissue of the mediators are all under biologic control.

The extent of activation of the mast cell is controlled by regulation of access of antigen to this cell, the amount of specific IgE antibody bound to the mast cell surface, and by the intensity of the stimulus. The mast cell itself might alter local permeability, allowing increased antigen contact, or by the H_2 action of released histamine may suppress lymphocyte recognition of antigen and thereby prevent immune response to invaders. In addition, the ratio of specific mediator generated may be dependent upon the intensity of the activating stimulus.

Following secretion of the mast cell granule, the release of performed mediators and the full expression of their activity is dependent upon the independent solubilities of each of the mediators. Thus β-glucuronidase, α-hexosaminidase, arylsulfatase A, histamine, eosinophil chemotactic factor of anaphylaxis (ECF-A), and ECF-oligopeptides are fully soluble in physiologic buffers, whereas the tryptase-heparin complex remains intact in such buffers. Although the mechanism(s) by which the mast cell granule is solubilized in vivo remains unknown, it is clearly an important step in regulating the activity of mast cell inflammatory mediators.

Regulation of the action of mast cell mediators upon target cells may derive from the interaction of several mediators, or their metabolites with the same target cell. Thus, histamine may be additive or inhibitory to ECF-A action upon eosinophils depending upon the ratio of the two activities present. As noted above, mediators may also be synergistic on smooth muscle.

The regulation of generation of unstored mediators has not been fully elucidated, but data suggest that the local cell population regulate their production. For example, LTC_4, PAF, and lipid chemotactic factors can all be generated from neutrophils and/or mononuclear leukocyte populations. The ratios of critical target cells thus may be crucial to the amount and type of mediator generated.

Finally, the persistence of the effect of mediators is also regulated. While this regulation may reflect the limited availability of mediators, tachyphylaxis, and excretion, it is also affected by enzymatic inactivation. As many mast-cell–derived chemotactic mediators are eosinophilotactic, the eosinophil content of mediator-inactivating enzymes may provide a feedback control of mediator effects. Notably, the eosinophil contains histaminase and phospholipase D, which inactivate histamine and PAF, respectively. SRS-A is inactivated by the intact eosinophilic granulocyte, presumably due to the action of oxygen metabolites. In addition, the eosinophil can generate prostaglandin E (PGE), which elevates mast cell cAMP and thereby inhibits further mediator release, and finally mast cell granules following their exocytosis may be ingested by eosinophils, thereby removing heparin-chymase complexes from the tissue fluids. Some other cells also contain mediator-inactivating enzymes. Neutrophils contain histaminase, and at least one mononuclear cell population is rich in histamine methyltransferase.

Summary

The mast-cell–derived preformed and newly generated mediators are released by IgE-dependent and independent mechanisms, and are biologically available during inflammatory events. Mediators of immediate hypersensitivity possess the ability to induce immediate tissue responses such as a wheal and flare, anaphylaxis, or rapid onset, brief duration alterations in pulmonary function, and mediate a prolonged inflammatory response. The fact that IgE and mast cells are relevant to prolonged inflammatory events has been documented by passive transfer with isolated IgE, of delayed inflammatory responses in skin, and by the dependence upon IgE antibody for similar delayed alterations in pulmonary mechanics following inhalation of antigen. In lung, these delayed responses are prevented by pretreatment with disodium cromoglycate, which supports a role for the mast cell. Histopathologic assessment of delayed responses reveals an influx of neutrophils, eosinophils, basophils, lymphocytes, and mononuclear leukocytes, the deposition of fibrin, and vascular abnormalities which may progress to frank vasculitis (Solley et al., 1976). Although some of the mediators responsible for the early and later phases of the IgE-mast cell reaction can be surmised from the kinetics of their in vitro effects, their absolute identification and participation in disease requires further definition.

The postulated role of the mast cell and its mediators in inflammation may provide insight not only into the clinical evolution of some allergic disorders, but also into the local homeostatic regulation of the host–environment interface. Although much remains to be clarified, the rapidly expanding understanding of target cell activation together with the identification of mast-cell-derived mediators provides a framework for definition of the complex processes engendered following IgE–antigen interaction.

LYMPHOKINES

Overview

Antibodies are by no means the only soluble products of lymphocytes. T lymphocytes, and to a lesser extent B lymphocytes, produce a class of soluble substances which interact primarily with other leukocytes. They differ from the mediators discussed above in that most have little, if any, effect upon the vasculature. These *lymphocyte mediators* or *lymphokines* play a crucial role in cell-mediated immunity by greatly amplifying the original interaction between antigen and a relatively small number of T cells. Some of these mediators have effects which we would define as inflammatory in nature, attracting or stimulating cells of the reticuloendothelial system. Other lymphokines are clearly immunoregulatory, influencing other lymphocytes and/or their secretion products.

The lymphokines are a poorly understood and characterized mediator group. This is due in part to the difficulty in obtaining them in sufficient quantities to permit standard biochemical assays. In addition, the heterogeneity of the lymphocyte preparations routinely used to produce lymphokines has obscured the questions of mediator origins. The recent development of lymphokine preparations from monoclonal T lymphocytes (Altman & Katz, 1982) has ameliorated, to some extent, both of these problems. However, lymphocyte mediators are still usually classified by their biological activities, as demonstrated in vitro or in vivo. Table 3-3 lists some of the better defined lymphokines and their properties, and some of the more important lymphokines are discussed below.

Lymphocyte Mediators

Migration inhibition factor (MIF)

The first lymphokine to be discovered was MIF, a substance which inhibits the movement of macrophages. MIF is produced by lymphocytes in response to antigen recog-

TABLE 3-3. Lymphokines

A. Mediators affecting macrophages
1. Migration inhibition factor (MIF)
2. Macrophage activating factor (MAF) (same as MIF?)
3. Chemotactic factors for macrophages
4. Antigen-dependent MIF

B. Mediators affecting polymorphonuclear leukocytes
1. Chemotactic factors
2. Leukocyte inhibitory factor (LIF)
3. Eosinophil stimulation promoter

C. Mediators affecting lymphocytes
1. Mitogenic factors
2. Factors enhancing antibody production
    Antigen-dependent
    Antigen-independent
3. Factors suppressing antibody production
    Antigen-dependent
    Antigen-independent

D. Mediators affecting other cells and systems
1. Cytotoxic factors, lymphotoxin (LT)
2. Growth inhibitory factors (same as LT?)
3. Osteoclastic factor
4. Collagen-producing factor
5. Colony-stimulating factor
6. Interferons
7. Immunoglobulin binding factor
8. Tissue factor (procoagulant factor)

---

nition. It is probably a protein, with a molecular weight (mol wt) between 25,000 and 55,000 in humans. There is evidence that MIF activity may represent more than one molecular species (Remold & Mednis, 1977). MIF interacts with a specific receptor on the macrophage surface at extremely low concentrations. It acts to increase the macrophage population at a site of antigenic challenge.

Macrophage activating factor (MAF)

Macrophages which have been incubated with lymphocyte mediator preparations develop a number of structural and biochemical changes which have been termed *activation.* Activated macrophages show an increase in their ability to phagocytize and destroy foreign material. MAF is indistinguishable in its physical characteristics from MIF, and it is suspected that they are in fact the same mediator. However, the activation of macrophages occurs two to three days after exposure to lymphokine preparations, while MIF activity is detectable within 24 hours.

Chemotactic factors

Lymphocyte mediator preparations have been shown to exhibit chemotactic activity directed toward monocytes, neutrophils, eosinophils, and basophils. The molecules exhibiting chemotactic activity for polymorphonuclear leukocytes fall in the 24,000 to 55,000 mol wt range, and it is not certain whether they represent one substance, or a separate factor for each cell type. Eosinophil chemotaxis by lymphocyte mediators is different from that for neutrophils and basophils in that it requires the presence of antigen–antibody complexes (Cohen & Ward, 1971). Chemotactic factor for monocytes and macrophages is similar in its physical characteristics to that for polymorphonuclear cells, but appears to be a separate substance.

Leukocyte inhibitory factor (LIF)

LIF is a soluble factor produced by lymphocytes, which inhibits the migration of neutrophils. The effects of LIF on neutrophils are analogous to the effects of MIF on macrophages, and in analogy to MAF it may also enhance the phagocytosis of neutrophils. LIF has no effect on macrophages, however. It appears to be an esterase with a molecular weight of about 68,000 (Rocklin, 1974).

Lymphocyte mitogenic factor

Lymphocytes can produce a soluble factor which nonspecifically stimulates other lymphocytes to undergo blast transformation and cell division. As with many other lymphocyte mediators, the ability to produce this lymphokine is a T-cell–dependent phenomenon, since it cannot be demonstrated in lymphocytes from neonatally thymectomized animals.

Regulation of antibody production

Ever since it was first determined that T cells collaborate with B cells in the antibody response, immunologists have been searching for soluble factors which might mediate such interactions. Following the initial report of Dutton et al. (1971), of a soluble helper factor produced by T cells, a wide variety of such soluble mediators have been reported. Both inhibitory and facilitative factors have been identified.

In both cases, factors which are specific to a particular antigen have been demonstrated. The specificity of these lymphokines appears to be mediated by a protein chain with an antigen recognition site, and yet which is different in structure from the immunoglobulin heavy chain. Some of the antigen-specific mediators also exhibit a second protein chain which contains Ia subunits, segments which are determined by the major histocompatibility complex (MHC) and can confer MHC specificity. Some antigen-specific mediators appear to act by coupling the bound antigen to B cells by the Ia regions of the molecule, since pretreating B cells with anti-Ia antibodies abolishes the mediator effect. Others, and specially antigen-specific suppressor factors, act upon T cells which in turn influence B cells (Altman & Katz, 1982).

Other factors are not antigen specific, but influence the production of many B cell clones. This is a more heterogeneous group than the antigen-specific lymphokines, both in their actions and structures. As with the antigen-specific factors, some non–antigen-specific lymphokine molecules contain Ia subunits and thus can express MHC specificity. Nonspecific factors fall into two major groups. One acts on B cells and macrophages by an as yet unelucidated mechanism. The other group influences antibody production by affecting T-cell intermediaries.

Cytotoxic mediators

Several lymphokines have been shown to be cytotoxic or cytostatic to target cells. These include not only the lymphotoxins, but also inhibitors of bacterial proliferation, colony formation, and DNA synthesis. These factors appear to be proteins in the 40,000 to 80,000 mol wt range. It has been suggested that all of the cytotoxic and cytostatic effects of lymphocyte mediators may be performed by one molecular species which exhibits different properties under different conditions and for different target cells, and which can be split into subunits which retain some biological activity (Rocklin, Bendtzen, & Greineder, 1980). Cytotoxic lymphokines are almost certainly involved in T-lymphocyte-mediated cell killing.

Interferon

The interferons are a family of glycoproteins which are characterized by non–virus-specific antiviral activity. It is now recognized that the interferons possess a wide spectrum of biological activities beyond their antiviral functions, as illustrated in Table 3-4. These include inhibition of cell proliferation, especially of neoplasms, and various aspects of immunoregulation. They appear to provide protection from viral infection not by affecting the virus itself, but by conferring host cell resistance to viral infection. It is presumably for this reason that they are often species-specific, being most effective in the organism from which they are derived. Interferon produced by lymphocytes is known as immune interferon, and in humans has a molecular weight of about 40,000.

Immunoglobulin binding factor

Lymphocytes produce a factor with a molecular weight of 150,000, which binds to IgG–antigen complexes. It is immunoregulatory in that it supresses IgG and IgM production. It also prevents the fixation of C1q, and thus protects against complement-mediated cell lysis. Its interference with complement function may act as a regulatory mechanism to control inflammation. There is evidence that immunoglobulin binding factor is in fact the Fc receptor of the T cell, shed from the cell surface under the appropriate conditions (Neauport-Sautes & Fridman, 1977).

TABLE 3-4. Biological Effects of Interferons

A. Effects on cell surfaces
    Increased expression of histocompatibility antigens
    Increased net negative charge
    Altered binding of Con A, TSH, and cholera toxin

B. Effects on cell division
    Inhibition of replication, especially of tumor cells

C. Effects on specialized cell functions
    Increased macrophage phagocytosis
    Enhanced prostaglandin synthesis

D. Effects on the immune system
    Enhanced cytotoxicity of sensitized lymphocytes against tumor cells
    Increased IgE-mediated release of mediators from basophils
    Inhibition of antibody response to T-cell–dependent antigens
    Inhibition of some delayed hypersensitivity reactions
    Inhibition of DNA synthesis in stimulated lymphocytes

E. Effects on viruses
    Inhibition of replication

Vasoactive lymphokines

While most lymphocyte mediators have little effect upon the vasculature, two vasoactive factors have been identified. Both skin reactive factor and vascular permeability factor increase vascular permeability. Tissue factor, while not affecting permeability, has potent procoagulant activity.

Lymphokine Production

The initial demonstration of lymphokine production involved the identification of soluble factors involved in delayed hypersensitivity. Thus, lymphokine production has traditionally been associated with T lymphocytes. As methods of separating T and B lymphocytes have improved, it has become clear that B cells can also, under the appropriate circumstances, produce lymphocyte mediators. While B cells can manufacture lymphokines in the absence of T cells, lymphocyte mediator production remains a T-cell–dependent phenomenon and is closely correlated with the status of cellular immunity of the host.

Thus, while B cells from normal humans can produce MIF, B cells from patients with T-cell deficiency cannot (Rocklin, Remold, & David, 1972). In contrast to the production of immunoglobulins, lymphocytes are not limited to the synthesis of a single lymphokine. A single lymphocyte clone usually produces several lymphocyte mediators (Altman & Katz, 1982). While lymphokine production is usually attributed exclusively to lymphocytes, other cell types have been shown to have the capacity for their manufacture. A substance with MIF-like activity is produced by dividing fibroblasts, especially those infected by viruses (Hammond et al., 1974). The ability of fibroblasts and other cell types to produce interferons is well documented.

Production of lymphocyte mediators can be stimulated by recognition of specific antigen. However, a number of nonspecific stimuli are also effective, including mitogenic factors and elements of the complement cascade. Macrophage participation appears to be important for lymphokine production, especially by T cells. This does not seem to be a function of antigen presentation, since macrophages are required for mediator production stimulated by nonspecific mitogens as well as by antigen recognition (Epstein, Cline, & Merigan, 1971).

Regulation and Interaction

There is relatively little information yet available regarding the regulation of mediator production by lymphocytes. However, there are several points at which such regulation can be postulated. Given the importance of macrophages to the production of lymphokines, factors which influence these cells could be expected to exert some control over lymphocyte mediators. Since MIF, MAF, and lymphocyte chemotactic mediators are such factors, it seems reasonable to assume that positive feedback plays a role in the amplification of lymphokine production. Similarly, lymphocyte-activating factors would tend to amplify lymphokine production in a nonspecific manner. Substances produced by other inflammatory systems which influence macrophages, such as C3b, could also enhance mediator production. Another potential point of regulation is via influences acting directly upon lymphocytes. Lymphokine production can be depressed or even prevented by histamine or corticosteroids, providing additional substrates for interaction between the lymphocyte mediator system and other inflammatory pathways. Factors which influence the mediators themselves could also play a regulatory role. Substances have been demonstrated in normal serum which break down MIF and chemotactic lymphokines. These could regulate both the duration and the spatial spread of lymphocyte mediator action. Finally, regulatory influence could be exerted upon the interaction between mediators and their target cells. For example, corticosteroids prevent the action of MIF and MAF on macrophages, but not the effect of chemotactic factor upon these same cells (Rocklin et al., 1980).

The Role of Lymphokines in Immune Responses

Enough is known about the biological activities of lymphokines to suggest a role for these mediators in immune responses. After activation of T or B cells by antigen, substances are produced to mobilize immune and inflammatory cells, by way of vascular permeability and by direct chemotactic activity on macrophages, neutrophils, basophils, and other lymphocytes. Once the inflammatory cells are recruited to the site, their random movements would be inhibited by MIF and LIF, so that they are retained at the focus of antigen recognition. They would also be activated to promote phagocytosis and destruction of bacteria, viruses, or tumor cells. Colony stimulating factors would increase production of leukocytes in bone marrow, to replenish cells drawn from the circulation. Lymphotoxins and interferons could participate directly in the attack on foreign material. Mitogenic factors would amplify the response by nonspecifically activating lymphocytes, so that they could produce more lymphokines. These nonspecific, essentially inflammatory lymphocyte mediators could play a role in virtually any response to antigen. They appear to be primarily responsible for the expression of many aspects of delayed hypersensitivity, and other facets of cell-mediated immunity.

Lymphokines would also act to recruit B-cell participation. Factors which promote antibody synthesis would mobilize the B-cell response to antigen, adding antibody to the response. The resolution of the response to antigen could also be affected by lymphokines. Suppressor factors would decrease or even terminate antibody production as need declined. Immunoglobulin bonding factor would tend to inhibit complement fixation. Mediators which enhance coagulation and collagen synthesis would promote tissue repair, and contribute to the healing phase.

In summary, while the role of the lymphokines during in vivo immune responses cannot accurately be assessed with our current level of understanding, it appears to be major. It seems likely that they play a pivotal part at two critical interfaces: between cell-mediated and humoral immunity, and between specific immunity and inflammation.

CONCLUSIONS

The accessory systems described in this chapter share one major purpose: to amplify the effects of specific antigen recognition by a relatively small number of lymphocytes or antibody molecules. In each, antigen recognition serves as a trigger which activates nonspecific inflammatory processes. In these systems, the specific portion of the immune response serves primarily to identify the location of foreign material, while the effector mechanisms are nonspecific inflammatory cells and/or molecules. The systems are characterized by self-regulation which tends to limit the inflammatory reaction to the site of initiation. In addition, components of each system can initiate and/or regulate aspects of other inflammatory pathways. For example, the lymphocyte mediator immunoglobulin binding factor can inhibit the cytotoxic effects of complement, while C3b opsonization can act to increase lymphokine production. These regulatory mechanisms presumably exist in order to maximize the effectiveness of evoked responses at the desired site of action, while minimizing the spatial and temporal extent of nonspecific events which cannot distinguish between host tissue and foreign material.

Each of these systems also serves a broader purpose as part of an integrated response to antigen. Mediators can enhance or suppress the function of lymphocytes, and thus become part of the specific immune response by which they are usually initiated. This is especially true of the lymphokines, which appear to be involved in many aspects of B lymphocyte regulation by T lymphocytes. The more complex aspects of immune/inflammatory regulation have only recently begun to be characterized. However, it is now clearly recognized that they play an important role in response to antigen. Normal function in the complex relationships between immune and inflammatory responses is a necessary adjunct to host defense. Breakdown of these interactions plays an equally major role in immunopathologic diseases.

REFERENCES

Altman A, Katz DH: The biology of monoclonal lymphokines secreted by T cell lines and hybridomas. *Adv Immunol* 1982; 33: 73.

Black DW, Duncan WAM, Durant CJ, Garielin CR, Parsons EM: Definition and antagonism of histamine H_2-receptors. *Nature (London)* 1972; 236: 385.

Boswell RN, Austen KF, Goetzl EJ: Intermediate molecular weight chemotactic factors in rat mast cells: Immunologic release, granule association and demonstration of structural heterogeneity. *J Immunol* 1978; 120: 15.

Center DM, Soter NA, Wasserman SI, Austen KF: Inhibition of neutrophil chemotaxis in association with experimental angioedema in patients with cold urticaria: A model of chemotactic deactivation *in vivo*. *Clin Exp Immunol* 1979; 35: 112.

Chenoweth DE, Goodman MG, Weigle WO: Demonstration of a specific receptor for human C5a anaphylatoxin on murine macrophages. *J Exp Med* 1982; 156: 68.

Chenoweth DE, Hugli TE: Demonstration of specific C5a receptor on intact human polymorphonuclear leukocytes. *Proc Natl Acad Sci* (USA) 1978; 75: 3943.

Chenoweth DE, Hugli TE: Human C5a and C5a analogs as probes of the neutrophil C5a receptors. *Mol Immunol* 1980; 17: 151.

Cohen S, Ward PA: In vitro and in vivo activity of a lymphocyte and immune complex-dependent chemotactic factor for eosinophils. *J Exp Med* 1971; 133: 133.

Dolovitch J, Hargreave FE, Chalmers R, et al: Late cutaneous allergic responses in isolated IgE-dependent reactions. *J Allergy Clin Immunol* 1973; 52: 38.

Dutton RW, Falkoff R, Hirst JA et al: Is there evidence for a nonantigen specific diffusable chemical mediator from the thymus-derived cell in the initiation of the immune response? *Prog Immunol* 1971; 1: 355.

Epstein L, Cline MJ, Merigan TC: The interaction of human macrophages and lymphocytes in the PHA stimulated production of interferon. *J Clin Invest* 1971; 50: 744.

Gomori C: Chloroacetyl esters as histochemical substrate. *J Histochem Cytochem* 1953; 1: 469.

Hammond ME, Roblin RO, Dvorak AM, et al: MIF-like activity in simian virus 40-transformed 3T3 fibroblast cultures. *Science* 1974; 185: 956.

Hugli TE, Muller-Eberhard HJ: The structural basis for anaphylatoxin and chemotactic functions of C3a, C4a, and C5a. *Crit Rev Immunol* 1981; 321.

Hugli TE, Muller-Eberhard HJ: Anaphylatoxins: C3a and C5a. *Adv Immunol* 1978; 26: 1.

Kaliner MA, Austen KF: A sequence of biochemical events in the antigen-induced release of chemical mediators from sensitized human lung tissue. *Exp Med* 1973; 138: 1077.

Kiernan JA: A pharmacological and histological investigation of the involvement of mast cells in cutaneous axon reflex vasodilation. *Quart J Exp Physiol* 1975; 60: 123.

Mikhail GR, Miller-Milinska A: Mast cell population in human skin. *J Invest Dermatol* 1964; 43: 249.

Muller-Eberhard HJ: Complement. *Ann Rev Biochem* 1975; 44: 697.

Neauport-Sautes C, Fridman WH: *J Immunol* 1977; 119: 1269.

Paterson NA, Wasserman SI, Said JW, et al: Release of chemical mediators from partially purified human lung mast cells. *J Immunol* 1976; 117: 1356.

Platshon LF, Kaliner MA: The effects of the immunological release of histamine upon human lung cyclic nucleotide levels and prostaglandin generation. *J Clin Invest* 1978; 62: 1113.

Remold HG, Mednis AD: *J Immunol* 1977; 118: 2015.

Roberts LJ, Lewis RA, Hansborough R, et al: Biosynthesis of prostaglandins, thrombaxanes and 12-hydroxy-5,8,10,14 eicosatetraenoic acid in rat mast cells, abstract. *Fed Proc* 1978; 37: 384.

Rocklin RE: Production of activated lymphocytes: Leukocyte inhibitory factor (LIF) distinct from migration inhibitory factor (MIF). *J Immunol* 1974; 112: 1461.

Rocklin RE, Remold HG, David JR: Characterization of human migration inhibition factor (MIF) from antigen-stimulated lymphocytes. *Cell Immunol* 1972; 5: 436.

Rocklin RE, Bendtzen K, Greineder D: Mediators of immunity: Lymphokines and monokines. *Adv Immunol* 1980; 29: 55.

Ryan GB, Majno G: Acute inflammation. *Am J Pathol* 1977; 86: 185.

Selye H: *The Mast Cell.* London, Butterworths, 1965.

Solley GE, Gleich GJ, Jordon RE, et al: The late phase of the immediate wheal and flare skin reaction. Its dependence upon IgE antibodies. *J Clin Invest* 1978; 58: 408.

Stossel TP: Phagocytosis. *N Engl J Med* 1974; 290: 717, 774, 833.

Tomita A, Patterson R, Suszko IM: Respiratory mast cells and basophiloid cells. *Int Arch Allergy* 1974; 47: 261.

Wasserman SI, Soter NA, Center DM, et al: Cold urticaria: Recognition and characterization of a neutrophil chemotactic factor which appears in serum during experimental cold challenge. *J Clin Invest* 1977; 60: 189.

APPENDIX

Mast Cell–Dependent Mediators:
Vasoactive and Bronchospastic Mediators

Histamine

Histamine is a product of decarboxylation of the amino acid histidine and it is ionically bound to the proteoglycan-protein backbones of mast cell granules. The effects of histamine are expressed as both direct and reflex constriction of smooth muscle, and increase the distance between endothelial cells of venules, thereby increasing the potential for transudation of serum and for extravasation of leukocytes.

The biologic activities of histamine are expressed by its interaction with either of two specific classes of receptors on target cells. Those receptors designated H_1 predominate in skin and smooth muscle and are inhibited by classic antihistamines, while H_2 receptors are selectively blocked by a group of compounds, including burimamide, metiamide, and cimetidine (Black et al., 1972). Pulmonary bronchoconstriction, vasodilation, and increased cGMP are H_1 effects, while H_2 effects include inhibition of both human lymphocyte-mediated cytotoxicity and IgE-mediated histamine release due to elevation in cAMP content. The wheal and flare response in skin is due to a combined effect of histamine on the H_1 and H_2 receptors. Histamine also inhibits chemotaxis through H_2, receptors presumably also by stimulating adenylate cyclase and increasing cAMP.

Slow reacting substance of anaphylaxis (SRS-A)

Slow Reacting Substance of Anaphylaxis (SRS-A) is not a single mediator as previously thought. It is now known to be a family of sulfido-peptide leukotriene metabolites of arachidonic acid, termed LTC, LTD, and LTE. Pure human mast cell preparations generate 100 to 200 μg of these potent mediators per 10^6 mast cells. SRS-A is active as a constrictor of peripheral airways to a much greater extent than of central airways, causes local edema and vasoconstriction, hypotension, and depression of cardiac contractility.

Other products of arachidonic acid oxidation

Arachidonic acid mobilized from cell membrane phospholipids by the action of phospholipases may be converted to prostaglandins (PGs) and thromboxanes via a cyclooxygenase-dependent pathway or by lipooxygenase enzyme to hydroperoxy fatty acids and thence to monohydroxy fatty acids and the leukotrienes (Fig 3-4). Several of these products have been described in vitro subsequent to noncytolytic activation of mast-cell–rich tissues and isolated rat mast cells. Specifically, PGD_2, PGI, and monohydroxy fatty acids have been generated by isolated rat mast cells. Human lung mast cells have been shown to generate PGD_2 and thromboxane, and $PGF_{2\alpha}$ and PGE_2 are present after IgE-dependent activation of human lung tissue (Roberts et al., 1978; Platshon & Kaliner, 1978). Animal and human smooth muscle is constricted by $PFG_{2\alpha}$, PGD_2, thromboxane A, and both cyclic endoperoxides PGG_2 and PGH_2. In skin PGD_2 causes wheal and flare reactions.

Platelet activating factor (PAF)

PAF is immunologically generated subsequent to IgE-dependent processes. PAF is a unique phospholipid termed acetyl ether glycerophosphocholine. PAF is a potent mediator of wheal and flare, vasopermeability, and systemic hypotension as well as its role in inducing platelet activation and subsequent release of thromboxane and serotonin. The latter both contract smooth muscle.

FIG 3-4. Pathways of generation of oxidative metabolites of arachidonic acid. The major mast cell products are surrounded by boxes. PG = prostaglandin, HETE = 12-L-hydroxy-5,8,10,14-eicosatetraenoic acid, HHT = 12-L-hydroxy-5,8,10 heptadecatrienoic acid.

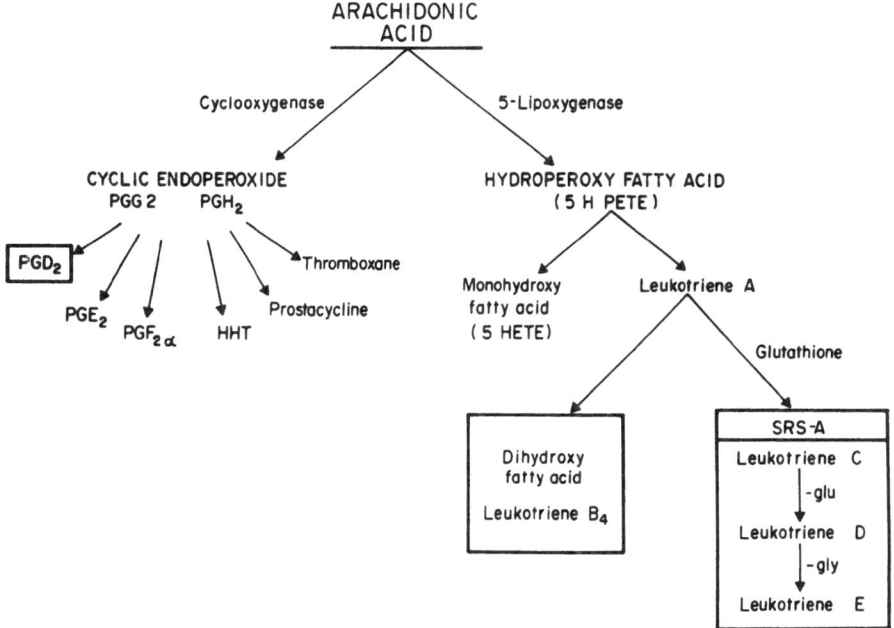

PAF also induces platelet aggregation and leads to the reversible sequestration of platelets in the lung and skin.

Chemotactic Mediators

Eosinophil chemotactic factor of anaphylaxis (ECF-A)

The first mast-cell–associated chemotactic factor described, ECF-A, small peptide, was identified in the anaphylactic supernatant of challenged guinea pig lung fragments and subsequently in the analogous human tissue and isolated mast cells (Paterson et al., 1976). This factor is preferentially chemotactic for eosinophils and deactivates this cell type to further migration.

Intermediate molecular weight eosinophil chemotactic peptide

In addition to low molecular weight ECF-A tetrapeptides, human lung and rat mast cells contain chemotactic factors of 1200 to 2500 mol wt with specificity for eosinophil polymorphonuclear leukocytes. These factors are preformed, immunologically releasable, and capable of deactivating eosinophils (Boswell, Austen, & Goetzl, 1978).

High molecular weight neutrophil chemotactic factors (HMW-NCF)

HMW-NCF has been described in rat mast cells, human lung fragments, and the sera of patients with physical urticaria or asthma following physical or antigen challenge. HMW-NCF appears in the circulation coincident with histamine following challenge of patients with asthma or cold urticaria. It has been characterized as a 750,000 mol wt neutral protein which attracts and deactivates neutrophils in vitro (Wasserman et al., 1977).

Histamine

In addition to its smooth-muscle–directed actions, histamine may modulate the migration of inflammatory leukocytes. Thus, via an H_1 mechanism, histamine enhances random and directed migration of eosinophils and neutrophils and is a weak chemotactic factor for human eosinophils in vivo and in vitro. By its H_2 actions, histamine inhibits both random and directed migration of neutrophilic and eosinophilic polymorphonuclear leukocytes.

Lipid chemotactic factors

The lipooxygenase products of arachidonic acid, and the dihydroxy fatty acid leukotriene B are potent chemotactic factors for both neutrophils and eosinophils. Equivalent effects on neutrophils have also been described for the cyclooxygenase product 12-L-hydroxy-5,8,10-heptadecatrienoic acid (HHT).

Structural Proteoglycans

Heparin

The sulfated, metachromatic, mucopolysaccharide heparin has been identified in human lung and skin and localized to the mast cells isolated from human lung tissue. Human heparin is a proteoglycan of approximately 60,000 mol wt. Human heparin interacts with human antithrombin III to accelerate anticoagulation. Heparin from other sources has been shown to inhibit the complement cascade at several key locations. In addition, heparin has been shown to bind to histamine and platelet factor IV, and to liberate lipoprotein lipase.

Granule-Associated Enzymes

Chymase

Chymase has been isolated from the mast cell of the rat and has been identified histochemically in the human mast cell (Gomori, 1953), and it is the major chymotryptic enzyme extractable from rat skin. This enzyme is minimally active as a protease while stored in the granule, probably because heparin and serotonin mask the active site; but once freed, its specific activity is comparable to that of pancreatic chymotrypsin. That chymotrypsin inhibitors have been shown to inhibit some inflammatory consequences of IgE-dependent activation in rabbit skin adds relevance to the hypothesis that this activity is mast cell dependent (Kiernan, 1975).

Tryptase

Tryptase, a 140,000 mol wt preformed enzyme, is released subsequent to antigen challenge of IgE-sensitized human lung fragments or mast cells. This activity can cleave C3 to generate C3a which may contract smooth muscle and increase vascular permeability.

Other hydrolytic enzymes

η-glucuronidase and *N*-acetyl-β-D-glucosaminidase (hexosaminidase) and arylsulfatase have been identified in human and rat mast cells and are released upon immunologic activation of the rat mast cell. These enzymes, when obtained from non–mast-cell sources, have been demonstrated to degrade ground substance mucopolysaccharides.

Chapter 4

Specific Immune Responses

Sharyn M. Walker
Michael G. Goodman

The authors thank Dr. William O. Weigle for reviewing and discussing the manuscript and Janet Kuhns, Mary Chalmers, and Alice Bruce for excellent secretarial assistance. This is a publication No. 3319IMM from the Department of Immunology, Scripps Clinic and Research Foundation, La Jolla, CA 92007. Sharyn M. Walker was supported in part by USPHS grant AI-07007 and AI-15284, American Cancer Society grant IM42-H, and Biomedical Research Support Program grant RRO-5514. She is a recipient of an American Cancer Society Junior Faculty Award and supported in part by NIH grant AI-16149. Her present address: Division of Research Immunology and Bone-Marrow Transplantation, Childrens Hospital of Los Angeles, Los Angeles, CA 90027. Michael G. Goodman was supported in part by USPHS grants AI-07007 and AI-15284, American Cancer Society Grant IM42-H, and Biomedical Research Support Program Grant RRO-5514. He is a recipient of USPHS Research Career Development Award AI-00374.

OUTLINE

INTRODUCTION

HUMORAL IMMUNITY
  B Lymphocyte Activation
    Antigen-specific activation
    Antigen-nonspecific activation
  Generation of the Primary Antibody Response
  Generation of the Secondary (Memory) Humoral Immune Response
  Regulation of the Humoral Immune Response

CELL-MEDIATED IMMUNITY
  Background
  Definition of T Cell Subsets
  T Cell Activation
    Major histocompatibility complex
    Mixed lymphocyte reaction (MLR)
    CMC (T-cell mediated)
      Recognition of virally infected tissue
      Mechanism of cytolysis
    Graft v host disease (GVH)
    Delayed hypersensitivity

INTRODUCTION

The immune response is the means employed by the body to protect itself from bacterial and viral disease and, probably, neoplastic disease. The immune system employs two basic lines of defense, humoral and cellular immunity. Humoral immunity is mediated by serum antibody produced by B cells, while cellular immunity is not mediated by antibody, but rather by cellular activity dependent upon T cells. In reality the immune response is rarely either exclusively cellular or humoral, but is a combination of both to a greater or lesser degree.

The immune system can perhaps best be characterized in terms of three features: specificity for antigen, memory, and capacity to distinguish self- from nonself-antigens. A hallmark of the immune response is the exquisite specificity in recognizing and neutralizing foreign substances, with T lymphocytes, for example, distinguishing trinitrophenylated antigens from dinitrophenylated. Memory, or the ability of the immune system to react more vigorously and faster upon reexposure to antigen, makes the immune system highly effective. Finally, the ability of the immune system to distinguish between self- and non-self-antigens enables it to attack foreign antigens effectively without becoming pathogenic.

It is becoming more and more apparent that the immune system depends upon a highly sophisticated interplay between various types of immune cells. For some time it was thought that lymphoid cells were homogeneous, until the T- and B-cell dichotomy was discovered (see chapter 1). After this discovery, it was thought that these two populations were homogeneous among themselves, but today both of these classes of lymphoid cells are divisible into numerous subpopulations, both functionally and in terms of surface antigens. This chapter discusses humoral and cellular immune responses in terms of the various cell types involved and how they function.

HUMORAL IMMUNITY

B Lymphocyte Activation

Antigen-specific activation

As discussed in chapter 1, bone-marrow–dependent or bursal-equivalent (B) lymphocytes are the precursors of antibody secreting cells and of lymphocytes maturing into morphologically identifiable plasma cells. The primary function of these cells is thus concerned with the production and secretion of immunoglobulin molecules, whose isotype, subclass, idiotype, antigen specificity, and affinity are governed by a host of genetic factors as well as the cells' prior antigen experience (reviewed by Katz, 1977). B lymphocytes can be activated by either antigen-specific or nonspecific mechanisms. Antigen-specific activation is the stimulation of a relatively small number of clones of B lymphocytes by antigen to secrete antibody specific for that antigen. Thus, the eliciting agent in this case is specific antigen, which is necessary but not sufficient.

The form in which antigen is presented to the immune system profoundly influences the ability of an organism to respond to that antigen. It was shown by Dresser (1961) that intravenous injection of soluble protein into experimental animals is an unreliable method for immunization. However, when the antigen is presented in monomeric form, as can be achieved by deaggregating the solution by ultracentrifugation, animals are rendered entirely unresponsive to the immunogen. On the other hand, when antigen is presented in an aggregated form, it inevitably evokes a strong antigen-specific humoral immune response. This situation has been investigated in great depth by Weigle and colleagues as an experimental model for the study of the induction, maintenance, and termination of tolerance to heterologous serum proteins, particularly human gamma globulin (HGG) (reviewed by Weigle, 1973). In the case of certain synthetic polymeric antigens, such as polyvinyl pyrrolidone (PVP), immunogenicity increases in direct proportion to molecular weight (Inaba et al., 1978).

The nature as well as the ultimate magnitude of the immune response mounted against a particular antigen is strongly influenced by the incorporation of antigen into adjuvant. An adjuvant is an exogenously administered substance which enhances the immunogenicity of a given preparation. Thus, administration of soluble bovine gamma globulin (BGG) emulsified in Freund's complete or incomplete adjuvant consistently evokes a significant immune response to an antigen which is otherwise of low immunogenicity (Dresser, 1961). In certain instances, when sufficient time elapses after exposure to antigen, adjuvant can suppress the immune response (Walker & Weigle, 1978). It has been demonstrated that the conformation of the protein surface is not appreciably altered by emulsification in such adjuvants. Theories pertaining to the mechanism of action of adjuvants center around the possibilities of delayed antigen release into the circulation, or of an altered circulatory pattern for lymphocytes, resulting in their concentration at sites of antigen localization.

Antigen, whether presented alone or in conjunction with adjuvant, is ultimately presented by mononuclear macrophages, the so-called antigen-presenting cells. Studies of antigen processing by macrophages indicate that these cells take up and metabolize most of the antigen to which they are exposed. However, a small pool of antigen is accumulated by these cells in a two-step process involving cell surface binding and subsequent compartmentalization of antigen (Waldron et al., 1974). Antigen-pulsed macrophages, containing only a minute fraction of the original antigen added to culture, when added to fresh macrophage-depleted cells in the absence of any other antigen, evoke a response comparable to that of cultures to which much greater amounts of antigen were added.

Another possible response of the immune system to antigen is a failure to respond. As mentioned above, this aspect of the immune system is critical to the avoidance of a chronic state of autoimmunity. Antigen-specific unresponsiveness can be induced in the humoral immune system, and is dependent upon the form of the antigen, the presence of T cells, the age of the host, and the immune competence of the host. Tolerance can be induced in both T cells and B cells, the former requiring lower doses of tolerogen and exhibiting longer duration of unresponsiveness (Weigle, 1973). Central unresponsiveness results from the deletion of antigen-reactive cells, while peripheral tolerance is the result of suppression, antigen blockade, or antibody-mediated inhibition. Central unresponsiveness is thought to mimic the state of tolerance to self-antigens enjoyed by the normal host. Study of the mechanisms of induction and termination of this type of tolerance is, therefore, directly relevant to the mechanisms involved in diseases of autoimmunity.

Antigens used to induce immune responses in experimental animals are generally divided into two classes: those dependent on the presence of functional T cells, and those independent of the influence of such cells. The response to thymus-dependent (TD) antigens (e.g., heterologous erythrocyte antigens, serum protein and glycoprotein antigens) can be abolished by treatments designed to eliminate T-cell function. Moreover, antigen-specific B cells must receive signals from a population of specific T cells in order to produce antigen-specific antibody. It was subsequently demonstrated that when spleen cells were depleted of a population of cells adherent to plastic surfaces, the ability of the remaining nonadherent cells to mount an antibody response was abolished. Thus, it appears that three distinct cellular populations are required for the production of antibody to thymus-dependent antigens: T cells, B cells, and adherent cells of the monocyte–macrophage lineage. The role of the macrophage in antigen presentation has been mentioned above. The involvement of T cells in this response appears to be a regulatory one, and is discussed at greater length in a later section.

The humoral immune response to a TD antigen such as sheep red blood cells (SRBC) involves the recognition of a large number of antigenic determinants on the cell surface of the erythrocyte. In order to study the response to an antigen with a single antigenic determinant, the hapten-protein conjugate model has been devised. A hapten is a small, chemically defined substance which is antigenic but not immunogenic (ie., it is unable to induce an antibody response by itself). For the induction of such a response, hapten must be coupled to an immunogenic macromolecule, termed a carrier. It has been demonstrated that in animals previously exposed to a particular hapten-protein conjugate, a secondary or memory response can be evoked only if the hapten is conjugated to the identical carrier. Elucidation of this so-called "carrier effect" indicated that the haptenic determinant reacts with specific B cells to produce hapten-specific antibody only when the antigenic determinants on the carrier interact with carrier-reactive T lymphocytes. Such cells, which do not actually produce antibody but are essential for its production by B cells, are referred to as T helper cells. Carrier effects can also be demonstrated to pertain to the antibody responses to complex, but unconjugated, antigen, such as heterologous erythrocytes. In this case, the T cells react with a helper determinant while the B cells react with an antibody-inducing determinant.

In the mouse, B cells can be divided into two compartments of approximately equal size on the basis of their expression or lack of expression of a surface differentiation marker referred to as Lyb 5. B cells bearing this surface marker can generate antibody responses to antigen in the absence of T cells so long as soluble helper factors derived from T cells are present. Hapten-carrier linkage is not required. Moreover, when helper T cells are involved, their recognition of antigen-presenting cells (but not of B cells) is restricted by the major histocompatibility complex (MHC). In contrast, B cells that lack the Lyb 5 determinant do not respond to antigen in the presence of helper factors, but rather require contact-mediated recognition of both antigen-presenting cells and B cells in a manner restricted by the MHC. This activation pathway requires linked recognition of hapten and carrier.

Activation of B lymphocytes by antigen under inductive circumstances leads to the production of antigen-specific antibody whose range of affinity is variable and depends upon the particular antigen used. In addition to measurement of antibody titers, B-cell activation can be monitored in terms of the number of antibody-producing cells or plaque-forming cells (PFC). The isotype of either the antibody or of the PFC response can be manipulated by choice of antigen or by prior antigenic experience of the B cells. Whether such antigen-specific B-cell induction is the result of one nonspecific signal or two separate signals, one specific and one nonspecific, has been vigorously contested (Bretscher & Cohn, 1970; Coutinho & Möller, 1975) and will not be dealt with in the current work. It must be noted, however, that recent work by Howard and Paul (1983) implicates an initiating stimulus followed by at least four auxiliary signals.

For one particular group of antigens, as mentioned above, induction of antibody responses appears to be essentially independent of the influence of helper T cells. These antigens are termed thymus-independent (TI). In general, IgG responses are more dependent upon the influence of T cells than are IgM responses, and conversely, most TI antigens induce primarily IgM responses. Induction of IgG responses to these antigens can be accomplished, but requires either repeated injections of antigen or unusual experimental conditions. The difference in the class of antibody produced may reflect differential TD v TI antigen binding to cell surface receptors of one or the other of these Ig classes, or alternatively, indicate a basic requirement for T cell help in the production of IgG antibody.

Thymus-independent antigens tend to be large polymers with a high frequency of a particular antigenic determinant. In the mouse, experimental evidence supports the existence of two distinct classes of thymus-independent antigen. The first of these, TI-1, includes haptens conjugated to *Brucella abortus,* to bacterial lipopolysaccharide (LPS), or to polyacrylamide beads. A distinct subset of B lymphocytes responds to antigens of this class. They arise early in ontogeny, display greater amounts of surface IgM than surface IgD, and are inhibited in their responses by antiserum to surface IgM but not to surface IgD. The other set of TI antigens (TI-2) includes substances such as polyinosinic-polycytidilic acid, type III pneumococcal polysaccharide, levan, and haptens conjugated to dextran or Ficoll. The B lymphocyte subpopulation reactive with this class of antigen arises late in ontogeny, displays greater amounts of surface IgD than surface IgM, and is sensitive to inhibition of its antibody responses by antisera to both surface IgM and surface IgD. TI-2 antigens are less T-independent than TI-1 antigens, and at low concentrations have been found to be entirely T-cell dependent. In man, the existence of thymus-independent antigens has not yet been demonstrated, perhaps owing to the newness of the assay for human PFC. Work with haptens conjugated to polyacrylamide beads (a TI antigen for the mouse) has demonstrated that while this agent is immunogenic for cultures of human peripheral blood lymphocytes, responses to it are entirely T-dependent (Galanaud, 1979)

Antigen-nonspecific activation

In contrast to antigen-specific activation, nonspecific activation of B cells involves the stimulation of a large proportion of all B-cell clones by a nonspecific stimulus (mitogen or polyclonal B-cell activator) to secrete antibody against a great diversity of antigenic determinants. Because of the heterogeneity of the B-cell clones involved, this form of activation has been termed polyclonal activation. In this case the eliciting agent is not antigen, but mitogen. Although such agents generally stimulate mitogen-reactive B cell clones both to proliferation and to polyclonal antibody production, this is not inevitably the case (Parker, 1975).

In the mouse, a large number of substances have been demonstrated to possess mitogenic or polyclonal activating capabilities. These agents include products of bacteria, viruses, and fungi, mitogens of plant origin, hydroxythiol compounds, derivatized nucleosides, agents which interact with characterized cell surface receptors (such as the Fc fragment of IgG), proteolytic enzymes, polyanions, and polyene antibiotics. The cellular requirements for induction of nonspecific responses vary with the particular mitogen used. For example, both the proliferative and polyclonal antibody responses evoked by LPS can be observed in the absence of adherent cells as well as T cells. However, whereas the polyclonal response to LPS can be augmented by helper T cells, the proliferative response cannot (Goodman & Weigle, 1979a). The Fc fragment of antibody molecules has also been found to induce proliferation of Fc receptor-bearing B lymphocytes. However, in this case, the proliferative response has been shown to be dependent on the presence of macrophages or macrophage-processed mitogen, while the polyclonal response is dependent on the presence of T cells. The proliferative response to hydroxy-thiol compounds involves both B and T lymphocytes, each of which in turn recruits the participation of uninvolved members of the reciprocal lymphocyte population. The polyclonal responses to these compounds are subject to the facilitative influences of T helper cells (Goodman & Weigle, 1979b). Recently, a new class of B-cell activator, the C8-substituted guanine ribonucleosides, has been shown to be taken up into the interior of the B cell and activate it intracellularly.

Pokeweed mitogen (PWM) stimulates the proliferation of both human B and T lymphocyte preparations. This response to PWM is amplified by synergistic interaction between human B and T cells insofar as T lymphocytes can facilitate the proliferation of B cells cultured with PWM. This phytomitogen has been found to stimulate the production of polyclonal antibody in cultures of human peripheral blood lymphocytes, tonsillar cells, and spleen cells. Such polyclonal activation is entirely dependent on the influence of T helper cells, and is regulated by a balance between helper cells and opposing T suppressor cells, as will be discussed in a later section.

Staphylococcus aureus (SpA) is a mitogen and a polyclonal B-cell activator for human lymphocytes. It has additionally been shown to activate human thymus cells. In contrast to PWM, SpA stimulates high-level proliferation in cultures of isolated human B lymphocytes. However, it has been found that human tonsillar T lymphocytes greatly potentiate the mitogenic response of tonsillar B cells to SpA, and conversely, human peripheral blood B cells can potentiate the responsiveness of peripheral blood T cells to the same mitogen.

Generation of the Primary Antibody Response

The primary humoral immune response may be defined as the antibody response mounted when an individual encounters a particular antigen for the first time. Subsequent experience with the same antigen leads to responses of greater magnitude and altered kinetic characteristics. There is a great degree of variability concerning the length of time which elapses between initial encounter with antigen and the subsequent peak of the primary antibody response to the eliciting agent. The lag period which elapses before the first detection of antibody is dependent upon the dose of antigen, the route of immunization, the physical form of the antigen, and the use of adjuvant. In general, antibodies to heterologous erythrocytes are usually first detected in vivo by day 3 to 4 and peak at day 4 to 6; responses to soluble protein are usually detected and reach maximal levels several days later. The duration of peak antibody levels is generally dependent upon the factors which determine the magnitude of that level and the lag time, particularly by incorporation of antigen into adjuvant.

Antigen-specific antibodies of the IgM class are generally detected earlier and in higher amounts than those of the IgG class. This in part is due to differential kinetics, and may in part be a reflection of increased avidity of IgM (containing 10 antigen-binding sites per molecule) with respect to IgG (containing two antigen-binding sites per molecule). As the IgG antibody titer rises, the IgM antibodies decline, an effect either directly or indirectly attributable to the presence of increasing quantities of IgG. The antibody initially synthesized against a given antigenic determinant has been shown to possess low binding constants (i.e., low binding affinity per antigen-binding site), whereas antibody synthesized later in the primary response is of higher affinity. This is particularly true for the IgG antibody response

Generation of the Secondary (Memory) Humoral Immune Response

The secondary or memory humoral immune response may be defined as the antibody response mounted by an individual who encounters a particular antigen which, when previously experienced, had evoked a normal immune response. This response can occur long after the primary response has subsided, at a time when antibody levels to the eliciting antigen are undetectable. However, the previous encounter with antigen has been found to induce a subpopulation of B cells termed memory B cells which are responsible for the secondary or anamnestic response. This response is elicited by considerably lower quantities of specific antigen and occurs after a significantly reduced lag period. The rate of increase in antibody titer is usually the same in primary and secondary responses. However, the ultimate magnitude of the secondary antibody response achieved is much greater than that seen in the primary response. The peak levels of antibody produced have been found to depend on a number of variables, including the length of time between antigen exposures, the serum titer of antibody to the eliciting antigen at time of exposure, the nature of antibodies formed in the primary response, and the nature of immunogen in question. Complexes between antigen and preexisting antibody, formed when antibody is present in excess, diminish immunogenicity and induce a transient drop in detectable antibody titers. However, formation of complexes between single antigen and high affinity antibody molecules has been found to enhance the immunogenicity of the antigen. The antibodies formed in the course of the secondary humoral immune response exhibit significantly higher affinity for antigen than antibody produced during the primary response. The quantity of IgM antibodies produced is generally either equivalent to or slightly greater than that seen in the primary response, whereas the major increase in titer is attributable to IgG antibody exhibiting much greater affinity for antigen. This qualitative shift in the nature of secreted antibody is felt not to reflect specificity or affinity changes in the products of individual B-cell clones; rather, it is felt to indicate a directed selection for clones producing high affinity antibody reactive with the range of determinants carried by a particular antigen molecule. This observation supports the conservative nature of variable gene product expression during the production of memory. In contrast, however, the expression of the constant heavy chain isotype shifts from primary responses (IgM) to secondary or memory responses (IgG) within single B-cell clones (Greaves & Hogg, 1971). The generation of memory B cells is dependent to a greater or lesser degree on the presence of T cells, with IgG memory being somewhat more T dependent than IgM memory. There is some evidence to suggest that the transition from memory cell to antibody-secreting cell is similarly T-cell dependent (Dresser & Popham, 1979). Moreover, although T-independent antigens can induce memory B cells, expression of their potential is T-cell dependent. The development of memory B cells has furthermore been shown to be dependent on the third component of complement (C3) and may involve formation of antigen-antibody–C3 complexes. However, once memory is generated, its expression does not depend on the presence of C3 (Klaus & Humphrey, 1977). Memory, or priming, of T helper cells generally requires much lower amounts of antigen than B-cell priming. These cells, moreover, are radioresistant in most experimental systems studied. Memory T cells are induced more rapidly than are memory B cells; memory in both cell types persists for at least a year.

Regulation of the Humoral Immune Response

The cell type most extensively and convincingly studied with respect to immunoregulatory properties is the T cell. These cells have been shown to possess regulatory capabilities for both antigen-specific and antigen-nonspecific responses. Regulation of specific responses is dependent upon cellular interactions (either direct or mediated by soluble factors), many of which are subject to genetic restriction. It has long been appreciated that antigen-specific regulation in the mouse involves both T helper cells and T suppressor cells (reviewed by Snell, 1978). These cells have been physically separated (Tse & Dutton, 1976) and have been distinguished by surface antigen phenotype (Lyt antigens) (Cantor & Boyse, 1977). These latter workers demonstrated that surface phenotype Lyt 1+ cells are programmed for helper function, and surface phenotype Lyt 23+ cells carry out suppressive and cytotoxic function. A third subset of T cells, bearing the phenotype Lyt 123+ is felt to constitute a pool of antigen-reactive precursor cells which are not yet committed to either the Lyt 1+ or the Lyt 23+ pathway. This precursor pool is receptive to activation by Lyt 1+ cells, resulting in the development of a profoundly suppressive T-cell subset (Eardley et al., 1978). This subset is felt to exert feedback suppression since their suppressive capacity is proportionate to the degree of antigen-induced T-cell help which is present. One important target of this Lyt 123+-associated suppression appears to be the T helper cell.

T cells can be activated nonspecifically to exert suppressor and helper function by incubation with a mitogenic lectin, concanavalin A (Con A). Such suppressor cells have been shown to diminish the responses to thymus-dependent, but not to thymus-independent, antigens. In contrast to the situation which pertains for many antigen-specific suppressors, Con A-induced suppressor cells manifest no requirement for H-2 compatibility in order to function. Con A-activated T cells produce a soluble immune response suppressor (SIRS) which inhibits the humoral immune responses of murine spleen cells in vitro (Nowowiejski-Wieder et al., 1984). Con A-induced helper cells have been separated from the suppressor cells on Ficoll velocity sedimentation gradients. These helper cells reconstitute the immune response of B cells to sheep erythrocyte antigens. Supernatants from Con A-stimulated cultures appear to contain a variety of helper factors, some of which have activity for T cells (interleukin 2) (Gillis & Watson, 1981), while others are directed at B cells (B-cell growth factors, B-cell differentiation factors) (Swain et al., 1983).

Evidence supporting the existence of a balance between the influence of helper and suppressor T cells in the immune responses of human lymphocytes to antigen has been obtained more recently. Moretta, Mingari, and Moretta (1979) separated T-cell subsets according to whether they have surface Fc receptors for IgG, IgM, or neither (T_γ, T_μ, and T_{null}). T_μ and T_γ cells exert diametrically opposed regulatory effects on antibody production by B cells, T_μ cells supplying helper function to B cells, and T_γ cells acting as functional suppressors. These authors studied the effects of various T-cell subpopulations on the polyclonal antibody responses of human lymphoid cells to pokeweed mitogen, a T-cell–dependent response. The suppressive function of T_γ cells was shown to be dependent upon their interaction with IgG immune complexes. Suppressive activity was also recovered in the supernatants of cultures of T_γ cells, provided they were exposed both to pokeweed mitogen and to immune complexes. In contrast, T_μ cells do not need to bind IgM immune complexes in order to exert helper function, although there is evidence in experimental animals that passive administration of IgM antibodies enhances the ultimate magnitude of the response achieved in a T-cell–dependent fashion. Furthermore, these authors have shown that patients with systemic lupus erythematosus have normal numbers of T_μ cells, but diminished numbers of T_γ cells, correlating with the disease activity observed in these patients. On the other hand, lymphocytes from patients with Hodgkin's disease contain a disproportionately high number of T_γ cells with essentially normal numbers of T_μ cells. These T_γ cells are capable of suppressing the activity of normal lymphocytes in mixed lymphocyte cultures, supporting the possibility that an increase in the proportion of these cells may be central to the disturbed cellular immunity seen in Hodgkin's disease.

Regulation of antigen-specific humoral immunity in man is subject to very similar immunoregulatory control. Dosch and Gelfand (1979) have presented evidence that T cells sensitive to 3 mM theophylline exert suppressor function with respect to antigen-specific responses, while those cells which are resistant to this agent exert potent helper effects. Moreover, theophylline-sensitive T cells carry Fc receptors for IgG, while theophylline-resistant T cells have Fc receptors for IgM. These investigators demonstrated negative restraints on the B-cell response to specific antigen at several levels. Removal of suppressor cells revealed the existence of an excess of simultaneously induced T helper activity. At the B cell level, removal of surface IgD by selective enzymatic digestion resulted in at least a 1,000-fold increase in antigen sensitivity. Schlossman and colleagues (1979) have defined a T-cell surface marker, TH_2, which is present on about 20% of the total circulating peripheral T cells. Suppressor cells activated by Con A contain this surface marker. Approximately 60% of all human peripheral blood T cells are negative for the TH_2 antigen. These cells exert helper activity for B-cell antibody responses. This group of investigators recently described a patient with hypogammaglobulinemia with normal numbers of B cells, but a vast excess of cells positive for the TH_2 marker. It thus appears that maintenance of a delicate balance between T-helper and T-suppressor cells is critical to the continued existence of a state of homeostasis in the normal host.

A more widely adopted group of T-cell surface markers has been developed (Reinherz and colleagues, 1979). These differentiation antigens (the OKT series) consist of a series of surface glycoproteins defined by monoclonal antibodies. Immature thymocytes first express only the OKT10 marker, followed by the appearance of OKT9. As these cells mature in the thymus, they acquire OKT4, OKT6, and OKT8. OKT4 is a 62,000-mol wt glycoprotein present on two-thirds of peripheral T cells and medullary thymocytes. These cells also bear OKT10, OKT3, and OKT1. Part of these cells also bear OKT8 (a 76,000-mol wt glycoprotein present on 30% of peripheral T cells and medullary thymocytes) and part of them lack OKT8. The OKT4+ cell is an inducer cell for T cells and B cells, driving B cells to antibody production and T cells to cytolytic activity under appropriate circumstances. The OKT8+ cell is suppressive in these situations, and counteracts the activity of OKT4+ cells. Most cytotoxic T lymphocytes (CTL) are OKT8+. In certain autoimmune diseases (lupus erythematosis, multiple sclerosis, Sjogren's syndrome, primary biliary cirrhosis, etc), OKT8+ cell numbers are diminished. In contrast, immunodeficiencies of different types may occur by virtue of defects at a number of different stages of maturation.

It has been proposed by Jerne (1974) that the immune system actually constitutes a vast, complex, interdependent network which is self-regulating. Fundamental to this concept is the observation that all antibody molecules of a given specificity possess a set of antigenic determinants, or idiotypes (i_1) which are adjacent or identical to the molecules' antigen-combining sites. Each antigen-combining site thus recognized not only its complementary antigen, but also a complementary idiotype (i_0) on another set of antibody molecules. The configuration of this latter idiotype is presumed to resemble that of the antigen very closely. When B cells (B_1) bearing the i_1 idiotype on their surface immunoglobulin encounter either antigen or complementary idiotype i_0, a stimulatory signal is received. Moreover, the antibodies produced by B_1 are inhibitory for the cells (B_0) producing antibody bearing the i_0 idiotype. Thus, when i_1-bearing antibodies encounter antigen, complex formation lowers the amount of free i_1 antibody, which in turn results in diminished antagonism toward B_0 and diminished stimulation of B_2, the set of cells antagonistic to B_1. Both of these effects allow B_1 to expand and produce increased quantities of specific antibody. However, as these changes occur, B_0 is suppressed and B_2 stimulated, restoring a state of equilibrium. Production of autologous anti-idiotypic antibody has been observed during the normal immune response (Brown & Rodkey, 1979). Idiotype specific cells can suppress humoral immunity, cell-mediated cytotoxicity, and mixed lymphocyte reactivity under appropriate experimental conditions. Stimulation of other lymphocytes by anti-idiotypic antibody has been demonstrated in lymphocyte proliferation assays.

CELL-MEDIATED IMMUNITY

Background

Cellular immunity is that arm of the immune system dependent upon cellular as opposed to humoral or antibody activity (Benacerraf & Unanue, 1979; Katz, 1977). Thymus-derived (T) cells are pivotal cells in cellular immune events, which can be grouped into two major categories, delayed hypersensitivity (DH) and cell-mediated cytotoxicity (CMC). DH is routinely manifested in vivo in response to infectious agents and CMC upon exposure to foreign tissue, such as transplanted organs or certain tumors.

While humoral immunity is highly successful in protecting against certain bacterial diseases and toxins, cellular immunity offers increased protection to diseases often insusceptible to control by antibody alone. For example, there are a number of pathogens, including certain bacteria, viruses, and parasites, which are not neutralized by antibody. This is because they are either refractive to complement, resistant to digestion by polymorphonuclear cells or macrophages, or require a relatively large number of phagocytic cells to control the infection. However, such pathogens can be controlled if macrophages, for example, are activated in some manner to increase metabolic and enzymatic activity, making formerly resistant organisms susceptible to digestion. Alternatively, if phagocytic cells can be attracted to an area of inflammation in large numbers, the pathogen can be controlled. In the last ten years, much evidence has shown that T cells upon recognition of invading organisms release substances called lymphokines, which not only activate macrophages to increased bacteriocidal capacity, but which are also chemotactic for various inflammatory cells, increasing their number at the site of infection (Cohen et al., 1977; Askenase & Lovern, 1983). Furthermore, reexposure of T cells to the same pathogen at a later time results in even a more vigorous and rapid elimination of the pathogen (Mackaness, 1969). This memory response can be transferred with sensitized cells, but not with serum, reconfirming the cellular nature of this type of immune response.

The other cellular phenomenon, CMC, may be important in the elimination of virally infected tissue and malignant tissue. There is much experimental evidence to suggest that T cells can be sensitized to kill cells which are sufficiently foreign to the host. In animals, the capacity to reject tissues has been transferred with T cells much more effectively than with antibody. Perhaps the best example is the rejection of tissues transplanted between various strains of animals or between humans, such as kidney and heart transplants.

Thus, in both DH and CMC, the key cell is the T cell. However, in DH this cell is a very small component of the inflammatory response, acting not as an effector cell, but as recruiter and activator of other cells, such as macrophages, which are equipped to digest invading organisms. The significance of T cells in control of infectious disease cannot be overemphasized, as experimental studies with thymectomized animals show high susceptibility to bacterial infection.

In contrast to DH in which the T cell recruits effector cells, in CMC the T cell is the effector cell, directly killing its target tissue. It is still controversial how CMC may function in vivo other than in the artificial situation of grafting. Cytotoxic T cells may carry out immunosurveillance of malignant tissue (Snell, 1978), but this is still debated. On the other hand, there is good evidence that cytotoxic T cells prevent viral infection through lysis of virally associated tissues (Snell, 1978). For example, individuals with congenital agammaglobulinemia who have optimal T-, but defective B-cell function are not abnormally susceptible to viral disease. Finally, the function of these cells may be to regulate the expression of other lymphoid cells, or in other words, to act as suppressor cells either through recognition of idiotype or antigen in association with lymphoid cells.

A relatively newly discovered cell may be a more likely candidate for effecting immunosurveillance. Because congenitally athymic nude mice are consistently found to reject certain tumors and do not have a higher than normal incidence of spontaneous tumors despite their T-cell deficiency, it was apparent that a cell other than a T cell might be suppressing the appearance of tumor cells. These mice were found to have cells which, unlike T cells, have little if any specificity for antigen, but have a propensity to kill tumor tissue. These cells, called natural killer cells, or NK cells, are neither T nor B cells, nor macrophages, but may be pre-T cells. NK cell activity can be enhanced in vivo with interferon inducers, BCG, and *Corynebacterium parvum* (Koren & Herberman, 1983).

Another form of CMC called antibody-dependent cell-mediated cytotoxicity or ADCC is mediated by lymphoid cells bearing receptors for the Fc end of immunoglobulin (reviewed by Forman & Möller, 1973). The effective cells are also neither T nor B cells nor macrophages and are called null cells or killer cells (K cells). They are assayed by their capacity to kill antibody-coated target cells. The specificity of killing is conferred only passively by the adsorbed immunoglobulin.

Definition of T-Cell Subsets

The area of T-cell research has blossomed and considerable information has been accumulated concerning T cells (reviewed by Miller & Mitchell, 1969; Cantor & Weissman, 1976; and Katz, 1977). Chapter 1 characterized T cells in detail. Briefly summarized, T cells can be categorized in three different ways. First, T cells have been divided functionally into T1 and T2 subpopulations (Cantor & Weissman, 1976), based on experiments in which it was found that lymphoid cells from various organs, such as spleen and lymph node, when mixed together, resulted in either enhancing or suppressing effects. T1 cells are relatively immature, nonrecirculating cells which are insensitive to antilymphocyte serum (ALS); they function as amplifier cells and usually reside in the spleen and thymus. T2 cells are mature, recirculating cells which are sensitive to ALS; they function as effector and regulatory cells and reside predominantly in lymph node and blood. Correlation of such functional differences with organ of origin resulted in the concept that lymphoid organs might serve purposes other than lymphocyte depots.

A system more commonly used in defining T lymphocytes today is based on antigenic differences between various T-cell subpopulations. The Ly antigen system of the mouse has been discussed in chapter 1. Basically, T cells mediating cytotoxicity are Ly 23 + and those mediating DH are Ly 1+. It should be reemphasized here that the Ly system defines only subsets of T cells and that T cells belonging to the Ly 1+ class, for example, are probably not all alike, but differ by other surface antigen markers and functions (Eardley et al., 1978; Benacerraf & Unanue, 1979; Katz, 1977; and Sullivan & Flaherty, 1979).

The systems used to define human T-cell subsets have been described earlier in this chapter.

T-Cell Activation

How antigen activates T cells, or even B cells, for that matter, is not known. Part of the confusion regarding T-cell triggering is that it has been difficult to define the T-cell receptor for antigen (Paul & Benacerraf, 1977; and Reinherz et al., 1983), while the B-cell receptor for antigen is well defined. The T-cell receptor may be classical immunoglobulin in extremely low density on the cell surface, a unique type of immunoglobulin, or some as yet undefined molecule. Because of the capacity of antigen or other ligands to cap surface receptor molecules, capping has been considered a mode of cell activation (Edelman et al., 1973). However, studies have shown that activation can occur without capping, although it is possible that patching, or slight lateral movement of receptors in the membrane, is sufficient to trigger the cell (Gunther et al., 1973). An influx of Ca++ into the antigen-triggered cell or a redistribution of Ca++ within intracellular compartments has been implicated in activation as a second signal, followed by changes in cyclic AMP and GMP ratios (Rasmussen & Goodman, 1977).

While the actual biochemical events involved in lymphoid cell triggering are still vague, it is appreciated that the form of the antigen is crucial to subsequent lymphoid cell activation. Initial sensitization of T cells requires that antigen be presented in association with antigen-presenting cells, such as macrophages. The mode of presentation has been detailed previously in this chapter. This association of antigen with the antigen-presenting cell is enhanced if the antigen is in particulate form, given with an adjuvant such as *Bordetella pertussis,* complete Freund's adjuvant, or bacterial endotoxin. Antigen in highly soluble or deaggregated form tends not only to fail to elicit an immune response, but leads to unresponsiveness or tolerance to the antigen. This has been shown with the antigen human gamma globulin (HGG) which, dependent on the amount of deaggregated HGG given, can result in T-cell tolerance extending nearly half the life span of the treated mouse (Weigle, 1973). It is assumed that for activation, T cells may require two signals, one involving binding the antigen, and the other from some interaction with the presenting macrophage. Without this second signal, the T cell may perceive a tolerogenic or "off" signal.

Major histocompatibility complex

Much has been learned about T-cell sensitization through transplantation of tissues. Initial study of tumors was done in mice without regard to strain, and due to strain differences some of the tumors were rapidly rejected. This has led to one of the most complex areas of immunological research today, immunogenetics. Basically, it was learned that individuals or various inbred strains of animals had unique molecules on the surface of many of their tissue cells that lymphocytes could recognize either as self or as foreign. More recent work suggests that these antigens may not only be involved in rejection of foreign tissue, but may also be involved in day-to-day immune responses. Animals bearing certain surface markers, or alternatively, lacking others, fail to respond to some antigens (McDevitt & Benacerraf, 1969), and both animals and humans bearing certain surface markers have a high propensity to certain diseases (Dausset & Contu, 1980). Several experimental systems are discussed to show how the histocompatibility complex may be important in T-cell sensitization in DH and CMC.

The histocompatibility complex in the mouse is called H-2, is located on the 17th chromosome, and is composed of five major regions: K, I, S, G, and D (reviewed by Benacerraf & Unanue, 1979; Katz, 1977; Shreffler & David, 1975). The analogous complex in the human is called HLA, is located on the 6th chromosome, and is composed of four major regions, HLA-D, HLA-B, HLA-C, and HLA-A (reviewed by Banacerraf & Unanue, 1979; Katz, 1977; and Shackelford et al., 1982). The I region of the mouse is probably equivalent to the human HLA-D region and the HLA-A, HLA-B, and HLA-C regions are similar to the H-2K and H-2D regions. The molecules coded for by these regions have been partially characterized. In general, the HLA-A, -B, and -C antigens are polymorphic glycoproteins of approximately 44,000 mol wt and are associated noncovalently with a 12,000 mol wt protein called β_2 microglobulin encoded on chromosome 15. The HLA-D region encodes for DR surface antigens, which are composed of two noncovalently linked glycoprotein chains of approximately 33,000 and 28,000 mol wt, and lack β_2 microglobulin. In the mouse, while most tissues bear H-2K and H-2D antigens, the Ia antigen is restricted to B cells and subsets of macrophages and T cells. These latter antigens are involved in recognition of antigen by amplifier or helper T cells (Lyt 1+ cells), which are involved in DH and antibody synthesis. The H-2K and H-2D encoded antigens are involved in sensitization of CMC-effector T cells.

Mixed lymphocyte reaction (MLR)

When lymphocytes from two different strains of mice or different individuals are mixed together, recognition of Ia (DR) antigens occurs and results in extensive lymphocyte proliferation after four to five days of culture. These proliferating cells, which can be assayed by their uptake of ^{3}H-thymidine, are Lyt 1+ and are a well-established source of T helper function. The MLR has been used as an indication of histocompatibility between various individuals to aid in tissue matching. However, as is seen below, the MLR does not measure the generation of cytotoxic T cells which are elicited.

CMC (T-cell mediated)

In the course of the MLR, cytotoxic T lymphocytes are generated. These are Lyt 23+ and constitute only a minor fraction of the proliferating cells. They are generated through recognition of H-2K and H-2D antigen differences between the two cell populations. The proliferating Lyt 1+ T cells serve as helper or amplifier cells to augment the generation of cytotoxic T cells, but are not necessary for their generation. Because H-2K and H-2D antigens are present on most tissues, cytotoxic T cells can be elicited by culture with other histoincompatible cell types, such as fibroblasts. However, extensive proliferation of amplifier cells does not occur, because fibroblasts lack Ia antigens. Thus, the MLR is elicited only in response to other lymphoid cells, while CMC is less tissue restricted.

In addition to recognition of H-2 antigens, T cells appear to be able to recognize tumor antigens and viral antigens. In the latter case, the virus must be in association with H-2 antigen to be recognized. Because tumor antigens have not yet been clearly defined, it is not certain if they, too, are recognized in association with an H-2 antigen or might themselves be modified H-2 antigens.

Recognition of virally infected tissue. Mice infected with virus generate T cells which can kill syngeneic, virally infected tissue cells in vitro (Doherty & Zinkernagel, 1975). The killer T cells are restricted to killing target cells bearing the H-2K or H-2D phenotype of the infected mouse. Thus, the killer cells which are syngeneic with the target "recognize" H-2 antigen (H-2K or H-2D) in association with viral antigen in some way in order to kill the target. Such H-2 restricted killing has led to several theories of recognition, one involving altered self (altered H-2 due to association with virus) and the other, a two-receptor model, with cytotoxic T cells bearing one receptor for viral antigen and another for H-2 antigen.

Mechanism of cytolysis. Cytotoxic T cells are most often assayed in vitro by using ^{51}Cr-labeled target cells, measuring the release of ^{51}Cr as an indication of cell death. Other assays are employed if killing takes more than 24 hours, because there is a high spontaneous release of ^{51}Cr from target cells (Lucas & Walker, 1974). When sensitization of killer T cells is optimized, for example, the use of peritoneal exudate T cells from in vivo allogeneic tumor sensitized animals, as much as 50% of the target cells can be killed in four hours with ratios as low as 2 lymphocytes per target cell. Thus, T-cell killing can be quite efficient. How T cells kill is not known, but killing has been most descriptively termed a "kiss of death". The lymphocyte contacts the target and firmly adheres, leaves the target, and shortly thereafter, the target cell lyses, due to an ionic imbalance (Martz, 1977). A soluble cytotoxin, called lymphotoxin, made by T lymphocytes, has been found and upon partial purification has been found to be a mixture of two different molecules varying in size and antigenicity (Walker et al., 1976). In certain cases antiserum to lymphotoxin has inhibited T-cell killing to varying degrees, but these experiments have not yet proved if lymphotoxin is the mediator of T-cell lysis.

Graft v host disease (GVH)

One could say that GVH is the in vivo analog of the MLR and CMC. It was found that when lymphoid cells from one strain of mouse are given to another mouse, splenomegaly results. This is the result of the large number of host spleen cells proliferating in response to the grafted spleen cells. If the host is irradiated first, the grafted cells survive, proliferate, cytotoxic cells are generated, and the grafted cells essentially reject the host, causing death, ie, GVH. GVH has been the problem in treating leukemia by whole body irradiation, followed by reconstitution with nonhost bone-marrow cells. Unless the cells are perfectly matched with the recipient, the grafted cells will attack the host. Various forms of immunosuppression have been used to reduce GVH, including selective irradiation such that all the host lymphoid cells are not killed (Strober, 1984) and elimination of mature T cells from the bone-marrow graft with monoclonal anti-T-cell sera (Reinherz et al., 1982).

Delayed hypersensitivity

Delayed hypersensitivity is elicited experimentally by immunization with antigen followed approximately 30 days later with an interdermal injection with a small amount of the same antigen. Or, if the antigen is chemically reactive, sensitization can be employed through painting substances on the skin which bind to skin proteins. This is called contact sensitivity and occurs naturally in response to poison ivy, for example, which contains a skin-sensitizing component, a catechol. The histological picture at the site of challenge with antigen after about 24 hours is normally a mononuclear cell infiltrate, predominantly macrophages, but in some cases polymorphonuclear cells are predominant. Experiments have shown that most of the infiltrating cells in the inflammation are not T or B cells, but phagocytic cells derived from the bone marrow with a small number of specific Ly 1+ T cells causing their recruitment. It has been assumed that the few T cells present release factors which lead to accumulation of phagocytic cells.

Numerous factors have been found by in vitro assay to be made by activated T cells, and these factors may be responsible for the histological picture of delayed hypersensitivity and contact sensitivity. Several substances have been described which influence macrophages, notably macrophage migration inhibitory factor (MIF). MIF is a glycoprotein of about 20,00 to 40,000 mol wt and has the capacity to inhibit macrophage movement (reviewed by Benacerraf & Unanue, 1979; Cohen et al., 1977). Another factor is macrophage activating factor (MAF) which increases enzymatic and metabolic activity of macrophages and may be the same as MIF. A factor chemotactic for macrophages has also been described and is distinct from MIF. Chemotactic factors have also been found which attract various polymorphonuclear cells, such as eosinophils and neutrophils. Injection of these various factors intradermally has duplicated their properties characterized in vitro, strongly implicating these substances as in vivo mediators of DH.

REFERENCES

Askenase PW, Lovern HV: Delayed type hypersensitivity: Activation of mast cells by antigen-specific T cell factors initiates the cascade of cellular interactions. *Immunol Today* 1983; 4:259–264.

Benacerraf B, Unanue ER: *Textbook of Immunology,* Williams & Wilkins Co, Baltimore, 1979.

Bretscher P, Cohn M: A theory of self-nonself discrimination. *Science* 1970; 169:1042–1049.

Brown JC, Rodkey LA: Autoregulation of an antibody response via network-induced auto-anti-idiotype. *J Exp Med* 1979; 150:67–85.

Cantor H, Boyse EA: Lymphocytes as models for the study of mammalian cellular differentiation. *Immunol Rev* 1977; 33:105-124.

Cantor H, Weissman I: Development and function of subpopulations of thymocytes and T lymphocytes. *Prog Allergy* 1976; 20:1-64.

Cohen S, David J, Feldman M, Glade PR, Mayer M, Oppenheim JJ, Papermaster BW, Pick E, Pierce CW, Rosenstreich DL, Waksman BH: Current state of studies of mediators of cellular immunity: A progress report. *Cell Immunol* 1977; 33:233-244.

Coutinho A, Möller G: The self-nonself discrimination: A one signal mechanism. *Scand J Immunol* 1975; 4:99-102.

Dausett J, Contu L: Is the MHC a general self-recognition system playing a major unifying role in an organism? *Human Immunol* 1980; 1:5-17.

Doherty PC, Zinkernagel RM: A biological role for the major histocompatibility antigens. *Lancet* 1975; I:1406-1408.

Dosch HM, Gelfand EW: Specific *in vitro* IgM responses of human B cells: A complex regulatory network modulated by antigen. *Immunol Rev* 1979; 45:243-274.

Dresser DW: Effectiveness of lipid and lipidophilic substances as adjuvants. *Nature* (London) 1961; 191:1169-1173.

Dresser DW, Popham AM: The influence of T cells on the initiation and expression of immunological memory. *Immunology* 1979; 38:265-274.

Eardley DD, Hugenberger J, McVay-Boudrea L, Shen FW, Gershon RK, Cantor H: Immunoregulatory circuits among T cell sets. I. T-helper cells induce other T cell sets to exert feedback inhibition. *J Exp Med* 1978; 147:1106-1115.

Edelman GM, Yahara I, Wang JL: Receptor mobility and receptor-cytoplasmic interactions in lymphocytes. *Proc Natl Acad Sci USA* 1973; 70:1442-1446.

Forman J, Möller G: Effector cells in antibody-induced cell mediated immunity. *Transpl Rev* 1973; 17:108-149.

Galanaud P: *In vitro* antibody response to trinitrophenyl-polyacrylamide beads. *Immunol Rev* 1979; 45:141-161.

Gillis S, Watson J: Interleukin-2 dependent culture of cytolytic T cell lines. *Immunol Rev* 1981; 54:81-110.

Goodman MG, Weigle WO: T cell regulation of polyclonal B cell responsiveness. I. Helper effects of T cells. *J Immunol* 1979a; 122:2548-2553.

Goodman MG, Weigle WO: Nonspecific activation of murine lymphocytes. V. Role of cellular collaboration between T and B lymphocytes in the proliferative and polyclonal response to 2-mercaptoethanol. *J Immunol* 1979b; 122:1433-1439.

Greaves MF, Hogg NM: Immunoglobulin determinants on the surface of antigen binding T and B lymphocytes in mice. In *Progress in Immunology* pp. 111-126, Ed. B. Amos, Academic Press, New York, 1971.

Gunther GR, Wang JL, Yahary L, Cunningham BA, Edelman GM: Concanavalan A derivatives with altered biological activities. *Proc Natl Acad Sci USA* 1973; 70:1012-1016.

Howard M, Paul WE: Regulation of B cell growth and differentiation by soluble factors. *Ann Rev Immunol* 1983; 1:307-333.

Inaba K, Nakano K, Muramatsu S: Regulatory function of T lymphocytes in the immune response to polyvinyl pyrrolidone. I. Two categories of suppressor T cells. *Cell Immunol* 1978; 39:260-275.

Jerne NK: Towards a network theory of the immune system. *Ann Immunol (Inst Pasteur)* 1974; 125C:373-389.

Katz, DH: *Lymphocyte Differentiation, Recognition and Regulation*, Academic Press, New York, 1977.

Klaus GGB, Humphrey JH: The generation of memory cells. I. The role of C3 in the generation of B memory cells. *Immunology* 1977; 33:31-40.

Koren H, Herberman H: The cryptic orphan NK cell. *Immunol Today* 1983; 4:97-99.

Lucas ZJ, Walker SM: Cytotoxic activity of lymphocytes. III. Standardization of measurement of cell-mediated lysis. *J Immunol* 1975; 113:209-224.

Mackaness GB: The influence of immunologically committed lymphoid cells on macrophage activity *in vivo. J Exp Med* 1969; 129:973-992.

Martz E: Mechanisms of specific tumor cell lysis by alloimmune T lymphocytes: Resolution and characterization of discrete steps in the cellular interaction. *Contemp Top Immunobiol* 1977; 7:301-361.

McDevitt HO, Benacerraf B: Genetic control of immune response. *Adv Immunol* 1969; 11:31-74.

Miller JFAP, Mitchell GF: Thymus and antigen reactive cells. *Transpl Rev* 1969; 1:3-42.

Moretta L, Mingari MC, Moretta A: Human T cell subpopulations in normal and pathologic conditions. *Immunol Rev* 1979; 45:163-193.

Nowowiejski-Wieder I, Aune TM, Pierce CW, Webb DR: Cellfree translation of the lymphokine immune response suppressor (SIRS) and characterization of its mRNA. *J Immunol* 1984; 132:556-558.

Parker DC: Induction and suppression of polyclonal antibody responses by anti-Ig reagents and antigen-nonspecific helper factors: A comparison of the effects of anti-Fab, anti-IgM, and anti-IgD on murine B cells. *Immunol Rev* 1980; 52:115-139.

Paul WE, Benacerraf B: Functional specificity of thymus-dependent lymphocytes. *Science* 1977; 195:1293-1300.

Rasmussen H, Goodman BP: Relationship between calcium and cyclic nucleotides in cell activation. *Physiol Rev* 1977; 57:421-509.

Reinherz EL, Meuer SC, Schlossman SF: The delineation of antigen receptors on human T lymphocytes. *Immunol Today* 1983; 4:5-9.

Reinherz EL, Geha R, Rappeport JM, Wilson M, Penta AC, Hussey RE, Fitzgerald KA, Daley JF, Levine H, Rosen FS, Schlossman SF: Reconstitution after transplantation with T-lymphocyte depleted HLA haplotype mismatched bone marrow for severe combined immunodeficiency. *Proc Natl Acad Sci USA* 1982; 79:6047-6051.

Reinherz EL, King PC, Goldstein G, Schlossman SF: Further characterization of the human inducer T cell subset defined by monoclonal antibody. *J Immunol* 1979; 123:2894-2896.

Shackelford DA, Kaufman JF, Korman AJ, Strominger JL: HLA-DR antigens: Structure, separation of subpopulations, gene cloning and function. *Immunol Rev* 1982; 66:133-187.

Shreffler DC, David CS: The H-2 major histocompatibility complex and the I immune response region: Genetic variation, function and organization. *Adv Immunol* 1975; 20:125-195.

Snell GG: Ir genes and T lymphocytes. *Immunol Rev* 1978; 38:3-69.

Strober S: Overview: Effect of total lymphoid irradiation on autoimmune disease and transplantation immunity. *J Immunol* 1984; 132:968-970.

Sullivan K, Flaherty L: The Qa-2 antigen in lymphocyte subpopulations. Mixed lymphocyte cultures and cell mediated lympholysis. *J Immunol* 1979; 123:2920-2924.

Swain SL, Howard M, Kappler J, Marrack P, Watson J, Booth R, Wetzel GD, Dutton RW: Evidence for two distinct classes of murine B cell growth factors with activities in different functional assays. *J Exp Med* 1983; 158:822-835.

Tse H, Dutton RW: Separation of helper and suppressor T lymphocytes on ficoll velocity sedimentation gradient. *J Exp Med* 1976; 143:1199-1210.

Waldron Jr, JA, Horn RG, Rosenthal AS: Antigen-induced proliferation of guinea pig lymphocytes *in vitro*: Functional aspects of antigen handling by macrophages. *J Immunol* 1974; 112:746–755.

Walker SM, Weigle WO: Effect of bacterial lipopolysaccharide on the *in vitro* secondary antibody response in mice. I. Description of the suppressive capacity of lipopolysaccharide. *Cell Immunol* 1976; 36:170–179.

Walker SM, Lee SC, Lucas ZJ: Cytotoxic activity in lymphocytes. VI. Heterogeneity of cytotoxins in supernatants of mitogen-activated lymphocytes. *J Immunol* 1976; 116:807–815.

Weigle, WO: Immunological unresponsiveness. *Adv Immunol* 1973; 16:61–122.

Chapter 5

Mucosal Immune Responses

Mario S. Nemirovsky

OUTLINE

HISTORICAL BACKGROUND

Since ancient times, man has tried to protect himself against epidemics. The Chinese, for instance, sniffed smallpox crusts as a preventive measure against the disease. This kind of protection was introduced from mideastern countries through diplomatic channels during the enlightened times of the 18th century (Silverstein & Miller, 1981). Undoubtedly, this procedure caused more sickness than protection.

During the post-Jenner era, the parenteral route of immunization was universally chosen. Meanwhile, some immunologists were interested in the possibilities offered by the natural way of contact with "foreignness"; the mucosae (respiratory, gastrointestinal, mammary, genitourinary) as a preferred way of immunization. One of the first microbiologists doing experimental work in this field was Kiyoshi Shiga, the discoverer of the dysentery bacillus. This was the etiological agent of dysentery, a disease with paramount gastrointestinal symptomatology. Besredka in 1927 introduced the concept of local immunity, stressing the usefulness of limited immunological reactions being initiated and carried out in mucosal tissues. Those structures are exposed to infectious agents, and it is precisely here where the mechanical barriers are weaker than in external teguments.

After World War II, the World Health Organization planned massive immunization programs as a way of eradicating epidemics. At this time, renewed interest in vaccination through mucosal contact appeared as an economical method of mass inoculation. One of the utmost successes in preventive medicine has been achieved by the virtual eradication of poliomyelitis using orally administered vaccines.

With the prodigious development of immunology in the last 2 decades, a clearer picture has emerged of the mucosal immune system. It possesses a full expression (from an immunological standpoint) of specific and nonspecific components, but with some differences both at the humoral and cell-mediated levels, when compared with parenteral immune responses. When the antigen is administered by subcutaneous, intradermal, intravenous, or intraperitoneal routes, the main centers of immune responses are the draining peripheral lymph nodes and/or the spleen. In the mucosal system, a largely expanded lymphoid tissue, closely in contact with the epithelial membranes, is responsible for the initiation of immune responses when antigens reach the mucosa.

These differences exist as a mechanism of adaptation to the constant and multiple antigenic stimuli to which we are exposed from birth. The reader must keep in mind that many questions in this area await answers. Among others: what is the precise relationship between "serum" and "secretory" immune response? How efficient is oral immunization as a way of obtaining systemic protection? Is systemic immunization expressed in secretions?

Another important aspect to be considered is the newness of the field. Many of the experimental results in this area have been obtained in laboratory animals and, therefore, cannot automatically be applied to the human situation without further investigation.

ROLE OF MUCOSA IN NONSPECIFIC HOST DEFENSE

Mucous Blanket (Mucin) and Other Mucosal Secretions

As pathogenic agents find intact skin a serious mechanical impediment to penetration and a disruption of its integrity is mandatory in order for such agents to obtain access to tissues. In contrast, mucosal epithelium appears to afford feeble protection to the respiratory, digestive, and genitourinary systems, which microorganisms or viruses should be able to overcome with relative ease. However, mucosae are not as defenseless as they appear at first glance: the mucosal blanket overlying the apical aspect of epithelial cells is the initial defense against infection (Florey, 1970).

The nose, for instance, serves as a preliminary but efficient barrier to the entry of foreign material. Its filtration capacity relies entirely upon the anatomical and physiological integrity of the mucociliary apparatus. Bacteria enter with the inspired air, and in general all particles bigger than 2μm can be trapped by the mucosal blanket, which is transported by the ciliary component of the epithelium to the pharynx, and swallowed. In the stomach, they are subjected to the chemical attack of acidic secretion. Those that survive are again trapped by the mucosal blanket, moved along by the peristaltic wave, and eliminated with the feces.

The mucous blanket forms a continuous shield covering the entire aerodigestive tract. The basic composition of the mucous blanket appears to be common to all mucosal surfaces, although differences have been described between and within species with regard to their exact chemical makeup. The nasal mucous blanket will serve as a descriptive example: the mucosal glands and goblet cells produce a highly viscous secretion that is diluted by the combined action of lacrimal gland secretions and transudate passing through epithelium. The mucous blanket consists of two layers: the inner one, a thinner film applied upon the apical aspect of epithelial cells, and the outer, a more viscous sheet. Mucin or "muco-substance" is formed by sulfated glycoproteins that have a highly efficient viscosity-raising property. The mucin, constituting only 2% to 3% of the total secretion, confers upon the mucous blanket its characteristic high viscosity. It is precisely this property that allows an effective trapping of foreign materials including bacteria.

Other components of the epithelium are also important to surface defense of mucosae contained within the mucous blanket.

Lysozyme

The presence of lysozyme, a bacteriostatic active enzyme, has been confirmed. This hydrolytic enzyme is able to lyse gram-positive microorganisms and appears to have a coadjuvant action in gram-negative germ lysis by means of specific antibodies and complement (Ganguly & Waldman, 1980).

Glucosidase

The lysis activity of lysozyme upon the microbial wall will not degradate it completely. The hydrolysis is completed by the enzymatic activity of an array of glucosidases. Their presence has been demonstrated in nasal secretions (Naumann, 1980).

Interferon and other viral inhibitors

Interferon, a substance that restricts intracellular virus replication, is synthesized by a variety of cells in vitro (fibroblasts, lymphocytes, epithelial cells, etc). To what extent epithelial cells produce interferon in vivo is unknown. Passively administered interferon protects nasal mucosa against virus attack (Ganguly & Waldman, 1980).

A number of nonspecific inhibitors of viral infectivity have been recognized for more than 40 years. These substances are complex in nature, of different molecular weight and sensitivity to heat. They are characterized by their capacity to agglutinate red cells. They are present in secretions, mainly in the upper respiratory tract and saliva (Naumann, 1980).

Lactoferrin

This iron-binding protein has antibacterial activity. Its localization inside the specific granules of the granulocyte allows it to be liberated during the phagocytic activity of these cells. Its action can be exerted by direct binding to iron contained within some microorganisms or by binding to iron necessary for the metabolism of some bacteria. Lactoferrin is found as a soluble factor in colostrum and milk. A significant protective role can be ascribed to this substance in the newborn's gastrointestinal tract (Ogra & Ogra, 1979).

Complement

Complement is capable of mediating the lysis or opsonization of a number of cells as well as bacteria and virus possessing a lipoprotein envelope. Even if the activation of the whole multienzymatic complex (common or classic pathway) is required for the lysis, many of its biological activities can be expressed early in the activation process (Colten & Alper, 1976). For instance, the activation of C1 and C4 by IgM antibodies can be enough to neutralize some viruses. In other instances, the activation process must proceed until C3 to effectively play a role in the neutralization process.

The alternate (or properdin) pathway can destroy virus-infected cells. This nonspecific mechanism can be highly effective in some secretions such as colostrum and milk (Waksman, 1979). In fact, the properdin pathway can be directly activated by parasites, without the involvement of antibodies, as required for the classical pathway. The parasites can release products that trigger the activation process, but this effect can be produced directly by components of their integument (Santoro, Bernal, & Capron, 1979).

The anaphylatoxins C3a and C5a are byproducts of complement activation causing smooth muscle contractions and increase in vascular permeability. Apparently, this action is mediated by histamine released by mast cells that are degranulated by direct action of anaphylatoxins. An additional effect is chemotaxis of leukocytes. All these activities, typical of an inflammatory reaction, can be effectively controlled by an enzyme called anaphylatoxin inactivator. Some proteolytic enzymes foreign to complement, such as plasmin, trypsin, and tissue and bacterial proteases, can generate C3a and C5a.

The enhancement of phagocytosis is one of the paramount functions of the complement system, especially in the struggle against bacteria. The contribution of complement in this matter is pluripotential; including some of the components of the classical pathway, especially C3. The properdin system is required for the most efficient disposal of pneumococci.

Immune adherence is a property first described in rabbit erythrocytes bearing C3 or C4 receptors, capable of attaching to a variety of cells, including macrophages. Antibodies against bacteria can activate, after binding to the specific antigenic determinant, the first four components of complement, and allow adherence. This mechanism can be exceedingly important in the in vivo clearance of blood bacteria as a prelude to phagocytosis.

The lytic activity of complement can be expressed in mucosal secretion (Etéviant et al., 1980). It is known that some of the complement proteins are synthesized by intestinal epithelium (Peltier, 1979) and that the alternate pathway can be activated by antibodies belonging to the secretory IgA isotype (Drutz, 1976).

Peptidase and peptidase inhibitors

Macrophages synthesize exopeptidases associated with plasma membranes and lysosomes, and endopeptidases of a broad proteolytic activity as well as of a highly restricted specificity such as complement proteinases. It has been shown that macrophages synthesize and secrete inhibitors of proteolytic enzymes. For instance, human macrophages synthesize C3b inactivator and B1H globulin which are regulators of the alternate pathway of complement activation (Werb, 1981). Macrophages elastases and collagenases can be neutralized by inhibitors secreted and synthesized by the same cell, which is also able to synthesize alpha-2 macroglobulin, an inhibitor of all endopeptidases. The latter, together with alpha-1 antitrypsin, appears to contribute to the modulation of the immune response by inhibition of natural killer activity and antibody-dependent cell-mediated immunity (Ades et al., 1982). Some microorganisms are able to synthesize proteases that cleave and inactivate IgA1 subclass of secretory IgA. This activity has been demonstrated for *Streptococcus sanguis*, group H streptococci, *Neisseria gonorrheae*, and *Neisseria meningitidis* (Drutz, 1976). The possibility of an in vivo counterpart of these mechanisms can have serious repercussions in mucosal immunity: as a consequence of the degradation of some secretory IgA antibodies, the mucosal surface colonization by some microorganisms can be enhanced.

Mucociliary Transport and Clearance

The mucous blanket consists of two layers: the inner one, a thinner film applied upon the apical aspect of epithelial cells, and the outer, a more viscous sheet.

It appears that the most effective protection is primarily afforded by the mechanical sweeping of epithelial cilia. Recently, it has been demonstrated that mucous secretion from goblet cells can be provoked by immune complexes as well as by antigens in orally immunized animals (Lake et al., 1980). In the cases where parasitic antigens are involved, this reaction appears to be a T-dependent phenomenon.

Pathogen/Antigen Penetration of Mucosal Epithelium

A good deal of experimental evidence indicates the capacity of mucosal epithelium to transport macromolecules able to provoke an immune response. For many years it has been known that the enterocytes of rodents are permeable to immunoglobulins contained in colostrum and milk, but this property disappears at weaning (Morris & Morris, 1978). Ultrastructural studies using ferritin (mol wt 750,000) and horseradish peroxidase (mol wt 40,000) indicate that these substances penetrate the intestinal epithelium of *adult* animals when introduced in the lumen of gut (Williams, 1978). Immunohisto-chemical techniques prove that these markers retain antigenic determinants, detected by specific antisera before and after cell passage.

There are no doubts about the participation of *lymphoepithelium*, ie, the epithelium overlying the nodular lymphoid tissue of GALT and BALT, in this mechanism of transport (Owen & Jones, 1974; Tenner-Racz et al., 1979). Environmental substances of antigenic nature could be transported from the apical to the basolateral aspect of epithelial cells and then reach the lymphoid tissue of mucosal membranes.

To what extent, if any, other mucosal epithelia participate in this mechanism of transport is still a matter of controversy. The exact nature of the cellular mechanisms governing this transport through epithelium is not known. This is an active mechanism, where the cells (or some putative receptors present at the apical aspect of them) exert some class of selection. It is clear that antigenicity of foreign material contacting epithelium is not necessary for transport.

For many microorganisms or parasites, a rupture on the continuity of mucosal epithelium is necessary for their access to mucosal lymphoid tissues.

Exotoxins may play an important role in this matter. Providing the potentially antigenic material has been able to cross the barrier put forward by the mucosal blanket and epithelium, the high concentration of macrophages wandering through the connective tissue of the mucosal lamina propria facilitate their trapping and the further processing of these substances (LeFevre, Hammer, & Joel, 1979).

In addition there are no physical barriers to exchange between mucosal segments of these cells, and the possibility has been raised that macrophages trapping antigenic material may present them to lymphoid tissue located elsewhere.

There are indications that the local immune response triggered by antigen may also regulate antigen uptake (Bienenstock & Befus, 1980).

Nonspecific Responses in Lamina Propria

Macrophages

When considering all factors involved in nonspecific responses, the role of *macrophages* has to be taken into consideration. These cells play an important role in both specific and nonspecific immune responses in lymphoid organs and, in general, in connective tissues where they are located. A considerable number are *free macrophages.* These wandering cells can travel long distances through blood vessels and use connective tissue fibers as support in extravascular tissues. Lung macrophages have been studied intensively (Bowden & Adamson, 1980). They are a part of the alveolar structure and as such are exposed to the inspired air and to all particulate matter contained in it, including bacteria. Because of continuous exposure, they are in a constant activated state. A number of enzymes released by activated macrophages can be identified in washings of bronchial secretions: cathepsin aryl-sulfatase, lipase, DNase, RNase, collagenase, β-glucuronidase

(Kaplan & Nielsen, 1979a,b). It is accepted that macrophages are temporary residents of other mucosal epithelia such as those of gastrointestinal or genitourinary systems. In mammary glands they can be identified in epithelial acini and in colostrum or milk (Ogra & Ogra, 1979). Milk cells contain phagocytosed immunoglobulins.

Experimental evidence indicates that after oral immunization, nonspecific protection afforded by macrophages can protect against microorganisms other than those used in priming (LeFevre et al., 1979).

Mast cells

Mucosal mast cells differ from those of connective tissue at several levels: morphological (both optical and electron microscopical), histochemical, biochemical, and responsiveness to degranulating agents (Befus et al., 1982; Bienenstock & Befus, 1980). They appear to be regulated by T cells. Their origin is uncertain: some evidence points to lymphocytes as precursors. A series of studies made in laboratory animals infected with *Trichinella spiralis* and *Nippostrongilus brasiliensis* helped to understand the participation of mucosal mast cells in immune reactions. The experimental helminthiasis provokes, after a brief period of decline, a dramatic increase in the number of mast cells infiltrating the lamina propria and mucosal epithelium. They are called "atypical" mast cells (Waksman & Ozer, 1976), intraepithelial mast cells or "globule leukocytes." There is evidence that these responses are under thymic control through an undefined set of long-lived T lymphocytes (Mayrhofer, 1979a,b). The mast cell proliferation is reminiscent of a basophil cutaneous hypersensitivity. Both mast cells and basophils are known to play an important role in delayed hypersensitivity reactions (Askenase, 1977), in addition to their well-known participation in immediate hypersensitivity reactions mediated by anaphylactic IgE antibodies.

Mast cell degranulation liberates vasoamines like histamine, and leukotrienes belonging to a family of arachidonic acid derivatives that play a central role as mediators of allergic reactions and inflammation (Samuelsson, 1981).

Hormones

Estrogens are known to increase clearance by the reticuloendothelial system (Sell, 1975). The influence of other hormones upon immune responses is an unsettled question. Humoral immunity appears to be regulated by pituitary hormones. Contact hypersensitivity is reduced in hypophysectomized rats and it can be restored by prolactin (Nagy & Berczi, 1981). The immunosuppressive effect of glucocorticoids is well known.

Blood vessels

Vasoamines liberated by mast cell degranulation modify the vascular bed, contributing to some of the characteristic features of inflammation. Blood vessel walls are the site of immune complex deposition in such diseases as periarteritis nodosa and glomerulonephritis (Sell, 1975). The consequence is thrombosis and obstruction of the blood vessels and the appearance of areas of necrosis and scarring.

Intercellular substance

The ground substance of the connective tissue is not merely the inert battleground of immune reactions, but appears to be influenced and affected by them: it has been shown that when guinea pigs are immunized with soluble proteins in such a schedule as to avoid anaphylactic reactions, an intraperitoneal challenge produces a local mast cell degranulation as well as mitogenic stimulation of normal connective tissue cells (Franzen & Norrby, 1982).

Autonomic nervous system

Agonists of the sympathetic nervous system known collectively as catecholamines (epinephrine, norepinephrine, and dopamine) and those of the parasympathetic system (acetylcholine) modulate the severity of allergic reactions by regulating the amount of mediator release from target cells (Frick, 1976). The close relationship of agonistic and antagonistic effects on autonomous nervous system is well exemplified in the pathogenesis of bronchial asthma (Reed, 1968). Receptors have been identified on the plasma membranes of target cells for acetylcholine and epinephrine. α-Adrenergic receptors respond to norepinephrine and in a much less degree to epinephrine or isoproterenol. β-Adrenergic receptors respond to isoproterenol and to a lesser degree to epinephrine or norepinephrine.

The hypothesis has been raised that catecholamines, acting as a first messenger, react with receptors such as adenylcyclase. This enzyme in its activated form activates a second messenger, cAMP. The latter induces the target cells to perform their physiological function (Sutherland, 1970).

SPECIFIC HOST DEFENSE IN MUCOSAE

Lymphoid Tissue in Mucosae

Mucosal membranes are seeded with great numbers of immunocompetent cells and macrophages. This wide distribution of lymphoid tissue serves as an anatomical framework for immune responses originating in or expressed in mucosal structures. A recent hypothesis suggests that there is a functional relationship between all mucosal lymphoid tissues with a common secretory immune system (Bienenstock & Befus, 1980).

The basic distribution of lymphocytes involved in mucosal immunity is as follows:

1. Lymphocytes distributed throughout the subepithelial lamina propria of mucosae as well as between epithelial cells (theleolymphocytes; Figs 5-1, 5-5, 5-6).

2. Collections of lymphocytes forming nodules in mucosal membranes of the respiratory and gastrointestinal systems.

Nodular lymphoid tissues are present in the small intestine and to a lesser extent in colon. The appendix contains a large collection of nodules (Fig 5-2). They are known

FIG 5-1. An intraepithelial lymphocyte * lying between columnar cells (C). (B) brush border. Mice jejunum, × 14,219. (Courtesy Prof. J. S. Hugon).

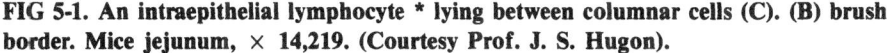

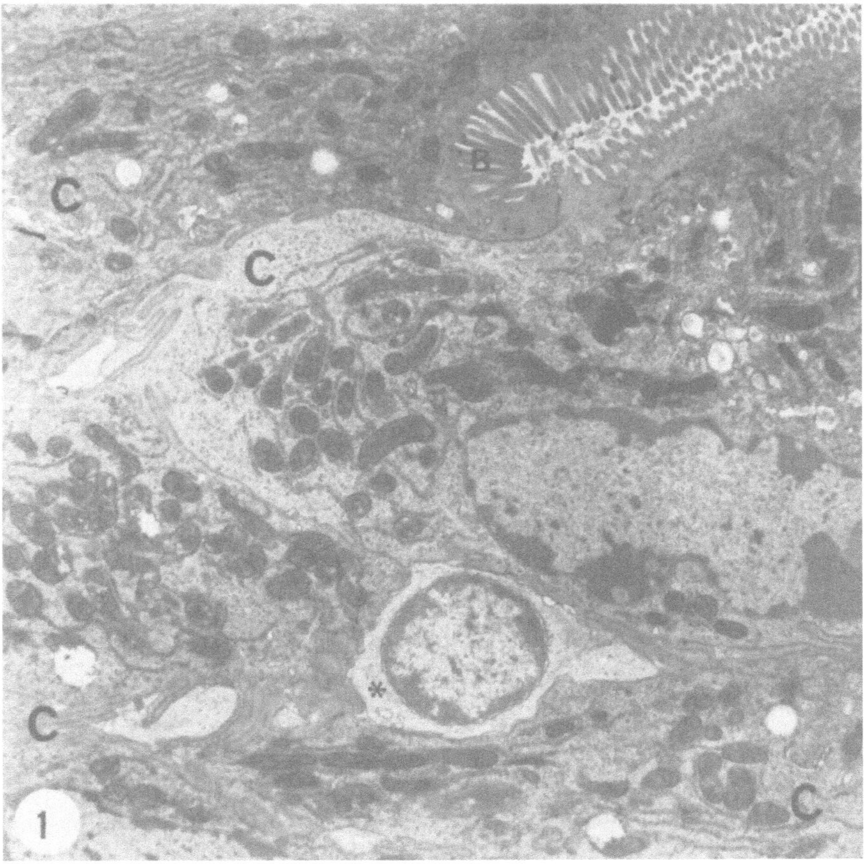

as gut associated lymphoid tissues (GALT). Much of our knowledge on mucosal immunity stems from experimental work on GALT.

An increasing amount of information is presently available concerning the nodular lymphoid tissue forming the Waldeyer's ring (adenoids and tonsils) at the entrance of the aerodigestive tract, and in general about the lymphoid tissue associated with the respiratory tree, known as bronchial associated lymphoid tissue (BALT).

The main histological features of Peyer's patches and tonsils are presented as examples of nodular lymphatic tissue associated with mucosa.

FIG 5-2. *Appendix.* **A lymphatic nodule of the lamina propria. (F) follicle; (C) corona; (D) dome; (TDA) thymus dependent area. Deep channels (arrows) are located at the periphery of the lymphoepithelium (L) (× 215).**

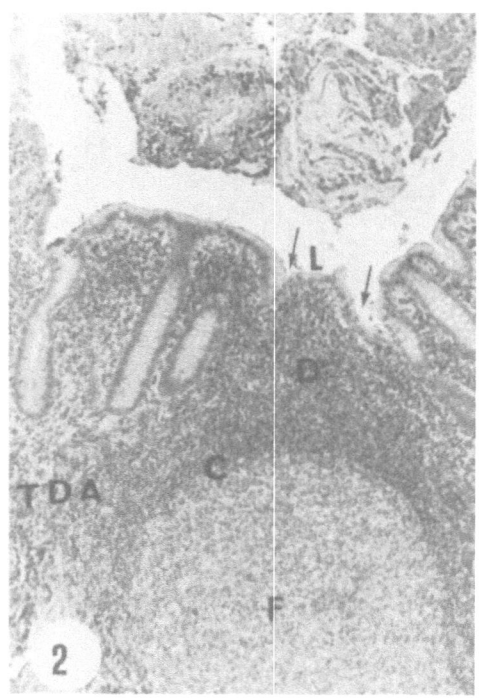

Peyer's patches

There is a great variability between species with regard to pre- and postnatal maturity of Peyer's patches as well as their distribution in the gut (Waksman & Ozer, 1976).

In humans, Peyer's patches can be identified during the last trimester of pregnancy. After birth, their development reaches a peak before puberty. Later on the tissue decreases in amount, but without complete atrophy even at advanced age. In young adults, each patch is formed by more than 300 lymphatic nodules. They are present throughout the intestinal tract, but the greatest number are located in the distal ileum.

The structure of each nodule (Fig 5-2) is characterized by the existence of a follicle or germinal center, similar to those in the lymph nodes (see chapter 1, Fig. 1-11) or spleen. A pale pole can be seen which contains sparse numbers of small lymphocytes. No mitotic figures are seen. Macrophages containing bacterial debris are easily identified. The dark pole is the site of an intense mitotic activity. There are numerous macrophages, blast cells, medium sized, and small lymphocytes. The latter appear to be concentrated at the periphery, in the vicinity of lymphatic capillaries. Macrophages within follicles are functionally different from those present in lymph nodes or spleen. For unknown reasons they appear to be unable to "process" antigens properly for presentation to B or T cells. Surrounding the follicle there is a crown or corona formed almost exclusively by small lymphocytes and some macrophages. In histological preparations it appears as a crescent formation. The periphery of the corona merges with lymphoid cells and macrophages densely concentrated in the lamina propria. This region is known as the dome. Here, all varieties of lymphocytes are found. The epithelium overlying the dome or lymphoepithelium (Owen & Jones, 1974) possesses a number of characteristics differing from those of the intestinal epithelium. Microvilli are scanty at the apical aspect of some epithelial cells. These cells, called M cells, form a membrane between lymphoid cells and the lumen. The lymphocytes are interposed between the basal lamina and plasmatic membrane of M cells. There are a considerable number of lymphocytes infiltrating the epithelium, but not lodging close to M cells. This lymphoepithelium lacks goblet cells, appears to be functionally different from mucosal epithelium elsewhere, and is more easily penetrated by antigenic material; especially through M cells. Deep channels are created between the periphery of dome lymphoepithelium and the surrounding mushroom-like intestinal mucosa not connected with lymphatic nodules. These channels facilitate the access and concentration of foreign materials (bacteria, debris, exfoliated cells) in the vicinity of the lymphoepithelium.

The periphery of the dome fuses with the lamina propria stretching between two lymphatic nodules. At this level there is no anatomic barrier such as connective tissue, which surrounds the follicle. This zone is known as TDA (thymic-dependent area) inhabited preferentially by T lymphocytes. Postcapillary venules which serve lymphocytes recirculation are easily identified in this area (Fig 5-2).

Tonsils

The tonsils are collections of lymphoid tissue which are distributed circumferentially in the oropharynx. The largest collection is organized with the palatine tonsils (Fig 5-3). They represent a considerable accumulation of lymphatic nodules closely related to the overlying stratified squamous epithelium. In fact, lymphocytes invade portions of this epithelium which has some of the characteristics of lymphoepithelium of Peyer's patches. The basal and lateral aspects of palatine tonsils are separated from the muscle walls of the pharynx by a dense connective tissue capsule.

The epithelial surface is irregular and contains deep invaginations or crypts, where antigenic material can accumulate. At this level, the epithelium is reduced to one of a few layers and is heavily infiltrated by lymphocytes (Fig 5-4).

The lymphatic nodules are similar to those found in Peyer's patches, but they are closer to the epithelium. Plasmocytes are particularly abundant in the corona. Dendritic macrophages, similar to those of germinal centers of lymph nodes and spleen, are seen in the follicles. The similarity is not only morphological but also functional: the handling of antigens allows the lymphatic tissue to mount an immune response in situ.

FIG 5-3. *Palatine tonsil*. Lymphoid nodules (L) localized close to the epithelium (arrows). (C) crypt (× 339).

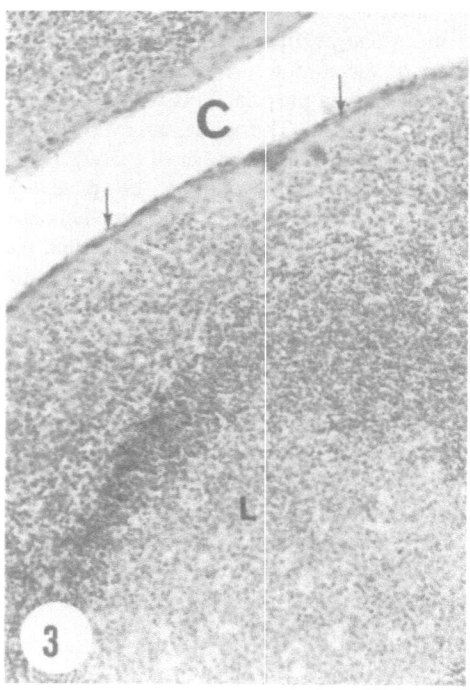

In general, the structure of the lymphoid tissue in tonsils is closer to that of lymph nodes or spleen than to that of Peyer's patches. The important difference is that only efferent lymphatic vessels can be identified; the epithelial crypts substitute for afferent lymphatics.

Circulation and Migration of Immunocompetent Cells in Mucosae

A good deal of attention has been focused on the nature of the cell populations forming the mucosal lymphoid tissues. Both T and B lymphocytes can be identified. The first are localized preferentially in the thymus-dependent areas of nodular lymphoid tissues and form the majority of those infiltrating the mucosal epithelium. B lymphocytes are the main components of the follicles of GALT and BALT. In fact, they form together an important part of the whole B-cell pool of the organism (Waksman & Ozer, 1976).

FIG 5-4. *Palatine tonsil.* **At higher magnification, lymphocytes (arrows) are infiltrating the thinner squamous epithelium (E)** ($\times$ **5,375).**

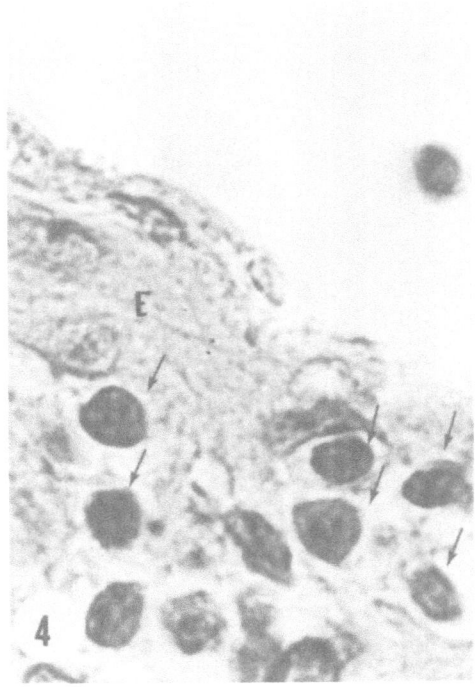

Those cells express membrane-bound immunoglobulins of the IgA isotype, and in a lesser proportion, IgM, IgG, and IgE. Studies in rabbits show that IgA-bearing B cells from the appendix are derived from IgM-bearing precursors.

Plasmocytes are localized in the lamina propria of mucosal membranes (Figs 5-5 and 5-6). No evidence of immunoglobulin synthesis in follicles of BALT and GALT has been demonstrated, with the exception of the tonsils (Ishizaka & Newcomb, 1970).

Immunologists have tried to follow the precursors of antibody-forming cells from the germinal centers of GALT to the site of localization and secretion beneath the epithelial membranes. Cell transfer experiments have shown that there is a population of precursor cells in Peyer's patches which are able to produce immunoglobulins in the intestine. These precursor cells possess membrane-bound IgA, and lack IgM attached to them or C3b receptors. The pathways followed by these cells are not completely known, but it appears clearly that the mesenteric lymph nodes are a necessary stop on their way to the mucosae.

FIG 5-5. *Nasal mucosa*. In the lamina propria can be identified plasmocytes (P), macrophages (M), lymphocytes (L), eosinophils (E). Arrows: basal lamina. C: columnar cells (× 5,375).

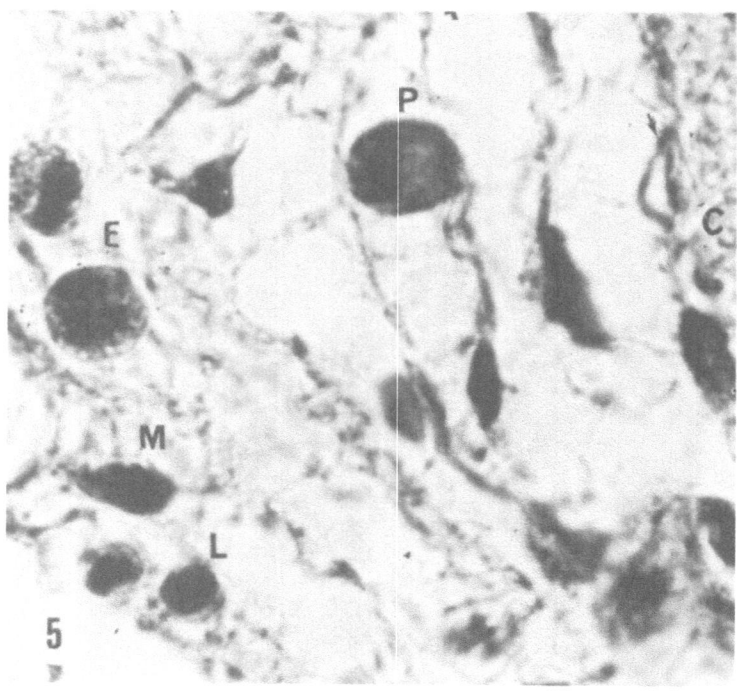

These precursor cells can also be isolated from thoracic duct lymph, indicating that the following sequence is likely to occur (Lamm, 1976):

germinal centers of GALT ⟶ mesenteric lymph nodes ⟶ duct lymph ⟶ blood circulation ⟶ lamina propria of the intestine.

These studies have also been extended to BALT. When lymphoid cells from lungs were injected to lethally irradiated rabbits, these cells were able to repopulate the intestine, spleen, and lung (Bienenstock & Befus, 1980). The predominant isotype identified in membrane-bound immunoglobulins of these cells was IgA.

Mesenteric lymph node cells transferred in rabbits have also been shown to home to mammary tissues and to secrete IgA.

Quantitative transfer studies were carried out with precursor cells from bronchial lymph nodes. The results obtained clearly indicated that these cells preferentially homed

FIG 5-6. *Ileum*. Chorion of the villi. Macrophages (M), plasmocytes (P), and eosinophils (*) are located near the basal lamina (arrows). (C) columnar cells (× 5,375).

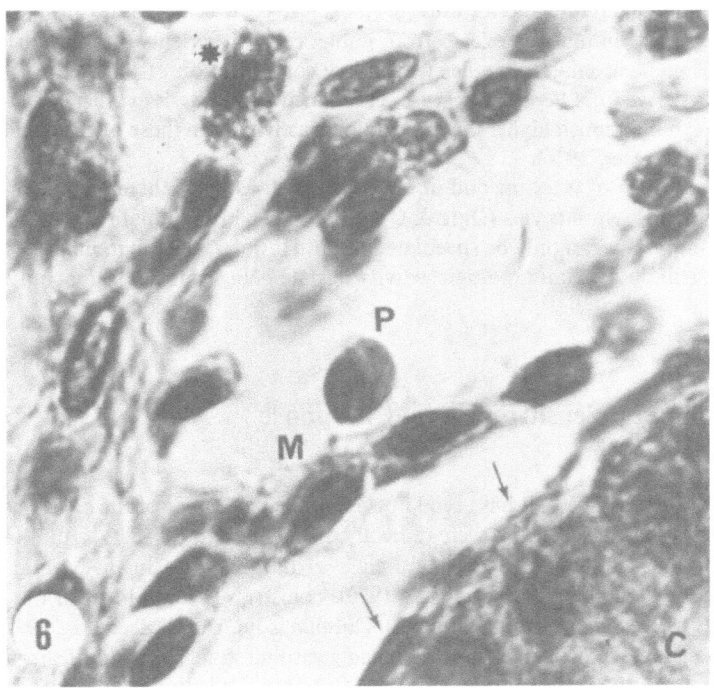

to the lungs and secondarily to the small intestine and mesenteric lymph nodes. It appears that the first priority goes to the organs of origin, and accessorily to other mucosal tissue (Bienenstock & Befus, 1980).

The factors responsible for homing are unknown, but a hormonal factor or cell-mediated receptor is suspected.

The IgA precursor cells have been stressed in this description, but it is important to mention the role of precursor cells belonging to other isotypes such as IgG or IgE. Even if representing only a small fraction of the entire humoral response in secretions, their physiological role could be much greater than their concentration, especially IgE (Izhizaka & Newcomb, 1970; Waksman & Ozer, 1976).

A much simpler pathway can be established for lymphoid cells in tonsils: immunoglobulin-synthesizing plasmocytes of all isotypes are present in germinal centers and infiltrate the surrounding tissues (Ishikawa, Wicher, & Arbesman, 1972).

Mucosal T cells

There is an important subpopulation of helper T cells in the lamina propria of mucosal membranes. Additionally, theleolymphocytes, lymphocytes which are found between mucosal epithelial cells, are almost exclusively T cells. These cells are suspected of playing a role in mucous release from goblet cells. In rodents they have been shown to possess metachromatic granules with a low concentration of histamine. In gut they apparently derive from Peyer's patches T cells. Functional analysis in other species indicates that they exhibit a much higher in vitro cytotoxic activity than those of the lamina propria (Waksman & Ozer, 1976).

In the lumen of intestine and in secretions such as milk, there are macrophages as well as T and B lymphocytes (Ogra & Ogra, 1979). The functional role of these cells in mucosal immunity can only be speculated upon. However, these lymphocytes have been shown to still possess immunologic activity despite being outside of the confines of the tissue.

Local Immune Sensitization and Response

Immunoglobulins

Since the early 1960s, it has been known that the percentage of the different immunoglobulin isotypes in secretions were radically different from those in serum (Heremans, 1974). Immunoglobulin A is the main class of immunoglobulin in parotid secretion (Brandtzaeg, Fjellander, & Gjeruldsen, 1970), colostrum, and milk (with the exception of bovines where the predominant immunoglobulin is IgG) (Tomasi & Grey, 1972). Similar observations were made in nasobronchial and gastrointestinal secretions, tears, and sweat. Table 5-1 shows the composites of different secretions. It is important to point out that IgM and IgE are also secretory immunoglobulins not only because they are present in secretions but also because they are synthesized by plasmocytes homing to the lamina propria of mucosal epithelium (Waksman & Ozer, 1976). The small proportion of IgG present in secretions (with the noted exception of bovine mammary secretion) is due to passive serum transudation through the mucosal epithelium and local synthesis (Table 5-1).

Considerable attention has been focused on IgA in secretory systems. Other immunoglobulins, while in considerable smaller concentrations, nevertheless may play an important role. Antibodies of IgM isotype have been postulated as being precursors of secretory antibody responses. Secretory IgM is the main isotype present in secretions of patients affected by a selective IgA immunodeficiency and in most instances, S-IgM can effectively replace S-IgA from a physiological standpoint (Tomasi, 1976; see chapter 10). Exact quantitation of immunoglobulins in secretions can be difficult due to technical reasons. For example, the presence of proteolytic enzymes in gastrointestinal secretions may rapidly degrade non-IgA immunoglobulins and therefore not accurately reflect the concentration. Additionally, there may be considerable variation in the flow rate (saliva and tears, for example), which may reflect the state of hydration, central nervous system

TABLE 5-1. Concentrations of Immunoglobulins in Human Serum and Secretions.

Biological fluid	IgA	IgM	IgG
Serum [a]	328	132	1,230
Colostrum[a]	1,234	61	10
Whole saliva [a]	30,4	0,6	4,9
Parotid saliva [b]	2,75	0,48	—
Jejunal secretions [a]	27,6	—	34,0
Colonic secretions [a]	82,7	—	86
Lower respiratory tract secretions [c]	0,86	—	0,31

NOTE: Concentrations are given in miligrams per 100 ml.

[a] From Vaerman, *Res Immunochem Immunobiol* 1973; 3:91.

[b] From Tomasi and Zigelbaum, *J Clin Invest* 1963; 42:1552.

[c] From Reynolds et al., *Adv Exp Med Biol* 1978; 107:553.

stimulation, or drug effect; all of these may affect the concentration of immunoglobulins contained in the secretions.

IgA in serum represents 5% to 10% of the total immunoglobulin concentration (Vaerman, 1973). The majority is constituted by monomers of 152,000 mol wt and a 7-S sedimentation coefficient. A small percentage of serum IgA is present as a dimer and even as a polymer. Secretory IgA (S-IgA) is composed of dimers. Additionally, there is one attached glycoprotein of mol wt 58,000 known as secretory component (SC). The tridimensional structure of S-IgA is not completely known but many studies indicate that secretory component combines with the Fc segment of each α-chain by disulfide bridges and covalent bonding, which extends over a considerable surface. At least four antigenic determinants have been identified in secretory component. The glycoprotein can be isolated as free SC in secretions of IgA immunodeficient patients, and also in colostrum and bile of immunologically competent individuals. A distinct polypeptide known as J chain has also been identified, in combination with S-IgM and S-IgA. The molecular weight of J chain is 23,000 to 26,000. This polypeptide is synthesized by the same plasmocytes making IgA and IgM in the lamina propria of mucosal membranes. They are suspected of functioning in the intracellular assemblage of H and L chains of

IgA or IgM and in the mechanism of liberation by exocytosis of the immunoglobulins from plasmocytes. The molecular weight of S-IgA is 390,000 and has an 11-S sedimentation coefficient. The complex formed by SC + J + $(\alpha L)_2$ may be an adaptive mechanism which enables these molecules to resist the effects of proteolytic enzymes (Hanson et al., 1980). There are also small percentages of IgA contained in secretions which are not linked to SC. These "free" IgA can be either monomers or polymers. IgA polymers constitute 10% of total IgA in colostrum. Between 5% and 20% of IgA in nasobronchial secretions are 7-S monomers. Higher percentages are seen in jejunal secretions and bile.

Origin of Serum IgA. Experimental work carried out in different species indicate that a considerable proportion of serum IgA is synthesized by resident populations of plasmocytes in the lamina propria of mucosal membranes and annex glands. This is nicely demonstrated by experiments in which protected mice, whose intestinal tract is shielded during total body irradiation, show no fall in serum IgA when compared to nonprotected mice (Cebra et al., 1976). Why a proportion of IgA remains a monomer and unassociated with SC or J chain and ultimately finds its way into the serum rather than the external secretion is still a mystery. It is known that in humans an important additional source of IgA is the bone marrow and that a definite percentage of lymphocytes bearing IgA on their surface can be found in the peripheral lymph nodes and spleen.

Origin of S-IgA. Studies utilizing radiolabeled amino acids and histochemical techniques have demonstrated that S-IgA is almost exclusively synthesized by plasmocytes located in the lamina propria of mucosae. More than 80% of plasmocytes in small intestine, colon, and rectum synthesize IgA (Fig 5-7). Other studies have shown a lesser percentage of IgA-synthesizing plasmocytes in the salivary glands, nasobronchial tissues, and mammary glands (Waksman & Ozer, 1976). The origin of precursors of those plasmocytes has been the subject of much experimentation (Hall, 1978). In rats it has been shown that intravenously injected ^{3}H-thymidine-labeled lymphocytes collected from thoracic duct (predominantly GALT derived) localize preferentially in the lamina propria of the gut. To what extent antigen absorbed by the lymphoepithelium plays a role in this "homing" is still a matter of controversy. The fact that homing is seen even in allografted fetal intestine tends to refute the role of antigen as the homing signal. Experiments carried out in mice have shown that lymphocytes from mesenteric lymph nodes transferred to syngeneic pregnant recipients preferentially seed and begin synthesizing IgA (Roux et al., 1977) in the mammary glands at the end of gestation and during lactation. In nonpregnant females of the same species, mesenteric lymphocytes labeled with ^{3}H-thymidine localized 24 hours after transfer in the intestine, cervix, uterus, vagina, and mesenteric lymph nodes (Bienenstock & Befus, 1980). Sixty percent of these cells had surface IgA. When the labeled lymphocytes originating in mediastinal lymph nodes were transferred to syngeneic animals, they localized preferentially in lungs. The predominant isotype present in these cells was also IgA.

On the contrary, labeled peripheral lymph nodes' lymphocytes localized preferentially in the organs of origin with the main isotype being IgG. It is of interest to point out that the few labeled lymphocytes which populated peripheral lymph nodes and originated in mesenteric lymph nodes exhibited IgG on their cell membrane.

FIG 5-7. Localization of IgA-producing plasmocytes in the lamina propria of rat colon (arrows). (C) columnar cells. Slide incubated with FITC-rabbit antirat IgA (technique of Husband & Gowans, *J Exp Med* 1978; 148:1146).

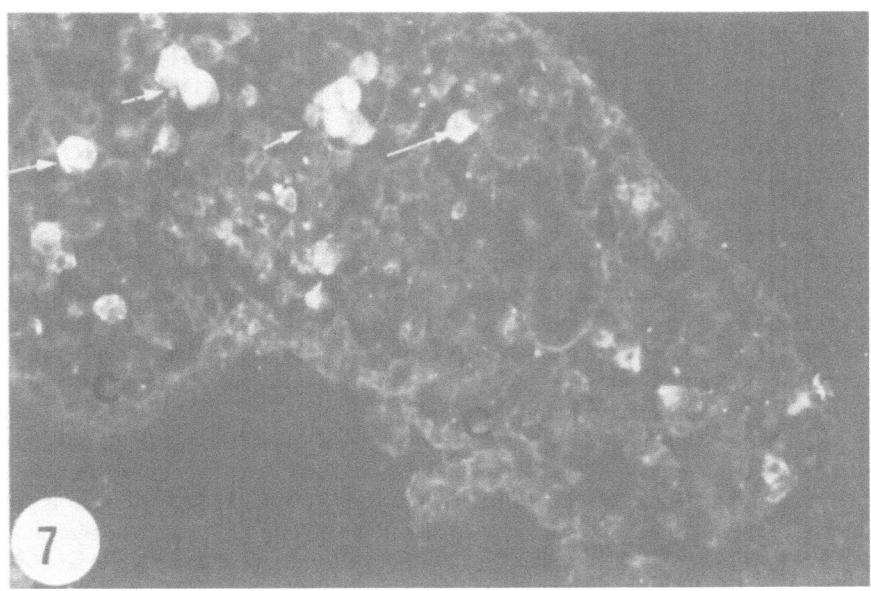

The precise role of GALT and BALT lymphoid cells in S-IgA formation is still unknown, but it is universally accepted that these nodular lymphoid tissues are the site of the expansion of a population of B cells seeding mucosal membranes via the mesenteric lymph nodes, thoracic duct lymph, arterial vessels, and arterial capillaries of the lamina propria of mucosal membranes. The reason for this circuitous route to their final destination is not completely clear. An attractive explanation is that this expansion multiplies the opportunities for these precursors of antibody-synthesizing cells to contact "their" antigen and follow the necessary steps to actively produce and secrete antibodies. This would occur irrespective of the site of first contact with the antigen, anywhere in the mucosal membranes.

L and H chains of IgA as well as J chain are synthesized in the endoplasmic reticulum of mucosal plasmocytes and possibly assembled before leaving the cell. From these subepithelial localization, $(L\alpha)^2 +$ J contact epithelial cells at their basal aspect. Once at the epithelial cell-membrane secretory component is thought to be the specific receptor for the IgA dimer coupled to J chain (Brandtzaeg & Baklien, 1976). However, entry of this molecule into the epithelial cell may occur as nonspecific endocytosis. Within the epithelial cells, these molecules become coupled to secretory component. This glycoprotein has been demonstrated by biochemical and immunohistochemical techniques to be synthesized by epithelial cells.

The ensemble, $(L\alpha)^2 + J + SC$, is transported to the apical aspect of the cells where they are then transported to the brush border by exocytosis. A similar mechanism is thought to occur for IgM pentamers (Brandtzaeg & Baklien, 1976).

It has been shown that Sc has a high affinity for mucin, the main component of the mucosal blanket. This affinity may facilitate the localization of S-IgA at the surface of epithelial cells. For unknown reasons, S-IgM appears to have less affinity for mucin.

Some recent studies have shown that dimeric IgA is transported through the hepatocyte from blood to bile. This transport is dependent upon the presence of free secretory component on the plasmatic membrane of the hepatocyte (Fisher et al., 1979). It is possible, but not yet proven, that pentameric IgM follows the same way.

The antibody nature of some of the "transhepatic" IgA has been shown (Hall et al., 1979). It is conceivable that dimeric IgA-J chain molecular complexes derived from submucosal plasma cells are absorbed into the blood or lymph channels instead of being transported into the external secretions. Once within blood these molecules are transported to the liver, subsequently linked to secretory component on the surface of the hepatocyte, and finally transported into bile. Incorporated into bile, the molecular complex enters the intestinal lumen to serve its protective role.

IgE. Until now, attention has been focused on IgA, the predominant immunoglobulin contained in the external secretion. However, IgE must also be considered as a "secretory" immunoglobulin (Hong, 1978). The physiological role of this immunoglobulin is still a matter of speculation, but its function appears to go beyond what occurs in immediate hypersensitivity states. Perhaps some of the functions attributed recently to IgE in secretory immunology can help to clarify their overall contribution to immunological function. In fact, there are suggestions that mucosal lymphoid tissue may control IgE antibody synthesis, in which exposure of mucosal membranes to allergens leads to a process of differentiation, migration, and localization of IgE precursor plasma cells (Fig 5-5). These locally active antibodies could trigger a localized anaphylactic reaction helping to eliminate the antigen-bearing foreign body (a parasite, for instance). In addition, exposure via mucosal surfaces to some antigenic substances may have other consequences. For instance, it is known that in some species neonatal oral exposure to some antigens leads to a serum response of predominantly IgE antibodies. The structure of IgE in secretions appears to be similar to that of serum IgE.

Recent studies identified a distinct mast cell population in mucosal membranes from those located in other connective tissues. These differences appear to be physiological and biochemical, as well as morphological. They may play a direct role in the release of mucous by goblet cells through anaphylactic mucosal reactions mediated by IgE.

Cases of experimental and human schistosomiasis have shown a mechanism of antibody-dependent cell-mediated cytotoxicity (ADCC) whereby the target cell is a peritoneal macrophage or a blood monocyte (considered to be a precursor of tissue macrophages). The addition of the serum from the parasitized animal to a suspension of macrophages and parasitic larvae (schistosomules) produces death of the larvae after three to 18 hours of incubation, through the release of hydrolytic enzymes from the now-activated macrophages. These macrophages appear to possess a specific receptor for the Fc segment of aggregated IgE (Capron et al., 1982). It has been clearly demonstrated by two series of experiments that the antibodies engaged in this reaction belong to the IgE class (Capron et al., 1975).

1. In rats, heating of the serum of parasitized animals for 30 minutes at 56°C eliminates their cytotoxic capacity, which cannot be restored by fresh complement. It is known that IgE is a thermolabile class of immunoglobulins, and is destroyed at that temperature.
2. The immunoabsorption of IgE from parasitized serum eliminates its cytotoxic activity.

It is tempting to conceive an in vivo mechanism of this kind as protection against reinfection by parasites having a mucosal portal of entry. This mechanism includes the participation of macrophages located in the lamina propria of mucosal membranes, as well as inside the epithelium and specific antibodies of IgE class. Eosinophils also appear to be the target cells of these cytotoxicity reactions and have been shown to possess Fc receptors for IgE. It has been determined that between 1.5% and 4% of peripheral human lymphocytes bear a receptor for IgE. The significance of this observation is still obscure, but it is possible that an ADCC with the participation of lymphocytes may exist. This subpopulation of lymphocytes may intervene in the regulation of IgE synthesis.

Antibody properties of secretory immunoglobulins. Antibody specificities against numerous bacteria and viruses have been detected in secretory immunoglobulins. Some of them are considered as "natural" antibodies because no previous antigenic exposure can be demonstrated. It is clear today that for a majority of them, their existence can be explained by cross-reacting specificities: bacterial or alimentary antigens provoke the formation of antibodies reacting in vitro with other antigens possessing some common or closely related antigenic determinants.

S-IgA molecules are endowed with agglutinating properties as effective as the 19S-IgM molecules. Their theoretical valence is 4 (two antibody-combining sites per monomer) but, as is the case with pentameric IgM, some of these combining sites may be inactive. This striking agglutinating property may impede adherence of bacteria to the epithelial walls and impede their colonization.

The neutralizing capacity of S-IgA of bacterial endotoxin or viruses has been demonstrated; however, their bacteriolytic or phagocytosis-promoting activities are still controversial (McGhee et al., 1978; Hanson et al., 1980).

S-IgA antibody complexes when artificially aggregated are able to activate the properdin of alternate pathway of the complement cascade; however, it is unknown whether these complement components are present in secretions, and at what concentration.

S-IgA also appears to afford protection against caries development in teeth (Lehner, 1976). Here the action is through inhibition of the enzymatic activity of glucosyltransferase. This enzyme is necessary for the synthesis of dextran, which adheres to the teeth and forms a dental plaque. Without these polysaccharides, the bacterial growth of different strains of *Staphylococcus* is considerably more difficult.

Cell-mediated immunity (CMI)

Our knowledge in the field of cell-mediated immunity in relationship with secretory immunology is still sketchy (Waksman & Ozer, 1976). Since 1970 it has been known that systemic immunization can induce a local CMI response upon subsequent mucosal challenge. This kind of reaction appears to be dependent on the nature of the antigen, and of the administered dose.

The mucosal lymphoid tissues have been extensively analyzed for identification of different lymphocyte subpopulations involved in cell-mediated immune reactions (transplantation immunity, graft-v-host reactions, mixed lymphocyte rections, response to mitogens). Possibly of great importance in this regard is the population of lymphoid cells not organized as nodular lymphoid tissue, but extensively distributed all over mucosal membranes.

It is known that intraepithelial lymphocytes are predominantly T cells with strong suppressor activity.

Those lymphoid cells localized in the lamina propria of mucosal surfaces or secretory glands appear to be endowed with predominantly helper activity. These functionally different T cells are locally produced and migrate from the thymus-dependent areas of GALT and BALT to the neighboring mucosa.

Immunization by respiratory or intestinal routes is associated with the appearance of cells capable of realizing lymphokines such as MIF. Their T-cell origin has not been confirmed.

The biological significance of other lymphokines being eventually liberated by lymphocytes in mucosae is still unknown.

It is possible to produce a local CMI, without any systemic manifestation following intranasal or aerosolized immunization, but the possible physiological activity of locally produced lymphokines and their protective or trophic effects are still a matter of speculation. Some of the milk cells present in colostrum or milk are known to be T lymphocytes and the possibility of transferring a CMI to the neonate through these cells has been recently raised (Ogra & Ogra, 1979).

Relationship between local and systemic immunity

Once the immune response is initiated by mucosal transport of antigen, this response can be mediated in the following ways:

1. a local immune response with secretory and/or cell-mediated specific response;
2. a local response as in 1 but accompanied by a specific antibody response in serum;
3. a systemic immune response, with participation of peripheral lymphoid organs.

One cannot predict which events of the above will be triggered by a given antigen. Most responses probably represent a combination of all of them.

The reader should be aware of the importance of this point when analyzing the possibilities offered by mucosal vaccination. The response is usually a combination of events, and we are currently unable to preferentially facilitate any of these responses. Despite this fact there have been outstanding results obtained by local mucosal immunization procedures.

Modulation of the Immune Response by Mucosal Access of Antigen

It has been known for more than 30 years that the oral administration of antigen can induce a state of immunological tolerance (Tomasi, 1980), demonstrated when the same antigen is later applied by parenteral route (Salzburger–Chase phenomenon).

When this experimental design was carried out in rats using human serum albumin as the antigen, an additional observation was that there was also an inhibition of intestinal absorption of the antigen.

This tolerant state can be induced in adult animals using a large variety of hapten-carrier mixtures, as well as particulate or soluble antigens.

The initial experiments were done using the intestinal route of tolerance induction, but later on it was demonstrated that a similar state could be obtained by respiratory sensitization.

Recent studies demonstrate that antigen-specific T suppressor cells are induced and they they localize in mesenteric lymph nodes, Peyer's patches, and spleen. They specifically suppress the IgG, IgM, or IgE response. It is not clear if a similar suppression of IgA synthesis occurs. A tolerant state of orally immunized animals has also been shown for cell-mediated immune reactions. Mice receiving sheep red blood cells by mouth were found to become tolerant to SRBC and showed a serum suppressor factor believed to be antigen-antibody complexes (Andre et al., 1975). Recent work indicates that antibodies of IgG class are present in serum of orally induced tolerant animals, and that they were able to suppress the in vitro primary immune response of mice normal spleen cells to SRBC.

The homeostatic role attributed to secretory immunoglobulins appears to be controlled by the entry of substances of antigenic potentiality contained in food through their disposal by specific S-IgA or S-IgM antibodies. Some indirect confirmation of this function has been previously mentioned in the cases of IgA immunodeficient patients who appear to be incapable of controlling antigenic uptake and therefore show high titers of serum IgG antibodies against many food antigens.

Vaccination by Mucosal Route

Successful outcome of vaccination through oral or respiratory routes appears to be predicated upon the existence of immunological memory by mucosal lymphoid tissues. Many early reports failed to substantiate long-term immunologic memory. However, when studies were confined to the upper respiratory tract, it was shown that nasal immunization was followed by a secondary humoral response in bronchial secretions after local challenge. It is also believed that priming by parenteral route can be followed by a strong anamnesic response after oral challenge.

The integrity of functionally active adenoids and tonsils appear to help generate secretory antibodies in the nasopharyngeal secretions. Children with adenoids and tonsils who received live-attenuated poliovirus showed a considerable rise in specific antibodies as compared with those adenoidectomized and tonsillectomized children.

Our knowledge of secretory immunity will continue to grow as we gain experience with successful oral immunization programs. By combining various priming techniques with differing antigen dosages our ability to produce long-term protection should improve; however, we must always be cognizant of the relative ease with which tolerance can be produced via the oral route.

REFERENCES

Ades EW, Hinson A, Chapuis-Cellier C, Arnaud P: Modulation of the immune response by plasma proteases inhibitors. I. Alpha²-macroglobulin and alpha¹-antitrypsin inhibit natural killing and antibody-dependent cell-mediated cytotoxicity. *Scand J Immunol* 1982; 15:109.

Andre C, Heremans JF, Vaerman J-P, Cambiaso CL: A mechanism for the induction of immunological tolerance by antigen feeding: antigen-antibody complexes. *J Exp Med* 1975; 142:1509.

Askenase PW: Role of basophils, mast cells, and vasoamines in hypersensitivity reactions with a delayed time course. *Progr Allergy* 1977; 23:199.

Befus AD, Pearce FL, Goodacre R, Bienenstock J: Unique functional characteristics of mucosal mast cells. *Adv Exp Med Biol* 1982; 149:521.

Bienenstock J, Befus AD: Mucosal immunology, *Immunology* 1980; 41:249.

Bowden DH, Adamson IYR: Role of monocytes and interstitial cells in the generation of alveolar macrophages. I. Kinetic studies of normal mice. *Lab Invest* 1980; 42:511.

Brandtzaeg P, Baklien K: Intestinal secretion of IgA and IgM: A hypothetical model, in Lachman PJ (ed): *Immunology of the gut.* Ciba Foundation Symposium 46 (new series), Elsevier/Excerpta Medica, 1979, 77.

Brandtzaeg P, Fjellander I, Gjeruldsen ST: Human secretory immunoglobulins. I. Salivary secretions from individuals with normal or low levels of serum immunoglobulins. *Scand J Hoematol* 1970; 12, Suppl 1.

Capron A, Dessaint J-P, Capron M, Bazin H: Specific IgE antibodies in immune adherence of normal macrophages to Schistosoma mansoni schistosomules. *Nature* (London) 1975; 253:474.

Capron A, Dessaint J-P, Capron M, Joseph M, Torpier G: Effector mechanisms of immunity to schistosomes and their regulation. *Immunol Rev* 1982; 61:41.

Cebra JJ, Kamat R, Gearhart P, Robertson SM, Tseng J: The secretory IgA system of the gut, in Lachman, PJ (ed): *Immunology of the Gut.* Lachmann, Ed., Ciba Foundation Symposium 46 (new series), Elsevier/Excerpta Medica, 1979, p 22.

Colten HR, Alper ChA: Complement, in Bach FH & Good RA (eds): *Clinical Immunobiology.* New York, Academic Press, 1976, vol 3, p 387.

Drutz DJ: Immunity & infection, in Fudenberg HH, Stites DP, Caldwell JL, Well JV (eds): *Basic and Clinical Immunology.* Los Altos CA, Lange, 1976, p 182.

Etéviant M, Chevance LG, Lesourd M, Ohayon H: Complement activation and cyto-immunological alterations of the respiratory mucosa. *Ann Immunol (Inst Pasteur)* 1980; 131D:13.

Fisher MM, Nagy B, Bazin H, Underdown FJ: Biliary transport of IgA: Role of secretory component. *Proc Nat Acad Sci USA* 1979; 76:2008.

Florey HW: The secretion of mucus and inflammation of mucous membranes, in Florey L (ed): *General Pathology.* New York, Academic Press, 1970, p 195.

Franzen L, Norrby K: Immunological challenge causes mitogenic stimulation in normal connective tissue cells. *Acta Patho Microbiol Scand* 1982; 90(A):385.

Frick OL: Immediate hypersensitivity, in Fudenberg HH, Stites DP, Caldwell JL, Wells JV (eds): *Basic and Clinical Immunology.* Los Altos, CA, Lange, 1976, p 204.

Ganguly R, Waldman RH: Local immunity and local immune responses. *Progr Allergy* 1980, 27:1.

Hall, JG: The traffic of lymphocytes through the gut of mammals, in Hemmings WA (ed): *Antigen Absorption by the Gut.* MTP Press, 1978, p 207.

Hall J, Orlans E, Reynolds J, Dean Ch, Peppard J, Gyure L, Hobbs S: Occurrence of specific antibodies of the IgA class in the bile of rats. *Int Arch Allergy Appl Immunol* 1979, 59:75.

Hanson LA, Ahlstedt S, Anderson B, Carlsson B, Dahlgren U, Lidin-Janson G, Mattsby-Baltzer I, Svanbord-Eden C: The biologic properties of IgA. *J Reticuloendothelial Soc* 1980, 28:1s.

Heremans JF: Immunoglobulin A, in Sela M (ed): *The Antigens Vol II,* New York, Academic Press, 1974, p 365.

Hong R: IgE as a secretory immunoglobulin, in Bach M (ed): *Immediate Hypersensitivity,* New York, Dekker, 1978, p 189.

Ishikawa T, Wicher K, Arbesman CE: Distribution of immunoglobulins in palatine and pharyngeal tonsils. *Int Arch Allergy Appl Immunol* 1972; 43:801.

Ishizaka K, Newcomb EW: Presence of IgE in nasal washings and sputum from asthmatic patients. *J Allergy* 1970, 46:197.

Kaplan J, Nielsen ML: Analysis of macrophage surface receptors. I. Binding of alpha-macroglobulin-protease complexes to rabbit alveolar macrophages. *J Biol Chem* 1979; 254:7323.

Kaplan J, Nielsen ML: Analysis of macrophage surface receptors. II. Internalization of alpha-macroglobulin-trypsin complexes by rabbit alveolar macrophages. *J Biol Chem* 1979; 254:7329.

Lake AM, Bloch KJ, Sinclair KJ, Walker WA: Anaphylactic release of intestinal goblet cells mucus. *Immunology* 1980; 39:173.

Lamm ME: Cellular aspects of immunoglobulin A. *Adv Immunol* 1976; 22:223.

LeFevre ME, Hammer R, Joel DD: Macrophages of the mammalian small intestine: A review. *J Reticuloendothelial Soc* 1979; 26:553.

Lehner T: Immunological responses to bacterial plaque in the mouth, in Lachmann PJ (ed): *Immunology of the Gut.* Ciba Foundation Symposium 46 (new series) Elsevier/Excerpta Medica, 1979, p 150.

Mayrhofer G: The nature of the thymus dependency of mucosal mast cells. I. An adaptive secondary response to challenge with Nippostrongilus brasiliensis. *Cell Immunol* 1979; 47:304.

Mayrhofer G: The nature of the thymus dependency of mucosal mast cells. II. The effect of thymectomy and of depleting recirculating lymphocytes on the response to Nippostrongilus brasiliensis. Cell Immunol 1979; 47:312.

McGhee JR, Mestecky J, Babb JL, eds: *Secretory Immunity and Infection.* New York, Plenum, Vol 107, Adv Exp Med Biol, 1978.

Morris B, Morris R: Macromolecular uptake and transport by the small intestine, in Hemmings WA (ed): *Antigen Absorption by the Gut.* MTP Press, 1978, p 23.

Nagy E, Berczi I: Prolactin and contact sensitivity. *Allergy* 1981, 36(6):429.

Naumann HH: On the defense mechanisms of the respiratory mucosa towards infection. *Acta Otolaringol* 1980; 89:165.

Ogra SS, Ogra PL: Components of immunologic reactivity in human colostrum and milk, in Ogra PL, Dayton DH (eds): *Immunology of Breast Milk.* New York, Raven Press, 1979, p 185.

Owen RL, Jones AL: Epithelial specialization within human Peyer's patches. An ultrastructural study of intestinal lymphoid follicles. *Gastroenterology* 1974; 66:189.

Peltier A: Complement, in Bach JF (ed): *Immunology.* New York, Wiley, 1979, p 235.

Reed ChE: The role of the autonomic nervous system in the pathogenesis of bronchial asthma. Is the abnormal bronchial sensitivity due to beta-adrenergic blockage? In Rose B, Richer M, Sephon A, Frankland AW (eds): *Allergology,* Amsterdam, Excerpta Medica 1968, p 402.

Roux ME, McWilliams M, Philips-Quagliata MJ, Weisz-Carrington P, Lamm ME: Origin of IgA-secreting plasma cells in the mammary glands. *J Exp Med* 1977; 146:1311.

Samuelsson B: Leukotrienes: Mediators of allergic reactions and inflammation. *Int Arch Allergy Appl Immunol* 1981; 66(Suppl.):98.

Santoro F, Bernal J, Capron A: Complement activation by parasites. A review. *Acta Tropica* 1979; 36:5.

Sell S: *Immunology, immunopathology and immunity.* New York, Harper & Row, 1975.

Silverstein AM, Miller G: History of immunology. The royal experiment on immunity: 1721-1722. *Cell Immunol* 1981; 61:437.

Sutherland EW: On the biological role of cyclic AMP. *JAMA* 1970; 214:1281.

Tenner-Racz K, Racz P, Myrwik QN, Ockers JR, Geister R: Uptake and transport of horseradish peroxidase by lymphoepithelium of the bronchus-associated lymphoid tissue in normal and baccilus Calmette-Guerin-immunized and challenged rabbits. *Lab Invest* 1979; 41:106.

Tomasi Jr, TB: *The Immune System of Secretions.* Englewood Cliffs NJ, Prentice Hall, 1976, chapter 10.

Tomasi Jr, TB: Oral tolerance. *Transplantation* 1980; 29:353.

Tomasi Jr, TB, Grey HM: Structure and function of immunoglobulin A. *Progr Allergy* 1972; 16:81.

Vaerman J-P: Comparative immunochemistry of IgA. *Res Immunochem Immunobiol* 1973; 3:91.

Waksman BH: Summary, in Ogra PL, Dayton DH (eds): *Immunology of the Breast Milk.* New York, Raven Press, 1979, p 257.

Waksman BH, Ozer H: Specialized amplification elements in the immune system. *Progr Allergy* 1976; 21:1.

Werb Z: Characterization and classification of macrophage proteinases and proteinases inhibitors, in Adams DO, Edelson PJ, Koren H (eds): *Methods for Studying Mononuclear Phagocytes.* New York, Academic Press, 1981, p 561.

Williams EW: Ferritin uptake by the gut of the adult rat: An immunological and electronmicroscopical study, in Hemmings WA (ed): *Antigen Absorption by the Gut.* MTP Pres, 1978, p 49.

Chapter 6

Tonsillitis and Adenoiditis

Marek Rola-Pleszczynski

OUTLINE

IMMUNOLOGY OF TONSILS AND ADENOIDS
  Humoral Immunity
  Cellular Immunity

MICROBIOLOGY OF TONSILS AND ADENOIDS

THERAPEUTIC CONSIDERATIONS

Several studies in the last decade have underlined the involvement of external mucosal membranes in the defenses of the body against pathogenic microorganisms or noxious substances. The nasopharynx constitutes the portal of entry of all inhaled and ingested agents and is endowed with abundant immunocompetent lymphoid tissue. Thus, because of its intimate contact with the external environment and its immunologic potential, the tonsillar lymphoid tissue has been attributed a "gatekeeper" role in local, and possibly systemic, immune defense mechanisms.

This chapter focuses on the immunology and the microbiology of nasopharyngeal lymphoid tissue and considers some therapeutic implications.

IMMUNOLOGY OF TONSILS AND ADENOIDS

The lymphoid tissue encircling the pharynx is known as Waldeyer's ring. It includes two faucial tonsils (tonsils), pharyngeal tonsils (adenoids), and lymphoid tissue at the base of the tongue (lingual tonsils), and that on the posterior wall of the pharynx. In the embryo, the tonsils develop next to the thymus from the first, second, and third pharyngeal pouches, and it has been suggested that tonsillar tissue may be more reactive than other developing lymphoid tissue in the first weeks of life (Godrick & Patt, 1971). At birth, the tonsils are devoid of germinal centers, which later develop immediately beneath the cryptal epithelium. They tend to be poorly vascularized, while the perifollicular areas contain a dense capillary network. Characteristically the tonsils have no afferent, but only an efferent, lymphatic circulation (Kobury, 1968).

Normal human tonsils consist predominantly (80% to 90%) of lymphoid cells, with variable numbers (5% to 20%) of plasma cells and a small number of monocytes and neutrophils (Zucker-Franklin & Berney, 1972). In contrast to the peripheral blood, where a predominance of T cells is normally found, tonsils and adenoids are composed of more than 50% B cells (Rynnel-Dagoo, 1976; Siegel, Grieco, & Gupta, 1976), except after a peritonsillar abscess when local T cells reach peripheral blood percentages (Siegel, 1978). Because of the numerous studies performed to elucidate the role of the tonsils in immunological responses, it may be useful to review separately the humoral and the cellular components and functions of these tissues.

Humoral Immunity

Early studies by Gitlin and Sasaki (1969) have shown that IgA-bearing cells, although fewer in numbers than IgG-bearing cells, produced five times as much immunoglobulin per unit time and per cell. The IgA was mostly of secretory (11S) type, although variable amounts of 7S IgA were also detected. In contrast, tissue culture experiments showed a ratio of 3.7:1 for tonsillar IgG:IgA synthesis (Brandtzaeg, Surjan, & Berdal, 1978) with most IgA being monomeric, without J chains. The vast majority of IgA-forming cells within the tonsils are found close to the basement membrane, in the glandular tissue of the epithelium, and in germinal centers. IgG- and IgM-bearing cells are scattered throughout the lymphoid tissue and so are IgE-containing cells. The tonsils have been reported to have the highest density of IgE-containing cells of all lymphoid tissues (Tada & Ishizaka, 1970), although subsequent studies (Brandtzaeg et al., 1978; Pesak, 1971) have indicated a virtual absence of this immunocyte class in palatine tonsils. Moreover, compared to tonsils and adenoids from nonatopic individuals, these tissues from atopic subjects were observed to harbor a much larger population of IgE-forming plasma cells (Ali, Fayemi, & Nalebuff, 1979). Most of the IgD-bearing cells within the tonsils are found in the mantle zone surrounding the germinal centers. A general predominance of IgG-producing cells followed by IgA, IgM, and IgD was observed in children as well as adults both in tonsils and adenoids. The percentage Ig class ratios of 64:30:4:2 in tonsils showed little variations in disease. In contrast, the ratios were changed from 54:35:8:3 in healthy adenoids to 70:23:5:2 in hypertrophy (Korsrud & Brandtzaeg, 1980). Although the overall immunocyte class ratios were similar in all age groups, the average number of cells per tissue unit decreased to almost 50% with increasing age, over 18 years (Brandtzaeg et al., 1978).

Not only can all five classes of immunoglobulins be synthesized in the tonsils, but specific antibodies to various antigens have been demonstrated both in vivo and in vitro (Ogra & Karzon, 1971; Pesak, 1971). When cultured in vitro with various antigens such as poliovirus, sheep red blood cells, or tetanus toxoid, lymphocytes from human tonsils have been observed to synthesize specific antibodies (Hoffman, Schmidt, & Oettgen, 1973;

Surjan & Surjan, 1971; Sloyer et al., 1973). The production of antibody was dependent on DNA synthesis in the cultured lymphocytes. B cells and their progeny appear to be generated locally in the tonsils by active de novo lymphopoiesis (Kobury, 1968). Ontogenetically, the human tonsils may be considered an integral functional component of the gut-associated lymphoid tissue (GALT) and humoral immunity, with a direct relationship between atrophy or absence of tonsils and deficiencies of GALT (Good, 1968).

Cellular Immunity

In contrast to locally generated B cells, tonsillar T cells probably originate from the peripheral circulation, although local sensitization and subsequent effector function is likely. Oettgen et al. (1966) carried out the first studies with cultured tonsillar lymphocytes by measuring their response to mitogens and antigens. Blastogenesis occurred when these cells were stimulated with phytohemagglutinin (PHA), poliovirus, *Bordetella pertussis*, and diphtheria and tetanus toxoids, but the responses to antigens were only observed when lymphocytes were derived from previously immunized children. Tonsillar lymphocytes were also found to proliferate in response to alloantigens in mixed leukocyte cultures (Schwartz, 1967). With the advent of more sophisticated approaches to differentiating lymphocyte populations, several studies have analyzed the participation of T cells in proliferative responses. Sugiyama et al. (1976) reported that tonsillar lymphocytes responded much less than blood lymphocytes to purified protein derivative (PPD) in the absence of adherent cells, whereas responses to PHA were similar. In contrast, tonsillar lymphocytes responded far better to pokeweed mitogen (PWM) than did blood lymphocytes, a finding that could be explained only in part by the higher content of tonsils in B cells. More recently, however, Mazuran et al. (1979) found proliferative response to PPD and concanavalin A (Con A) to be higher in tonsillar cell cultures than in blood cell cultures, whereas tonsillar cells reacted less than blood cells to PHA. In another study (Delespesse et al., 1976), tonsillar B cells, even when depleted of adherent cells or treated with mitomycin to inhibit their proliferation, were found to exert a striking enhancing effect on the T cell responses to PHA and Con A.

Lymphocytes from adenoids have been shown to react less than peripheral blood lymphocytes to mitogens, PPD, and to heat-killed *Hemophilus influenzae* (Mogensen, Meistrup-Larsen, & Anderson, 1979).

Antiviral immunity has also been studied and compared between local tonsillar and systemic immunocytes (Hurtado et al., 1975; Morag & Ogra, 1975). Tonsillar lymphocytes readily responded with in vitro blastogenesis when stimulated with rubella or mumps antigens following natural infection with the corresponding virus, or intranasal immunization (Morag et al., 1975). In contrast, subcutaneous immunization induced no local but adequate systemic responses to these antigens. During the same period, independent work by Hurtado et al. (1975) showed evidence of another activity of tonsillar lymphocytes, namely cytotoxicity against virus-infected cells, potentially similar to that ascribed to peripheral T cells (Rola-Pleszczynski et al., 1975). Discrepancies were found, however, between local and systemic cytotoxic activities, in that some subjects exhibited one without the other, thus lending further support to immune compartmentalization in regard to antiviral defense mechanisms.

Production of lymphokines, such as migration inhibitory factor (MIF), has also been described in tonsillar lymphocytes in response to viral (Morag et al., 1975) or bacterial antigens (Mazuran et al., 1979). In addition, both classical type I and immune type II interferon can be produced by tonsillar lymphocytes (Sugiyama et al., 1977), again suggesting a potentially important role for these cells in local defenses against viruses.

MICROBIOLOGY OF TONSILS AND ADENOIDS

In contrast to adenoids, which seem to react as other lymphoid organs to local antigenic stimulation, tonsils have the additional property of harboring potential or actual pathogens. Evidence has accumulated which suggests that at least one type of tonsillar infection, namely exudative tonsillitis, may be caused by bacteria, viruses, mycoplasma, toxoplasma, and yeasts. These organisms include *Streptococcus pyogenes, Corynebacterium diphtheriae, Mycoplasma hominis,* Epstein-Barr virus (Veltri et al., 1975), adenovirus, and herpes simplex virus (Sprinkle et al., 1977) as well as *Toxoplasma gondii* and perhaps *Candida albicans.*

Various other viral, bacterial, and fungal organisms have been cultured from tonsils and adenoids, but their pathogenic potential and role remain doubtful at best.

The importance of viral latency in the nasopharynx is still controversial. Since Epstein-Barr virus (EBV) selectively infects B cells and these cells are predominant in tonsillar tissues, much interest has been focused on the involvement of latent EBV infection of the tonsils in human infectious and neoplastic diseases.

THERAPEUTIC CONSIDERATIONS

In the early 1970s, approximately 1 million adenotonsillectomies were performed in the United States each year, at a cost of close to half a billion dollars to the American public. In Canada, the cost to the health insurance plan was estimated at 11.4 million dollars per year (Shan & Carr, 1974). More recently, efforts to identify specific indications for this operation have gradually restrained its use.

General statements that adenotonsillectomy is never justified in contemporary medical practice is probably just as illogical as past pronouncements that the mere presence of lymphoid tissue in the nasopharynx was sufficient reason for its removal. Therefore, indications for the operation are still subjective but can be rationally formulated on an individual basis using the following guidelines:

1. Important airway obstruction, especially as seen in the rare patient with secondary cor pulmonale.

2. Malignancy, especially lymphoma.

3. Peritonsillar abscess.

4. Recurrent middle ear disease or complicated sinusitis secondary to nasopharyngeal obstruction, although controversy persists about the benefit of adenoidectomy v adenotonsillectomy or tonsillectomy alone (Hibbert & Stell, 1978). In these cases, allergy, if present, should be treated before resorting to operation.

5. Speech pathology and orofacial deformities when the operation is agreed to by dentists, oral surgeons, and speech therapists.

6. Children with three or more genuine laboratory proven episodes of bacterial exudative tonsillitis. On this aspect, past history has been shown not to be reliable and prospective follow-up is needed (Paradise et al., 1978).

Dysphagia, large cryptic tonsils, cervical adenitis, recurrent nonstreptococcal sore throat or upper respiratory infections, or snoring should *not* constitute valid indications for either adenoidectomy or tonsillectomy, or both.

In spite of these guidelines, the controversy about the effects of removal of tonsils and adenoids on the microbial defense and local immune functions of the host is still present. Although nasopharyngeal lymphoid tissue has been shown to be immunologically active, its removal causes little effect on systemic immunity (Veltri et al., 1972). Local immunity, however, is markedly affected as demonstrated by Ogra (1971); local specific antipolio secretory IgA declined sharply after operation in all children studied. Similarly, de novo production of these antibodies was two to four times lower in children whose tonsils had previously been removed. An increased incidence of paralytic poliomyelitis following adenotonsillectomy has been demonstrated through epidemiologic studies and should probably be correlated with Ogra's observations.

In contrast to local antibody-mediated immune defenses, nasopharyngeal cell-mediated immunity has been insufficiently studied to permit evaluation of its role in either anti-infectious or antineoplastic defenses. One study suggested that tonsillectomized individuals had a higher incidence of Hodgkin's disease (Vianna et al., 1971) but other well-controlled studies failed to discern such an association (Gutensohn et al., 1975; Johnson & Johnson, 1972; Reuskanea et al., 1971). It thus appears that additional epidemiologic and immunologic studies will be required before one can ascertain an association between tonsillectomy, malignancy, and any other modifications of the immune system. In turn, these studies will be dependent on additional data being gathered at the present time, in many laboratories, on actual functions of immunocytes from tonsils and adenoids in health and disease.

REFERENCES

Ail M, Fayemi AO, Nalebuff DJ: Localization of IgE in adenoids and tonsils. *Arch Otolaryngol* 1979; 105:695.

Brandtzaeg P, Surjan L Jr, Berdal P: Immunoglobulin systems of human tonsils. I. Control subjects of various ages: Quantification of Ig-producing cells, tonsillar morphometry and serum Ig concentrations. *Clin Exp Immunol* 1978; 31:367.

Delespesse G, Duchateau J, Gausset P, Govaerts A: In vitro responses of subpopulations of human tonsil lymphocytes. I. Cellular collaboration in the proliferative response to PHA and ConA. *J Immunol* 1976; 116:437.

Gitlin D, Sasaki T: Immunoglobulins G, A and M determined in single cells from human tonsils. *Science* 1969; 164:1532.

Godrick EA, Patt GR: A comparison of the immune response of tonsils with the appendix and spleen in neonatal rabbits. *Atca Otolaryngol* 1971; 71:357.

Good RA: The immunological deficiency disease of man: Consideration of some questions asked by these patients with an attempt at classification. *Immunologic Deficiency Diseases of Man* 1968; IV, 17.

Gutensohn N, Li FP, Johnson RE, Cole P: Hodgkin's disease, tonsillectomy and family size. *N Engl J Med* 1975; 292:22.

Hibbert J, Stell PM: Critical evaluation of adenoidectomy. *Lancet* 1978; 1:489.

Hoffman MK, Schmidt D, Oettgen HF: Production of antibody to sheep red blood cells by human tonsil cell in vitro. *Nature* (London) 1973; 243:408.

Hurtado RC, Rola-Pleszczynski M, Merida MA, Hensen SA, Vincent MM, Thong YH, Bellanti JA: The immunologic role of tonsillar tissues in local cell-mediated immune responses. *J Pediat* 1975; 86:405.

Johnson SK, Johnson RE: Tonsillectomy history in Hodgkin's disease. *N Engl J Med* 1972; 287:1121.

Kobury E: Cell production and cell migration in the tonsil, in Cottier N (ed): *Germinal Centers in the Immune Response.* New York, Springer-Verlag, 1968, p 176.

Korsrud FR, Brandtzaeg P: Immune systems of human nasopharyngeal and palatine tonsils: Histomorphometry of lymphoid components and quantification of immunoglobulin-producing cells in health and disease. *Clin Exp Immunol* 1980; 39:361.

Mazuran R, Rabatic S, Sabioncello A, Dekaris D: Particulary of local immunity in the nasopharynx. *Allergy* 1979; 34:25.

Mogensen HH, Meistrup-Larsen K-I, Andersen V: Lymphocytes from adenoid vegetations: Proliferative responses in vitro as compared to blood lymphocytes. *Acta Path Microbiol Scand Sect C* 1979; 87:197.

Morag A, Ogra PL: Immunologic aspect of tonsils. *Ann Otol Rhinol Laryngol* 1975; 84 (Suppl 19):37.

Oettgen HF, Silbec R, Miesher PA, et al: Stimulation of human tonsillar lymphocytes in vitro. *Clin Exp Immunol* 1966; 1:77.

Ogra PL: Effect of tonsillectomy and adenoidectomy on nasopharyngeal antibody response to poliovirus. *N Eng J Med* 1971; 284:59.

Ogra PL, Karzon DT: Formation and function of poliovirus antibody in different tissues. *Progr Med Virol* 1971; 13:156.

Paradise JL, Bluestone CD, Backman RZ, et al: History of recurrent sore throat as an indication of tonsillectomy. *N Engl J Med* 1978; 298:409.

Pesak V: The localization of IgA and IgE globulins in the palatinal tonsils, nasal muccous membrane and nasal polypi. *Folia Microbiol (Praha)* 1971; 16:323.

Rola-Pleszczynski M, Hurtado RC, Woody JN, et al: Identification of the cell population involved in viral-specific cell-mediated cytotoxicity in man: Evidence for T cell specificity. *J Immunol* 1975; 115:239.

Reuskanea O, Vanka-Perttala T, Kowalainen K: Tonsillectomy, appendicectomy and Hodgkin's disease. *Lancet* 1971; 1:1127.

Rynnel-Dagoo B: The immunological function of the adenoid. *Acta Otolaryngol* 1976; 82:196.

Schwartz MR: Response of thymus and other human lymphoid tissues to PHA PWM and genetically dissimilar lymphoid cells. *Proc Soc Exp Biol Med* 1967; 125:701.

Shan CP, Carr LM: Tonsillectomies: In dollars and cents. *Can Med Assoc J* 1974; 110:301.

Siegel G: Characterization of clinical tonsil stages by their T-cell count. *Acta Otolaryngol* 1978; 86:469.

Siegel I, Grieco MH, Gupta S: Fc and complement-receptor rosette-forming cell ratios in human tonsils and peripheral blood. *Int Arch Allergy Appl Immunol* 1976; 50:488.

Sloyer JL, Veltri RW, Sprinkle PM: In vitro IgM antibody synthesis by human tonsil-derived lymphocytes. *J Immunol* 1973; 111:183.

Sprinkle PM, Veltri RW: The tonsils and adenoids. *Clin Otolaryngol* 1977; 2:153.

Sugiyama M, Yamamoto K, Kinoshita Y, Kimura S: Studies on difference in cellular immune response between the human tonsil and blood lymphocytes. *Acta Otolaryngol* 1976; 82:440.

Sugiyama M, Yamamoto K, Kinoshita Y, Kimura S: Studies on the capacity of human tonsillar lymphocyte subpopulations to produce interferon. *Acta Otolaryngol* 1977; 84:296.

Surjan L, Surjan M: Immunological role of human tonsils. *Acta Otolaryngol* 1971; 71:190.

Tada T, Ishizaka K: Distribution of IgE forming cells in lymphoid tissue in human and monkey. *J Immunol* 1970; 104:377.,

Veltri RW, Sprinkle PM, Keller SA, Chickll JM: Immunoglobulin changes in a pediatric otolaryngic patient sample subsequent to T and A. *J Laryngol Otol* 1972; 86:905.

Veltri RW, Sprinkle PM, McClung JE: Epstein-Barr virus associated with episodes of recurrent exudative tonsillitis. *Arch Otolaryngol* 1975; 101:552.

Vianna NJ, Greenwald P, Daview JNP: Tonsillectomy and Hodgkin's disease: The lymphoid tissue barrier. *Lancet* 1971; 1:431.

Zucker-Franklin D, Berney S: Electron microscopy study of surface immunoglobulin bearing human tonsil cells. *J Exp Med* 1972; 135:533.

Chapter 7

Immunology of Otitis Media

Robert W. Veltri
Philip M. Sprinkle

OUTLINE

GENERAL INTRODUCTION

IMMUNOLOGY OF ACUTE OTITIS MEDIA
Humoral Immune Response in Acute Otitis Media
Cellular Immune Response in Acute Otitis Media With Effusion
Animal Models in the Study of Pathogenesis of Acute Otitis Media
Specific Immunotherapy to Prevent Acute Otitis Media

IMMUNOLOGY OF NONACUTE, NONPURULENT OTITIS MEDIA
WITH EFFUSION
Introduction
Mechanisms of Immunopathogenesis

GENERAL INTRODUCTION

Fundamental studies of gross anatomy, morphology, and histopathology of the eustachian tube and middle ear have provided a sound basis for understanding inflammation in the middle ear. In an excellent summary of eustachian tube and middle ear anatomy Dr. David Lim has indicated that both local mucosal and systemic defense mechanisms are available (Lim, 1976a,b). The mature eustachian tube is lined with epithelium extending from the nasopharynx, and its cellular composition is approximately 20% goblet cells and 80% ciliated cells. In addition, there are an abundance of glands which empty into the lower two thirds of the tubal lumen. The secretions of the surface goblet cells and glands provide mucous and serous products which form the substance of a mucociliary blanket mobilized by the cilia. This mucociliary transport system is similar to the one that exists in the upper respiratory tract.

The physiological surface and subsurface features of the middle ear create a unique and sophisticated niche for local inflammatory processes to develop (Lim, 1979). In Lim's review the middle ear defense system was divided into distinct categories based on histological structure: (a) a mucociliary surface barrier which is biochemically characterized as being rich in mucopolysaccharides and glycoproteins; (b) a secretory immune system producing secretory immunoglobulin-A (IgA), as well as antibacterial enzymes (lysozyme) and surface active factors; (c) the resorptive system, which is made up of epithelial cells as well as vascular and lymphatic channels providing the sole portal of exit for inflammatory exudates and transudates; (d) the phagocytic and immune system located in the submucosal layer beneath the basement membrane consisting of macrophages, mast cells, T and B lymphocytes, and plasma cells. Hence, all the elements of local mucosal and systemic humoral and cell-mediated immunity are available to the middle ear.

The host's response to infectious agents and/or allergens in the above-described ecosystems provides the basis of this review of immunity in the middle ear. This review specifically excludes otitis media with effusion relating to defective eustachian tubes, cleft palate, barotrauma, or tumors obstructing normal eustachian tube function.

Any discussion of immunity in the middle ear further necessitates a definition and classification of the middle ear effusion (MEE) in terms of clinical, physical, cellular, and biochemical parameters. Several national and international meetings on otitis media have considered this subject (Lim et al., 1976a, b; Senturia et al., 1970, 1980; Wiet et al., 1979). The consensus opinion for classification is as follows:

1. purulent effusion—may be acute or chronic inflammatory exudate with numerous bacteria and polymorphonuclear cells.
2. serous effusion—an amber, low-viscosity fluid with few cellular elements and containing many of the constituents of serum, also present are small numbers of bacteria and numerous leukocytes.
3. mucoid effusion—a thickened inflammatory secretion rich in locally produced polysaccharides, secretory IgA, and glycoproteins but with fewer leukocytes and bacteria.
4. mixed effusions—combinations of types 2 and 3.

The above-mentioned effusions may become recurrent or chronic in nature and may represent a continuum in which one or more of the early events (acute otitis media with effusion) may progress to more chronic or recurrent inflammatory processes represented by 2, 3, or 4 in the classification system and involving the host's immune response at all levels (local and systemic) (Giebink, 1978b; Juhn et al., 1977).

IMMUNOLOGY OF ACUTE OTITIS MEDIA

Humoral Immune Response in Acute Otitis Media

The concept of an immune response capability in the middle ear originated with experiments described by Hopp et al. (1964). Hopp sensitized guinea pigs peripherally by immunization with bovine serum albumin and subsequently challenged the animals by transtympanic innoculation of the immunogen into the middle ear producing a serous-type effusion. Similar experiments have been performed in other experimental animals using other antigen-antibody systems and more sophisticated immunologic measurements but yielding the same ultimate result (Giebink et al., 1979d; Juhn et al., 1977; Miglets, 1973; Paparella et al., 1970).

Acute otitis media is primarily a disease of bacterial etiology whose natural history has changed very little over the years (Giebink et al., 1978; Helander-Brandefors et al., 1975; Howie, 1979). *Streptococcus pneumoniae* and *Hemophilus influenzae* are the primary etiological agents followed by Group A *Streptococcus pyogenes, Staphylococcus aureus*, enteric gram-negative bacilli, *Neisseria catarrhalis* (Coffey et al., 1967), and rarely viruses (Berglund et al., 1966; Berglund et al., 1967; Klein et al., 1976) may produce an acute otitis media during epidemics. In man this disease is completely reversible with proper chemotherapy (Giebink & Quie, 1978; Juhn et al., 1977; Laxdal et al., 1970) but untreated can lead to serious complications (Diamont et al., 1974).

A specific immune response to the bacterial pathogens causing the acute otitis media is well documented. The best available data on the humoral and cell-mediated immune response in humans have employed acute- and convalescent-paired blood and acute middle ear effusions. Sloyer et al. (1974) have reported on the nature of the humoral immune response to *pneumoniae* and *influenzae* serotypes in peripheral blood and MEE samples obtained from patients with microbiologically confirmed acute otitis media. Specific antibody to the above bacteria produced in the serum is commonly found in the IgG and IgM classes of immunoglobulin, whereas it may be found in all three major classes of Ig in the MEE. Branefors et al. (1979) recently confirmed these observations during natural infections with *influenzae* type B and four types of *pneumoniae* using an enzyme-linked immunoadsorbent assay. He demonstrated also that reinfection occasionally occurred in children sustaining high serum antibody titers to the infecting bacteria. The IgA in MEE is of local origin (Mogi, 1976; Ogra et al., 1974; Sloyer et al., 1975) while the IgG and IgM specific antibodies originate from the serum.

Another important factor is that the frequency of detection of specific antibodies to offending bacterial pathogens differs with age. Only 10% of patients under 1 year of age and 50% of patients over 2 years of age respond serologically to their infecting agent (Sloyer et al. 1974). In an attempt to relate the humoral immune response of acute otitis media to clearing of the disease process Sloyer et al. (1976) measured specific antibody in MEE at diagnosis and monitored clinical evidence of complete recovery. The found a significant ($p < .005$) correlation between presence of specific antibody in MEE at the time of diagnosis to returning of middle ear cavity to its normal pressure status. Hence, it appears that antibody of offending pathogens of otitis media when detected in MEE play an important role in resolution of infection as well as resistance of subsequent infections.

Sloyer et al. (1979) also made the observation of specific IgE antibodies to pneumococcal C-carbohydrate in MEE of two thirds of the patients studied. The data indicated a tendency for the MEE IgE-specific antibody titers to exceed the paired serum levels. This high incidence of an IgE-specific immune response may be a characteristic of the age of the patient sample as well as the nature of the specific antigens involved (carbohydrate). Sloyer postulated that the IgE-specific antibodies may be the "gate keeper antibody" (Steinberg et al., 1974) providing local resistance to infection by means of IgE-mediated hypersensitivity-type reactions at the local level. This consideration of local IgE-specific immunity is relevant to vaccination against otitis media. Also, the recent data demonstrating a specific local IgA response to oral and systemically administered viral vaccines (Sloyer et al., 1977) is of great value in establishing the efficacy of vaccination against acute otitis media.

Cellular Immune Response in Acute Otitis Media with Effusion

Local immunity in the middle ear during acute otitis media also involves the cell-mediated limb of the immune response. The MEE from acute otitis media patients are known to be rich in polymorphonuclear (PMN) cells, as well as T and B lymphocytes (Sloyer et al., 1976). The percent active rosette (T cells) was lower in MEE than paired peripheral blood of patients. Likewise, the PHA stimulation index was decreased in these same patients. Since no data from other laboratories is available to corroborate these findings on acute otitis media we must consider the results tentative. It is emphasized by the author of the above work that the depressed CMI results may reflect immuno-regulation at the cellular level (Waldman et al., 1978). Just as likely, however, is production of humoral modulators from the complement cascade as well as lymphokines (Lichtenstein et al., 1974) and immune complexes (Sinclair, 1978) that could affect the numbers as well as functional capabilities of immunologically competent cells.

Also, approaching the problem from the cellular level, Hill et al. (1977) made the observation that 14 children with recurrent otitis media and chronic diarrhea had a polymorphonuclear (PMN) leukocyte dysfunction as assessed by chemotaxis. In a more comprehensive study Giebink et al. (1979c) employed chemotaxis, chemiluminescence, and phagocytosis to evaluate possible PMN dysfunctions in systemic circulation of 102 children age 6 months to 12 years with persistent MEE and chronic otitis media. At the time of surgery for placement of ventilation tubes about one-fifth of the patients sampled showed PMN dysfunction by one or more of tests utilized. However, subsequent to surgery the PMN dysfunction assay results were normal, indicating a transient effect possibly precipitated by the persistent MEE. He since has repeated these studies in chinchillas and showed PMN dysfunction in 7/7 animals in acute phase, which persisted for 1 week and resolved in 2 weeks in 5/6 survivors (Giebink et al., 1979d). In a review by Johnston (1981) it was suggested that antibody C3b-dependent opsonization, and process of ingestion, which result in destruction of *S pneumoniae*, are also responsible for the majority of local pathology caused by resulting inflammation of acute otitis media. These data point to a possible central role of PMN function and the interaction of antibody with the complement cascade and its mediators in otitis media with effusion, an area of research emphasis for future consideration to better understand pathogenesis of acute otitis media.

Animal Models in the Study of Pathogenesis of Acute Otitis Media

A recent approach to studying acute otitis media and resultant MEE is the use of animal models. The experiments dealing with acute otitis media and purulent effusions involve the use of chinchillas. The model was first described for producing serous-type effusions in cats and chinchillas (Juhn et al., 1977). Using *S pneumoniae* serotypes 3,6,7,18, and 23 Giebink et al. (1979d) produced purulent MEE in chinchillas by direct trans-tympanic inoculation of as few as ten bacteria per ear (Giebink et al., 1979d). The MEE persisted 3 to 4 weeks and cleared spontaneously. Type-specific antibody was demonstrated in serum and MEE of most animals. These same authors also reported several oxidative and hydrolytic enzymes in the MEE after infection, and noted that only lysozyme persisted after clearing of MEE from the middle ear. Employing this same model Giebink et al. (1978) produced seroconversion in 63% of his animals by subcutaneous peripheral immunization with a polysaccharide pneumococcal vaccine. A transtympanic bacterial challenge with the vaccine strain *S pneumoniae* type 7 was attempted in 23 seropositive and seronegative chinchillas. Both seropositive and seronegative chinchillas were susceptible to infection but the immunized animals had a lower incidence of bacteremia, fewer pneumococci in their MEE, and lower mortality rates. Subsequently, Giebink et al. (1979d) demonstrated that of 23 immunized and 42 nonimmunized chinchillas whose nasopharynges were colonized with virulent type 7F *S pneumoniae*, only 7% of the immunized animals developed acute otitis media whereas 63% of unimmunized animals developed middle ear infections. Their elegant experiments prove the efficacy of peripherally administered vaccines of proper potency to modify the morbidity of pneumococcal otitis media in this animal model and have provided impetus for similar studies in humans (Howie et al., 1976).

From the studies in man and experimental animals on acute purulent otitis media with effusions it becomes obvious that the immune response to the host is important to both resolution and prevention of the disease. However, the age of first attack, intensity of immune response, presence of selective immune dysfunctions, and complex microchemical environment of the middle ear may determine whether recurrence of a purulent or nonpurulent MEE will occur. Not considered in my review on immunity is the significant and complex role of antimicrobial therapy in altering both the pathogenesis and possibly immunopathogenesis of otitis media with effusion. However, at least one recent animal model study using chinchillas suggests that ampicillin treatment of pneumococcal acute otitis media will block the development of an immune response, since animals were susceptible to reinfection with the homologous strain (Lewis et al., 1979). Although the effect of antimicrobial therapy on immunity is real, the subject of efficacy of antimicrobial therapy in man cannot be questioned, as evidenced by its role in prevention of serious complications such as bacteremia, mastoiditis, meningitis, and labyrinthitis (Giebink et al., 1978).

Specific Immunotherapy to Prevent Acute Otitis Media

A final consideration in this discussion of immunity in acute otitis media involves the current status regarding vaccination to alter the natural history of acute otitis media in man. The animal experiments described above demonstrated the possible value of pneumococcal vaccines in reducing morbidity, recurrence rates, and complications of acute otitis media (Giebink et al., 1978; Howie et al., 1976) and also for proving the importance of local immunity (Lewis et al., 1979). In a study by Howie et al. (1976) 60 infants 2 to 19 months of age were given an octavalent pneumococcal purified polysaccharide (PCP) vaccine containing types 1,3,6,7,14,18,19,23. The results indicated that of 34 children immunized at 2 to 5 months of age, ten experienced vaccine type otitis, whereas in the other 26 children immunized at 6 to 19 months, only one child suffered a breakthrough episode of vaccine type otitis. Hence, in that age group the vaccine showed good promise.

The problem of poor immunity of young infants given PCP vaccines has been confirmed in a later study by Sloyer et al. (1979b). This study also demonstrated that the PCP vaccination did not alter NP carrier status; the primary immune response was almost uniformly IgG rather than IgM, and evidence for a protective effect of the vaccine against accute otitis media by vaccine type strains was indicated. In a pneumococcal polysaccharide (PCP) trial in Finland, 781 children, aged 3 to 83 months, were monitored (Karma et al., 1979). The vaccine contained 14 pneumococcal types and the immune response intensity increased with age of vaccine recipient. Response to PCP types 1,6, and 12 were generally poor. During the first 13-month follow-up there were 45 vaccine type pneumococcal recurrences in 456 vaccines and 45 recurrences occurred among 288 controls. The protective efficacy of the PCP vaccine was 37% for the first 6 months. Hence, it appears that the vaccine can reduce recurrence rates of otitis media caused by pneumococcal types in PCP with the exception of type 6.

A subsequent follow-up at 2 years reported by Sloyer et al. (1981) has confirmed that immunization of infants under 12 months of age with the PCP vaccine for acute otitis media does not protect this age group against subsequent exposure to target *S pneumoniae* types. It is apparent that an ineffective immune response in this age group (Sloyer et al., 1979b) is a factor involved in this vaccine failure. Studies of pneumococcal pathogenesis of pneumonia in man and mice further attest to the requirement to stimulate at least a twofold serological rise in serum antibodies to provide protection (Schiffman, 1981) in normal as well as immunologically compromised hosts. Specifically, in regard to acute otitis media, Giebink (1981) has confirmed the same seroconversion quantitative response requirement following immunization of chinchillas to protect against experimental acute pneumococcal otitis media. It is, therefore, apparent that protection of children against acute otitis media will require a vaccine which is strongly immunogenic in the age group under 6 months of age in order to significantly alter the epidemiology of acute otitis media in children.

IMMUNOLOGY OF NONACUTE, NONPURULENT OTITIS MEDIA WITH EFFUSION

Introduction

The matter of serous, mucoid, and seromucoid MEE is a more complex issue in immunology. Progress in this important area of otolaryngology is focused on research conducted in the decade of the 1970s and reviewed at least four times in national and international conferences on otitis media with effusion (Lim et al., 1976; Senturia et al., 1970, 1980; Wiet & Coulthard, 1979). To provide a didactic formula to review this complex area we employ the classification system of Coombs and Gell (1968) to categorize current knowledge. Table 7-1 summarizes the system in terms of target organs or tissues, clinical manifestations, immune effector mechanisms, immunodiagnosis, and treatment. It is important to realize that this system of classification is chosen to organize information and does not imply that more than one of these immune injury mechanisms may not be operating in immunopathogenesis of middle ear diseases.

Mechanisms of Immunopathogenesis

Type I immune injury is the classical immediate type hypersensitivity involving specific antibodies of the IgE class directed against allergens of microbial surface antigens. This mechanism has thoroughly been reviewed (Ishizaka et al., 1975; Plaut et al., 1977). In regard to otitis media with serous and mucoid type effusions several laboratories have reported increased levels of IgE in MEE compared to serum (Bernstein et al., 1974, 1979a; Lim et al., 1976b; Mogi, 1976; Mogi et al., 1974). Such elevations in IgE concentrations observed in mucoid or serous type MEE may be due to contamination from the nasopharyngeal secretions loaded with IgE (Bernstein & Reisman, 1974; Mogi et al., 1977) and the poor clearance of such fluids due to their physical and biochemical characteristics (Wiederhold et al., 1979; Juhn & Huff, 1976), rather than local production in the middle ear (Lim et al., 1976a,b). As for the specificity of the IgE antibodies found in MEE of man several recent reports are available. Sloyer et al. (1979a) in a very young patient sample

TABLE 7-1. Immune Injury

Type I — Anaphylactic reactions (Immediate hypersensitivity)	
Target organs/tissues	GI tract, skin, lungs, nose.
Clinical Manifestations	GI inflammation, atopic dermatitis, urticaria, rhinitis, asthma, hives, etc.
Immune effector mechanism	IgE + allergen or antigen target cells (tissue mast cell or basophil) → Release of pharmacologically active mediators (histamine, serotonin, bradykinin, slow reactive substance, prostaglandins, etc) cause vasodilation, inflammation.
Immunodiagnosis	Serum IgE levels, Serum IgE specific antibody levels for selected allergens or antigens, skin testing with allergens and the Prausnitz-Kustner reaction.
Treatment	Antihistamines, epinephrine, aminophylline, or desensitization via allergen immunotherapy.
Type II — Cytotoxic reactions	
Target cells	Circulating blood cell elements (white blood cells, platelets, red blood cells) and organ specific antigens (eg, basement membrane).
Clinical manifestations	Hemolytic anemia (A,B,O,Rh), Thrombocytopenic purpura, lymphocytopenia, leukopenia, Goodpasteur's disease.
Immune effector mechanism	IgG or IgM antibodies combine with antigenic determinants on host cell membranes. Complement binds to the antigen-antibody cell bound complex thus activating the complement cascade and resulting in inflammation and necrosis. Alternatively, circulating antigen or haptens may adsorb to the target tissue eliciting the same final result. The presence of Fc receptor on target cells may play a key role in this type of immune injury.
Immunodiagnosis	Coombs test (direct or indirect), In vitro cytotoxicity assay (^{51}Cr release assay) versus specific target cells, Platelet aggregation in target tissues such as the kidney or lung

TABLE 7-1. Immune Injury continued

Immunodiagnosis continued	using the direct immunofluorescence procedure with fluorocein-tagged anti-IgG. Also, measurements of total complement or individual complement components are of value.
Treatment	Immunosuppressive drugs, transfusions of whole blood or cellular fractions.

Type III — Immune complex injury (Arthus-type)

Target organs/tissues	Blood vessels, skin, joints, kidneys, lungs.
Clinical manifestations	Serum sickness, acute immune vasculitis, polyarteritis nodosa, acute/chronic glomerulonephritis, rheumatoid arthritis, hepatitis, recurrent serous otitis media.
Immune effector mechanism	Antigen-antibody + complement + platelets; attraction of polymorphonuclear cells (contain Fc receptors) →release of lysosomal enzymes. Activation of the alternate pathway or complete complement pathway resulting in more inflammation.
Immunodiagnosis	Depressed CH^{50} (total complement, C) specific C components. Detection of circulating soluble immune complexes (Raji cell test, C1q binding, etc), fluorescent antibody studies for C3, IgG, antigen in situ.
Treatment	Plasmapheresis, antiflammatory agents. (corticosteroids), prostaglandin inhibitors (indomethacin, aspirin, etc, or administration of excess antigen.

Type IV — Delayed hypersensitivity (cell-mediated immunity)

Target organs/tissues	Transplanted organs, lung (Tuberculosis, TB), skin, brain, etc.
Clinical manifestations	Pulmonary cavitation of TB, overreaction to parasitic infestation, berylliosis, asbestosis, chemical contact dermatitis, graft rejection, postinfectious encephalitis.
Immune effector mechanism	Thymus dependent antigen-sensitized T lymphocytes directly attack affected tissues

TABLE 7-1. Immune Injury continued

Immune effector mechanism continued	(cytotoxic killer T cell), releasing lymphokines causing destruction of tissue. Also, sensitized T lymphocytes may encounter free antigen, releasing soluble lymphokines attracting more inflammatory cellular mediators causing additional tissue necrosis. Host v graft 1st and 2nd set rejections shows infiltration with small T lymphocytes.
Immunodiagnosis	Skin testing with appropriate antigen or hepran, passive transfer of sensitivity with lymphoid cells only (adoptive immunization). Detection of killer T lymphocytes by an in vitro cytotoxic ^{51}Cr release assay with specific target cells, measurement of lymphokines (mediators) such as lymphocytoxin, migration-inhibitory factor (MIF), interferon, or even quantitation of prostaglandins and cyclic AMP.
Treatment	Administration of immunosuppressive drugs which reduce the intensity of the CMI reaction (ie, corticosteroids), or find means to turn on immunoregulatory cells, such as suppressor T cells or macrophages.

with acute otitis media and some sterile serous type MEE detected IgE-specific antibodies to type-specific C-pneumococcal polysaccharide in paired-serum and MEE. Bernstein et al. (1979a) studying recurrent serous type MEE demonstrated binding of IgE antibody to *Staphylococcus epidermidis,* and *Corynebacterium* present in such MEE. Mogi et al. (1977) detected IgE-specific antibodies to the allergen, *Dermatophygoides farinae* (house mite), in nasal secretions of patients with respiratory allergy. In an animal model, Miglets (1973) sensitized squirrel monkeys passively by administering human serum positive for IgE ragweed antibodies. He performed a transtympanic challenge with ragweed and obtained a classic serous type MEE which he felt was primarily a transudative reaction in the middle ear.

Clinically in man, data strongly support a role for type I immediate hypersensitivity in contributing to production of a persistent MEE (Siegel, 1979). Placing a statistic on this role is most difficult since reports range from 28% to 85%. However, a good point is made by Reisman and Bernstein (1975), suggesting that serous otitis media is not an allergic disease but rather a complication of nasal allergy spilling over into the middle ear. In conclusion, type I immune injury can be considered a major contributing factor to the persistent MEE and, hence, must be considered in the differential diagnosis and treatment regime.

A type II mechanism of immune injury involves an antibody (IgG or IgM), complement cascade, and target cell interaction resulting in tissue destruction by the combined effects of cytotoxic antibody and inflammatory mediators produced via the complement pathway. The most classical examples involve autoimmune reactions in immunohematology, allergic encephalomyelitis, Hashimoto's thyroiditis, and the connective tissue diseases (Borel et al., 1976; Burnet, 1972; Rose, 1979). The presence of complement components (Bernstein et al., 1978; Maxim et al., 1977; Veltri & Sprinkle, 1976) and inflammatory mediators (Bernstein, 1976) and lysosomal enzymes (Veltri & Sprinkle, 1973, 1976) in MEE is well documented. However, the likelihood that their source is the result of a cytotoxic type II immune mechanism lacks sufficient evidence in the way of detection of autoantibodies to middle ear tissue elements. One problem with such data, if it were available, is the fact that some of these antibodies may be the result of an immune response to heterogeneic (cross-reactive) antigens on microorganisms that are involved in the pathogenesis of otitis media (Neter & Milgrom, 1975; Nowotny, 1972) and, hence, would be a result and not a cause of any pathology. To implicate this mechanism in the immunopathogenesis of chronic MEE would require demonstration of autoantibody to a target antigen in the middle ear (ie, epithelium, basement membrane, etc). Such has not been the case and is unlikely based on the normal clinical course and pathology observed in chronic or recurrent otitis media with effusion.

A type III immune complex mechanism of immune injury would require a source of antibody (immunoglobulins) and cellular effector elements (lymphocytes, plasma cells, macrophages), availability of the complement cascade (both classical and alternative pathway), soluble immune complexes, a source of soluble antigens, and a means or site of trapping and localization of all these elements (Williams, 1980). The serum-like qualities of MEE were deduced from natural and experimentally produced otitis media with effusion (Hopp, Elvitch, & Pumghrey, 1964; Juhn et al., 1977; Lim et al., 1976a,b; Miglets, 1973; Mogi et al., 1974; Veltri & Sprinkle, 1973, 1976).

In 1973, our laboratories identified and quantitated IgG, IgM, IgA, and IgD levels in paired-serum and MEE of patients with a history of chronic serous otitis media (Veltri & Sprinkle, 1973). Also, at this time we reported lysozyme to be elevated in MEE. We subsequently confirmed these observations in 1976 (Veltri & Sprinkle, 1976).

Mogi et al. (1974) demonstrated IgE levels in MEE and later Lim et al. (1976a) confirmed the findings. Mucoid MEE were shown to contain higher levels of IgE than paired-serum samples. However, the data were based on volume and not protein content of the MEE which may have led to an erroneous conclusion. In any event, the IgE is present often and in significant amounts and Mogi (1976), Sloyer et al. (1979a), and Bernstein et al. (1979a) have demonstrated antigen specificity for IgE found in MEE. Mogi (1976) and Ogra et al. (1974) demonstrated secretory IgA in MEE. The former group (Mogi, 1976) also demonstrated IgA-specific antibodies to staphylolysin and streptolysin in MEE and these antibody levels were higher in the MEE than in paired-serum samples indicating local production.

Thus, all serum immunoglobulins as well as secretory IgA have been found in the middle ear during inflammation. The amounts vary depending on the nature of the MEE (serous, mucoid, seromucoid), the chronicity of the problem, and the methods of quantitation and standardization. A specific immune response in the middle ear is also well established experimentally in animal models (Giebink et al., 1978; Giebink et al., 1979a; Juhn et al., 1977; Lewis et al., 1979; Miglets, 1973) as well as in artificial immunization studies (Sloyer et al., 1974; Sloyer et al., 1977) in humans.

The presence of T and B lymphocytes, macrophages, and PMNs has also been established in MEE (Bernstein et al., 1978; Goycoolea et al., 1979; Palva et al., 1979; Palva et al., 1976). Table 7-2 shows microbiological and cytological data on MEE from 14 patients. The bacteriology results were obtained after a 1:50 dilution of the MEE was made in physiological saline similar to the method of Liu et al. (1976). Note how few colonies of bacteria were obtained from positive MEE and that the cytological picture provided by the differential is one predominated by PMNs and lymphocytes. All the data indicate that these nonpurulent MEE are rich in leukocytes and macrophages, a fact of fundamental importance to any discussion of immune injury.

Regarding the complement cascade in MEE, in our 1976 article (Veltri & Sprinkle, 1976) we reported lysosomal enzymes, complement, C3, and C3PA in MEE. Subsequently, these data were confirmed by Maxim et al. (1977) and Bernstein et al. (1978b). Hence, there is ample evidence for an operational complement system (both pathways) in chronic MEE. In 1977, Maxim et al. (1977) demonstrated soluble immune complexes in MEE but not paired serum samples of patients with recurrent serous otitis media. At the Second National Conference on Otitis Media held March 3-5, 1978, in Scottsdale, Arizona, we reported on the purification of soluble immune complex from MEE (Veltri et al., 1979). We employed the method of Chenais et al. (1977) which combine Sephadex G-200 and protein-A Sepharose affinity chromatography to isolate IgG-type soluble immune complex. Recently, Mravec, Lewis, & Lim (1978) have been able to produce inflammatory changes in the middle ear of chinchillas using artificially constructed soluble immune complex.

To further solidify a type III immune complex mechanism a search for inflammatory enzyme systems was essential. Our laboratory identified lysosomal enzymes (Veltri & Sprinkle, 1976), and Juhn & Huff (1976) reported other pathologically relevant enzymes. Bernstein et al. (1976, 1979, 1976) demonstrated biological mediators of cellular immunity, the fibrinolysin system and prostaglandins in chronic MEE, also an important consideration for a type III immune injury hypothesis. The latter are important biochemical immunoregulators in this complex hypothesis and investigators have demonstrated increased levels of prostaglandins in MEE (Bernstein, Okazaki, & Reisman, 1976; Jackson et al., 1975). The importance of these prostaglandins to middle ear immunopathogenesis was evaluated by Jung et al. (1979) in animal experiments and suggests a direct role for this chemical in regulation of inflammation.

A final actor in this play is the microorganism. Liu et al. (1976) and other laboratories, including ours, have detected microorganisms in chronic serous and mucoid MEE. The

TABLE 7-2. Cytologic Examination of MEE

Age (Years)	Bacteria	No. of Colonies	Lymphs (%)	Differential			
				PMN (%)	RBC	Macrophage (%)	Degenerative Cells
5	S mitis	2	50	75	few	—	several
4	S epidermidis	3	16	79	many	5	several
5	S pneumoniae	2	21	79	many	—	many
7	No growth	—	60	40	several	—	—
6	S pneumoniae	28	65	50	few	—	several
5	S epidermidis	1	60	40	few	—	—
1	S epidermidis	2	85	10	many	5	several
6	No growth	—	60	35	few	5	many
6	S pneumoniae	3	33	67	few	—	many
45	S epidermidis	15	20	80	few	—	—
14	No growth	—	0	100	few	—	—
60	No growth	—	0	100	few	—	—
Adult	No growth	—	15	85	few	—	many

— = None.

source of these microorganisms is undoubtedly the nasopharynx (Veltri & Sprinkle, 1976; Lundgren & Rundcrantz, 1976). These microorganisms provide a rich source of antigenic surface structures as well as soluble antigens (polysaccharides) to bind antibodies of all classes to form particulate and soluble immune complexes. Finally, the proven negative pressure status of the middle ear and poor eustachian tube function during otitis media and the lack of a ready portal of exit except via resorption are the final factors of importance to this hypothesis.

Figure 7-1 summarizes the complex series of events involved in type III immune injury and complement-mediated inflammation (Lichtenstein & Henney, 1974; Frank, 1979; Piper, 1974), as well as the feedback control mechanisms necessary to tune this biological amplification system. Note that cell-mediated immunity, the clotting mechanism, antigens, microbial byproducts, antibodies, including IgE, all interact in this mechanism to produce inflammation without infection. An IgE-allergen complex may react with C3 activator and turn on the alternative complement pathway via C3PA (Muller-Eberhard, 1974) and Sloyer et al. (1976a), as well as Mogi et al. (1976) and Bernstein et al. (1979b), have detected IgE-specific antibodies in MEE. Maxim et al. (1977) have shown that killed *S pneumoniae* and *H influenzae* can nonspecifically activate the alternative complement pathway without the need for specific antibody, and other mechanisms exist to set off this pathway (Giebink et al., 1979). In either case the biological amplification system, once triggered, results in inflammation in the absence of bacterial proliferation (Goldstein, 1974).

Additional opportunities to trigger the complement occur via the classical IgG (subclasses 1,2, and 3) combining with one of innumerable antigens available in the nasopharynx (Veltri & Sprinkle, 1976; Lundgren & Rundcrantz, 1976), forming an immune complex, and setting into motion the classical pathway in Figure 7-1. Both the classical and alternative complement pathways generate a variety of pharmacologically active byproducts, including vasoactive amines and prostaglandins (Goldstein, 1974; Lichtenstein & Henney, 1974; Muller-Eberhard, 1974; Piper, 1974). Certain of these compounds have profound regulatory effects on metabolic regulators such as cyclic AMP (cAMP) levels of PMNs and T lymphocytes (Piper, 1974; Figure 7-1). Such compounds stimulate adenyl cyclase activity, which in effect blocks the release of lysosomal enzymes from PMNs and T lymphocyte activation with its concomitant release of lymphokines, essentially abrogating the continuum of inflammation. Another endogenous homeostatic mechanism illustrated in Figure 7-1 is the fact that enzymatic cleavage products generated from early steps in the complement cascade have an autoregulatory effect, resulting in a controlled flow rate for the pathway (Lichtenstein & Henney, 1974; Muller-Eberhard, 1974), a relevant matter of type III pathogenesis of recurrent otitis media with effusion. To further complicate matters, a mechanism exists to trip the complement pathway in which soluble immune complex binds to Fc receptors (FcR) of the C3 receptors of PMNs, lymphocytes, and/or macrophages causing activation of lysosomes and release of their enzymes (Goldstein, 1974).

Hence, all the ingredients of this complex mechanism have been described, but the final product depends on several positive and negative interactions of the components. The take-home lesson in this mechanism is that it is too complex to control with a single

FIG 7-1. A summary of mechanisms of induction of nonpurulent immunopathogenesis (inflammation).

The oropharynx harbors microbial pathogens and allergens, which provide a source of antigenic stimulation. The middle ear cleft and adjacent mucosa and submucosal lymphoid elements provide the source of immunologically competent immunocytes (both B and T cells). Specific antibodies present in B lymphocytes and harbored in submucosal middle ear tissue enter the middle ear cleft and react with microbial antigens. This brings into play the classical as well as alternate complement cascades and all ancillary reactions and feedback controls. Ultimately, the result is inflammation without the proliferative infectious state, which can be perpetuated and even establish a recurrent status as long as the pathogenic microflora in the oropharynx is not controlled. It should be apparent that such a mechanism calls into play both humoral (B lymphocytes) and cell-mediated (T lymphocytes) immune compartments via an immune complex reaction which may involve IgG, IgM, IgE-antigen complexes, or microbial antigen direct-complement activation via the alternative complement pathway.

It obviously would be important to segregate any allergic component in this process and treat this clinical state separately. The remaining and possibly the larger patient sample will necessitate immunomodulatory drugs which can reach the middle ear submucosal lymphoid apparatus and effectively reverse the progressive inflammatory process. Alternatively, well-directed chemotherapy, tonsillectomy, and adenoidectomy or active artificial immunization should be employed to modify the pathogenic oral microflora. The goal should be to interrupt the pathologic process as its most key steps, which should be source of effector immune reactions (submucosal lymphoid apparatus).

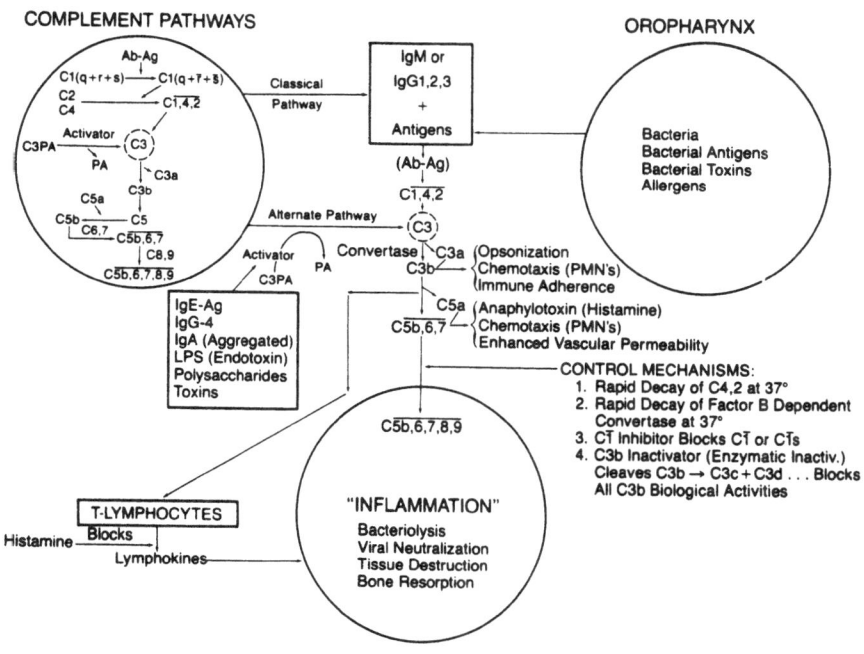

surgical or chemotherapeutic modality, but as our understanding of control mechanisms improve we may be better able to either prevent or modify the entire inflammatory sequence. Our inability to control this process could lead to chronic destructive ear disease such as tympanosclerosis, or the inflammatory mediators could spill over into the inner ear causing pathology if the otitis media with effusion is not contained.

The type IV mechanism of immune injury requires antigen-sensitized T lymphocytes (cytotoxic or killer (K)-cells), null cells (devoid of lymphocyte surface markers), antibody to a specific antigen and a target organ or tissue (Borel et al., 1976; Burnet, 1972; Rose, 1979). The mechanism of immune injury has been most classically associated with diseases mentioned in Table 7-1. In the case of immunopathology, the elimination of the inert antigen (beryllium of other chemical contact allergen) or microorganism (virus, tubercle bacillus, etc.) causing an innocent bystander reaction whereby inflammatory cells and mediators cause the destruction of normal as well as diseased tissues. Good illustrations of this phenomena would be postinfectious encephalitis of viral origin or pulmonary cavitation in tuberculosis. The necessary cellular elements, T-, B-, and null cells have been demonstrated in MEE (Bernstein et al., 1978b; Goycoolea et al., 1979; Palva et al., 1976, 1979; Veltri et al., 1979). Inflammatory mediators (Bernstein, 1976; Bernstein et al., 1979b; Bernstein et al., 1976; Jackson et al., 1975) and lysosomal enzymes (Juhn & Huff, 1976; Liu et al., 1976; Veltri & Sprinkle, 1976) are also present. It is highly conceivable that antibody directed cell-mediated cellular cytoxicity (ADCC) and cytotoxic T-lymphocytes interact on the mucosal surface resulting in some tissue destruction by this mechanism. The mechanism is not incompatible with the type III immune injury, and might fall under its regulatory influence (Frank, 1979; Goldstein, 1974; Muller-Eberhard, 1974; Piper, 1974) during inflammation in the middle ear. I believe we can keep the door open as to the role of delayed-type hypersensitivity as a contributing factor to the pathogenesis of otitis media with effusion.

In summary, the current status of our understanding of the immunopathogenesis of chronic or recurrent otitis media with effusion has vastly improved during the decade of the 1970's. The likelihood that a single mechanism of immune injury is the sole means for production of a chronic MEE is quite small. We have good evidence to suggest type I and III are important and type IV may also play a role in causing persistence of MEE in man. The evolution of the disease process from the time of sensitization (early childhood attacks of acute otitis media and how they were managed), to the eventual development of a serous, mucoid, or seromucoid type MEE remains an enigma. However, there is hope for management through intelligent differential diagnosis, artificial immunization, allergenic desensitization, and by means of employing well-defined pharmacologic antagonists targeted to specific inflammatory events described in this review.

REFERENCES

Berglund B, Salmivalli A, Groonoos JA: The role of respiratory syncytial virus in otitis media in children. *Acta Otolaryngol* 1967; 63:454–457.

Berglund B, Salmivalli A, Toivanen P: Isolation of respiratory syncytial virus from middle ear exudates of infants. *Acta Otolaryngol* 1966; 61:475-487.

Bernstein, JM: Biological mediators of inflammation in middle ear effusions. *Ann Otol Rhinol Laryngol* 1976; 85 (Suppl 25): 90-96.

Bernstein JM, Myers D, Nisengard R, Kosinski D, Wicher K: Antibody-coated bacteria in otitis media with effusions. *Ann Otol Rhinol Laryngol* 1979a; 89 (Suppl 68):104-109.

Bernstein JM, Okazaki T, Reisman RE: Prostaglandins in middle ear effusions. Arch Otolaryngol 1976; 102:257-258.

Bernstein JM, Reisman R: The role of acute hypersensitivity in secretory otitis media. *Trans Amer Acad Ophthalmol Otolaryngol* 1974; 78:120-127.

Bernstein JM, Schenkein HA, Gence RJ: Complement activity in middle ear effusions. *Clin Exp Immunol* 1978a; 33:340-346.

Bernstein JM, Steger R, Back N: The fibrinolysin system in otitis media with effusion. *Amer J Otolaryngol* 1979b; 1:28-33.

Bernstein JM, Syzmanski C, Albini B, et al: Lymphocyte subpopulations in otitis media with effusion. *Pediat Res* 1978b; 12:786-788.

Borel Y, Cunningham AJ, Datta SK, et al: Autoimmunity and self-nonself discrimination. *Transplantation Reviews* 1976; 31:1-285.

Branefors P, Dahlberg T, Nylen O: Study of antibody levels in childhood with purulent otitis media. *Ann Otol Rhinol Laryngol* 1979; 89: (Suppl 68):117-120.

Burnet FM: *Autoimmunity and Autoimmune Disease.* Philadelphia, FA Davis Co, 1972.

Chenais F, Virella G, Patrick CC, et al: Isolation of soluble immune complexes by affinity chromatography using staphylococcal protein-A sepharose of substitute. *J Immunol Methods* 1977; 18:183-192.

Coffey J, Martin A, Booth H, et al: *Neisseria catarrhalis* in exudative otitis media. *Arch Otolaryngol* 1967; 86:403-406.

Coombs RRA, Gell PGH: Classification of allergic reactions responsible for clinical hypersensitivity and disease; in Gell, Combs (ed): *Clinical Aspects of Immunology,* ed 2, Oxford, Blackwell Scientific Publ, 20, pp 575-596.

Diamont M, Diamont B: Abuse and timing of use of antibiotics in acute otitis media. *Arch Otolaryngol* 1974; 100:226-232.

Frank M: The complement system in host defense and inflammation. *Reviews of Infectious Diseases* 1979; 1:483-501.

Giebink GS: The pathogenesis of pneumococcal otitis media in chinchillas and the efficacy of vaccination in prophylaxis. *Reviews of Infectious Diseases* 1981; 3:342-352.

Giebink GS, Berzins IR, Huff J, et al: Polymorphonuclear leukocyte function during otitis media. *Ann Otol Rhinol Laryngol* 1979a; 89 (Suppl 68):139-142.

Giebink GS, Berzins IK, Schiffman G, et al: Experimental otitis media in chinchillas following nasal colonization with type 7F *Streptococcus pneumoniae:* Prevention after vaccination with pneumococcal capsular polysaccharide. *J Infect Dis* 1979b; 140:716-723.

Giebink GS, Mills EL, Huff JS: Polymorphonuclear leukocyte dysfunction in children with recurrent otitis media. *J Pediat* 1979c; 94:13-18.

Giebink GS, Payne EE, Mills EL, et al: Experimental otitis media due to *Streptococcus pneumoniae*: Immunopathogenic response in the chinchilla. *J Infect Dis* 1979d; 134:595-604.

Giebink GS, Schiffman G, Petty K, et al: Modification of otitis media following vaccination with the capsular polysaccharride of *Streptococcus pneumoniae* in chinchillas. *J Infect Dis* 1978; 138:480-487.

Giebink GS, Quie PG: Otitis media: The spectrum of middle ear inflammation. *Ann Rev Medicine* 1978; 29:285–306.

Goldstein IM: Lysosomal hydrolases and inflammatory materials, in Weisman G (ed): *Mediators of inflammation.* New York, Plenum Press, 1974; 51–58.

Goycoolea MM, Paparella MM, Juhn SK, et al: Cells in the middle ear defense system. *Ann Otol Rhinol Laryngol* 1979; 89 (Suppl 68):121–128.

Helander-Brandefors P, Dahlberg T, Nylen O: Acute otitis media: A clinical, bacteriological and serological study of children with frequent episodes of acute otitis media. *Acta Otolaryngol* 1975; 80:399–409.

Hill HR, Book LS, Hemming VG, et al: Defective neutrophil chemotactic responses in patients with recurrent episodes of otitis media and chronic diarrhea. *Amer J Dis Child* 1977; 131:433–436.

Hopp ES, Elvitch FR, Pumghrey RE: Serous otitis media—Immune theory. *Laryngoscope* 1964; 74:1149–1159.

Howie VM: Natural history of otitis media, in Wiet RJ, Coulthard SW (eds): *Proc of the Second National Conference on Otitis Media,* Columbus, Ohio, Ross Laboratories, 1979; 8–13.

Howie VM, Ploussard JH, Sloyer JL: Immunization against recurrent otitis media. *Ann Otol Rhinol Laryngol* 1976; 85 (Suppl 25):254–258.

Ishizaka T, Ishizaka K: Biology of immunoglobulin E, in Kallos P, Waksman GH, DeWeck P (eds): *Progress in Allergy* 1975; 19:60–121.

Jackson RT, Waitzman MB, Pickford L, et al: Prostaglandins in middle ear effusions. *Prostaglandins* 1975; 10:365–371.

Johnston RB Jr: The host response to invasion by *Streptococcus pneumoniae:* Protection and the pathogenesis of tissue damage. *Reviews of Infectious Diseases* 1981; 3:282–288.

Juhn SK, Huff JS: Biochemical characteristics of middle ear effusions. *Ann Otol Rhinol Laryngol* 1976; 85 (Suppl 25):110–116.

Juhn SK, Paparella MM, Goycoolea MV, et al: Pathogenesis of otitis media. *Ann Otol Rhinol Laryngol* 1977; 86:481–493.

Jung TTK, Smith DM, Juhn SK, et al: Effect of prostaglandin on the composition of chinchilla middle ear effusion. *Amer Otol Rhinol Laryngol* 1979; 89 (Suppl 68):153–160.

Karma P, Luotonen J, Pukander J, et al: Efficacy of pneumococcal vaccination against recurrent otitis media. Preliminary results of a field trial in Finland. *Ann Otol Rhinol Laryngol* 1979; 89 (Suppl 68):357–362.

Klein JO, Teele DW: Isolation of viruses and mycoplasmas from middle ear effusions: A review. *Ann Otol Rhinol Laryngol* 1976; 85 (Suppl 25):140–144.

Laxdal OE, Merida J, Jones RJH: Treatment of acute otitis media: A controlled study of 142 children. *Can Med Assoc J* 1970; 102:263–268.

Lewis DM, Meadema SJ, Schram JL, et al: Experimental otitis media in chinchillas. *Ann Otol Rhinol Laryngol* 1979; 89 (Suppl 68):344–350.

Lichtenstein LM, Henney CS: Adenyl cyclase-linked hormone receptors: An important mechanism for the immunoregulation of leukocytes, in Brent L, Holobrow J (eds): *Progress in Immunology II.* New York, American Elsevier Publ Co, 1974; pp 51–60.

Lim DL: Anatomy and functional morphology of the middle ear and eustachian tube: A review, in Wiet RJ, Coulthard SW (eds): *Proceedings of the Second National Conference on Otitis Media,* Columbus, Ohio, Ross Laboratories, 1979, pp 35–39.

Lim DL: Functional morphology of the mucosa of the middle ear and eustachian tube. *Ann Otol Rhinol Laryngol* 1976; 85 (Suppl 25):36–43.

Lim DL, Bluestone CD, Saunders WH, et al (eds): Recent advances in middle ear effusions, Ohio State University, May 29-31, 1975. Proceedings published in *Ann Otol Rhinol Laryngol* 1976b; 85 (Suppl 25):7-299.

Lim DL, Liu YS, Schram J, et al: Immunoglobulin E in chronic middle ear effusions. *Ann Otol Rhinol Laryngol* 1976a; 85 (Suppl 25):117-123.

Liu Y, Lim D, Long R, et al: Chronic middle ear effusions: Immunochemical and bacteriological investigations. *Arch Otolaryngol* 1976; 202:278-286.

Lundgren K, Rundcrantz H: Microbiology in serous otitis media. *Ann Otol Rhinol Laryngol* 1976; 85 (Suppl 25):152-155.

Maxim PE, Veltri RW, Sprinkle PM, et al: Chronic serous otitis media: An immune complex disease. *Amer Acad Ophthal Otolaryngol* 1977; 84:234-238.

Miglets AW: The experimental production of allergic middle ear effusions. *Laryngoscope* 1973; 83:1355.

Mogi G: Secretory IgA antibody activities in middle ear effusions. *Ann Otol Rhinol Laryngol* 1976; 85 (Suppl 25):97-102.

Mogi G, Honjo S, Maeda S, et al: Immunoglobulin E (IgE) in middle ear effusions. *Ann Otol Rhinol Laryngol* 1974; 83:393-398.

Mogi G, Maeda S, Yoshida T, et al: IgE in respiratory tract allergies. *Tran Amer Acad Ophthalmol Otolaryngol* 1977; 84:272-284.

Mravec J, Lewis DM, Lim DL: Experimental otitis media with effusion: An immune complex mediated response. *Trans Amer Acad Ophthalmol Otolaryngol* 1978; 86:258-268.

Muller-Eberhard HJ: Patterns of complement activation, in Brent L, Holobrow J (eds): *Progress in Immunology II*, New York, Amer Elsevier Publ Co, 1974, Vol 4, pp 173-182.

Neter E, Milgrom F (eds): *The Immune System and Infectious Diseases.* Basel, S Karger, 1975.

Nowotny A (ed): Cellular Antigens. New York, *Springer-Verlag,* 1972.

Ogra PL, Bernstein JM, Yurchak PR, et al: Characteristics of secretory immune system in human middle ear: Implications in otitis media. *Immunol* 1974; 112:488-495.

Palva T, Hayry P, Ylikoski J: Lymphocyte morphology in middle ear effusions. *Ann Otol Rhinol Laryngol* 1979; 89 (Suppl 68):143-146.

Palva T, Holopainen E, Karma P: Protein and cellular pattern of blue ear secretion. *Ann Otol Rhinol Laryngol* 1976; 85 (Suppl 25):103-109.

Paparella MM, Hiraide F, Juhn SK, et al: Cellular events involved in middle ear fluid production. *Ann Otol Rhinol Laryngol* 1970; 79:766-779.

Piper P: Mediators of anaphylactic hypersensitivity, in Brent L, Holobrow J (eds): *Progress in Immunology II*, New York, Amer Elsevier Publ, 1974, vol 4, pp 51-60.

Plaut M, Lichtenstein LM: Cellular and chemical basis of the allergic inflammatory response: Component parts and control mechanisms, in Middleton E, Reed CE, Ellis EF (eds): *Principles and practice*, St Louis, Miss, CV Mosby Co, 1977.

Reisman RE, Bernstein J: Allergy and secretory otitis media. *Pediat Clin North America* 1975; 22:251-255.

Rose NR: Autoimmune diseases, in Rose NR, Milgrom F, vanOss CJ (eds): *Principles of Immunology* ed 2. New York, Macmillan Publ Co, 1979, chap 25, 436-452.

Schiffman G: Immune responses to pneumococcal polysaccharide antigens: A comparison of the murine model and the response in humans. *Reviews of Infectious Disease,* 1981; 3:224-231.

Senturia BH (chairman): *Symposium on the Histopathology and Pathophysiology of the Middle Ear.* Held at the AFIP in Washington, DC, December 7-9, 1970. Proceedings published in abbreviated form in *Ann Otol Rhinol Laryngol* 1971; 80:305-475.

Senturia BH, Bluestone CD, Lim DL, et al (eds): *Second International Symposium on Recent Advances in Middle Ear Effusions.* Held at Ohio State University, May 9-11, 1979. Proceedings published in *Ann Otol Rhinol Laryngol* 1980; 89 (Suppl 68):1-362.

Siegel SC: Allergy as it relates to otitis media, in Wiet RJ, Coulthard SW (eds): *Proceedings of the Second National Conference on Otitis Media,* Columbus, Ohio, Ross Laboratories, 1979, pp 25-29.

Sinclair St CNR: Immunoregulation by antigen-antibody complexes. *Transplantation Proc* 1978; 349-353.

Sloyer JL, Cate CC, Howie VM, et al: The immune response to acute otitis media in children II. Serum and middle ear fluid antibody in otitis media due to *Hemophilus influenzae. J Infect Dis* 1975; 136:685-688.

Sloyer JL, Howie VM, Ploussard JH, et al: Immune response to acute otitis media in children I. Serotypes isolated and serum and middle ear fluid antibody in pneumococcal antibody. *Infection and Immunity* 1974; 9:1028-1032.

Sloyer JL, Howie VM, Ploussard JH, et al: Immune response to acute otitis media in children III. Implications of viral antibody in middle ear fluid. *J Immunol* 1977; 118:248-250.

Sloyer JL, Howie VM, Ploussard JH, et al: Immune response to acute otitis media: Association between middle ear fluid antibody and clearing of clinical infection. *J Clin Microbiol* 1976a; 4:306-308.

Sloyer JL, Ploussard JH, Howie VM: Efficacy of pneumococcal polysaccharide vaccine in preventing acute otitis media in infants in Huntsville, Alabama. *Reviews of Infectious Diseases* 1981; 3 (Suppl): 119-123.

Sloyer JL, Ploussard JH, Howie VM: Immunology and microbiology in acute otitis media. *Ann Otol Rhinol Laryngol* 1976b; 85 (Suppl 25):130-135.

Sloyer JL, Ploussard JH, Karr LJ: Otitis media in the young infant: An IgE mediated disease. *Ann Otol Rhinol Laryngol* 1979; 89 (Suppl 68):133-137.

Sloyer JL, Ploussard JH, Karr L, et al: Immunologic response to pneumococcal polysaccharide vaccine in infants. *Ann Octol Rhinol Laryngol* 1979; 89 (Suppl 68):351-356.

Steinberg P, Ishizaka K, Norman PS: Possible role of IgE-mediated reaction in immunity. *J Allergy Clin Immunol* 1974; 54:359-366.

Veltri RW, Maxim PE, Sprinkle PM, et al: Immune mechanisms related to pathogenesis of serous otitis media with effusion, in Wiet RJ, Coulthard SW (eds): *Proceedings of the Second National Conference on Otitis Media,* Columbus, Ohio, Ross Laboratories, 1979, pp 29-34.

Veltri RW, Sprinkle PM: Secretory otitis media: An immune complex disease. *Ann Otol Rhinol Laryngol* 1976; 85 (Suppl 25):235-239.

Veltri RW, Sprinkle PM: Serous otitis media immunoglobulin and lysozyme levels in middle ear fluids and sera. *Ann Otol Rhinol Laryngol* 1973; 85 (Suppl 25) 82:297-301.

Waldman TA, Blaese MR, Broder S, et al: Disorders of suppressor immunoregulatory cells in the pathogenesis of immunodeficiency and autoimmunity. *Ann Internal Med* 1978; 88:226-238.

Wiederhold ML, Zajtchuk JT, Vap JG, et al: Hearing loss in relation to physical properties of middle ear effusions. *Ann Otol Rhinol Laryngol* 1979; 89 (Suppl 69):185-189.

Wiet RJ, Coulthard SW (eds): *Second National Conference of Otitis Media.* Held in Scottsdale, Arizona, March 3-5, 1978, Proceedings published by Ross Laboratories, Columbus, Ohio, 1979.

Williams, RC: *Immune Complexes in Clinical and Experimental Medicine.* Cambridge, Mass, Harvard University Press, 1980.

Chapter 8

Nasal Allergy

Bram Rose
Diana Marquardt

OUTLINE

INTRODUCTION
Nasal Physiology

BASIC MECHANISMS
Immunoglobulins
Mast Cells and Basophils

CHEMICAL MEDIATORS
Primary Mediators
Secondary Mediators

IMMUNOPHARMACOLOGY
Cyclic Nucleotides

THE EOSINOPHIL

ROLE OF T AND B CELLS IN THE IGE RESPONSE

STUDIES OF NASAL SECRETIONS AND BIOPSIES

GENETICS OF ATOPIC DISEASE

ALLERGENS

INFECTION

CLINICAL DIAGNOSIS AND MANAGEMENT OF RHINITIS
Classification

ALLERGIC RHINITIS

NONALLERGIC RHINITIS
Rhinitis Medicamentosa
Hormonal Rhinitis
Rhinitis and Nasal Polyps
Aspirin Sensitivity

DIAGNOSTIC PROCEDURES
Skin Testing
Late Phase IgE-Mediated Reactions (LPR)
Nasal and Conjunctival Tests
Nasal Smears
Hemogram
Radioimmunosorbent Test for IgE (RIST)
Radioallergosorbent Test (RAST)

TREATMENT
Allergen Elimination

SYMPTOMATIC TREATMENT OF ALLERGIC RHINITIS
Antihistamines
Combination of Antihistamines with Pseudoepinephrine or
    Norepinephrine
Sympathomimetic Amines
Cromolyn Sodium (INTAL)
Corticosteroids
Immunotherapy
Standardization of Allergens
Forms of Treatment
Precautions
Tolerance or Ceiling

COMPLICATIONS
Intranasal Immunotherapy
Effect of Immunotherapy
The Mode of Action of Immunotherapy
Some Controversial Tests and Procedures for Diagnosis and
    Treatment for Allergic Diseases

NEWER APPROACHES TO IMMUNOTHERAPY
Alum-Precipitated Extracts
Pyridine-Treated Extracts
Chemically Modified Extracts
Tolerogens

REFERENCES

INTRODUCTION

The symptoms of sneezing, itching of the nose, eyes, profuse watery nasal discharge, and congestion occurring at a particular season of the year have been recognized for over a century as "hay fever" (Bostock, 1819). Although the major form of treatment, namely immunotherapy, has been in vogue since 1911 following its introduction by Noon (1911), it is only in recent years that the basic mechanisms have become clarified and have provided a better understanding both for nonspecific management and immunotherapy. This chapter deals with allergic rhinitis in particular as well as other forms of recurrent or chronic nasal congestion from which it must be differentiated.

Although the fundamentals of immunology and immunopharmacology have been described in previous chapters, some of these are repeated briefly, not only because the allergic diseases and their specific treatment are based on immunologic mechanisms, but because the mode of action of nonspecific management, both for the allergic and nonallergic forms, is based on immunopharmacology.

Nasal Physiology

The nasal airways are complex in terms of their surface area and are endowed with various functions. Under normal circumstances, the nose behaves as a magnificent air conditioner. It prepares the ambient air for the lungs so that particulate matter greater than 5 mm and most noxious gases are removed; it adds a liter of fluid every 24 hours, and up to 10% of body heat may be utilized to warm it adequately in the same period. The nasal mucosa is richly supplied with blood vessels which supply subepithelial and periglandular capillary networks. Two types of glands are found in the submucosa. These consist of small seromucous and large serous glands found in the anterior portion of the nose. The large serous glands are not found in the bronchi, and could explain the copious watery nasal discharge characteristic of rhinitis (Mygind, 1979). The vascular tissue is erectile and supplied both by sympathetic and parasympathetic fibers. Stimulation of the sympathetic fibers results in vasoconstriction, reduction in the volume of erectile tissue, and widening of the airways. The opposite effect occurs with stimulation of the parasympathetic fibers, namely vasodilatation, increase in size of the erectile tissue, and narrowing of the airways. Both histamine and β-adrenergic receptors have been identified in the nasal vasculature of the cat (Hiley, Wilson, & Yates, 1978).

BASIC MECHANISMS

Many of the basic mechanisms had been recognized in earlier investigations including reagin or skin sensitizing antibody, its susceptibility to heat, ability to be passively transferred (Prausnitz & Kustner, 1921), when combined with allergen to induce the release of mediators including histamine, the existence of a "blocking antibody" (Cooke et al., 1935), and the probability that atopic disease was inherited or genetically transmitted (Alexander, 1975; Coca & Cooke, 1923). It was not until the newer concepts of immunology as we now understand them were described and methods for the purification of allergens introduced, that a clearer picture began to emerge. Without doubt a major advance was the description of reagin as a fifth class of immunoglobulin and named IgE by the Ishizakas (1967) leading to methods for measuring not only total serum IgE but also specific IgE antibody (Aas & Johansson, 1971).

Immunoglobulins

IgE

Of all the immunoglobulin classes, IgE has the lowest serum concentration in the physiologic state. Normally it is approximately 100 IU/mL with a range of up to 150 IU/mL (Ishizaka, Ishizaka, & Hornbrook, 1966; Sears et al., 1980). It also has the lowest rate of synthesis, the shortest half life, of 2.3 days, is heat labile, and can remain fixed to tissue cells such as mast cells and basophils for long periods of time (Lichtenstein & Mamburger, 1978).

The chemical configuration of IgE is similar to that of the other classes of immunoglobulins, consisting of two heavy and two light chains, as well as two Fab and one Fc portions. Synthesis of IgE occurs primarily in the lymphoid tissues of the respiratory and gastrointestinal tracts (GI), which are also the sites of IgA synthesis. IgA and its secretory piece is an important factor for the maintenance of mucosal immunity both in the respiratory and GI tracts (Tomasi et al., 1980).

The control of IgE production in man is not well understood. However, it is clear from animal experiments and clinical observations that T lymphocytes exert a major influence, in that the level of production by the B lymphocyte (plasma cell) can be depressed

FIG 8-1. Allergen (Δ) combination showing bridging of Fab portions of two adjacent IgE molecules attached to Fc receptor sites of mast cell.

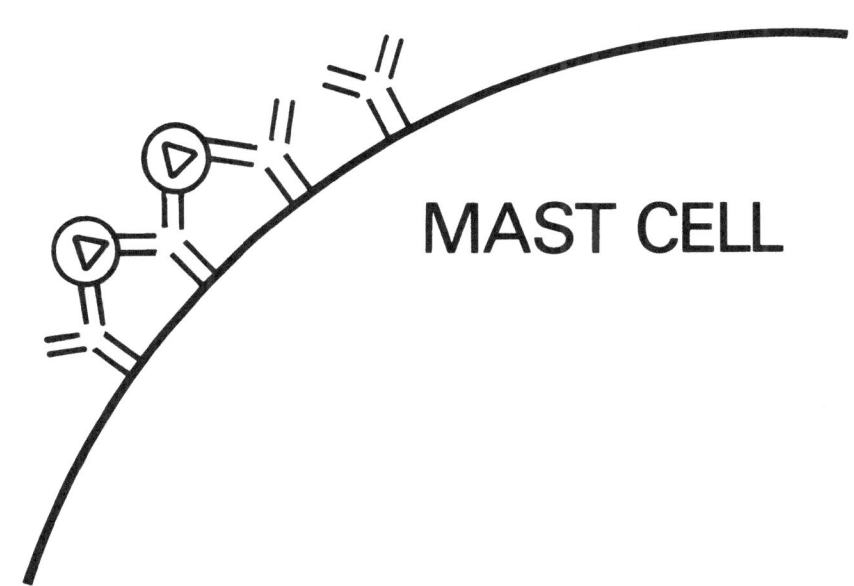

or maintained at a given level by T suppressor lymphocytes, or augmented by T helper cells (Harper et al., 1980; Geha et al., 1981).

IgE differs remarkably from all other immunoglobulin classes in that the Fc portion has an affinity for receptor sites on mast cells and basophils. Once this occurs, the two Fab portions are free to combine with an allergen provided that the IgE molecule has specific antibody activity for that specific allergen. It is now generally accepted that combination takes place in a particular fashion which is dependent on the fact that most allergens are divalent—they have two combining sites. In this case, the allergen combines with one Fab portion of one IgE molecule and with the Fab portion of an adjacent IgE molecule forming a bridge between the two (Fig 8-1).

Once the bridge is formed, the mast cell is activated, and a complex series of events ultimately leads to the release of chemical mediators (Ishizaka, 1976; Austen, 1978a). It is of some interest and importance that if a monovalent allergen can be produced which can combine with only one Fab fragment, the mast cell is not activated, but the IgE combining sites are effectively blocked. This method has been used for the prevention of sensitivity to penicillin (de Weck et al., 1973). It is also possible to induce mediator release from mast cells by the use of antihuman IgE antibody since combination occurs in the same manner as that of an allergen. The concept that two adjacent IgE molecules must be bridged or interconnected is supported by experiments on the isolation of mast cell IgE Fc combining sites (Conrad & Froese, 1976; Ishizaka et al., 1978). Thus, if an antibody prepared against IgE Fc receptor sites is added to rat mast cells, the events leading to the subsequent release of mediators is initiated.

The release of chemical mediators from either actively or passively sensitized tissues from various animal species has been extensively studied. Although early attempts to demonstrate the release of histamine into the blood of patients during an attack of asthma were unsuccessful owing to the lack of sensitive enough methods, (Rose et al., 1950) the release of histamine could be demonstrated in the blood of patients with allergy to cold (Rose, 1948). With modern techniques, this has now been shown in a variety of allergic conditions, primarily asthma (Lee et al., 1982).

Fc IgE Receptors

Initially, Fc receptors for IgE were thought to be confined to mast cells and basophils. Earlier studies had established that Fc receptors specific for IgG could be identified on monocytes and macrophages (Gonzales-Molina & Spielgelburg, 1977; Unkeless & Eisen, 1975; Walker, 1976), and that the class of immunoglobulin could induce various inflammatory reactions. Thus, when IgG_1 or IgG_3 is bound, the resulting reaction is phagocytosis. It is of considerable interest that Fc receptors for IgE have now been demonstrated on various monocytes including human lymphocytes (Melewicz & Spiegelberg, 1980) and, in particular, mouse and rat macrophages (Unkeless & Eisen, 1975). That the number of lymphocyte Fc IgE receptors appears to be modulated by the presence of specific antigen and IgE itself is suggested by the studies of Yodoi and Ishizaka (1980). In a recent study by Boltz-Nitulescu, Bazin, and Spiegelberg (1981), it appears, however, that the various Fc receptors are specific for immunoglobulin classes. These observations were carried out on mouse macrophages, and Anderson and Spiegelberg (1981) have recently demonstrated specific IgE Fc receptors on a human macrophage cell line. Of particular interest is the report of an increase in peripheral blood monocytes with Fc receptors for IgE in patients with severe allergic disorders (Burka & Paterson, 1980). The potential significance of these observations is considerable in terms of the production of allergic manifestations, because it is established that the macrophage can form and release slow reacting substance of anaphylaxis (SRS-A) (Bach & Brashler, 1978; Orange et al., 1980; Rouzer et al., 1980a,b).

IgG

In addition to IgE, there is evidence that other classes of immunoglobulins have reaginic properties (Richter et al., 1957). In 1970, Parish demonstrated the existence of a second type of antibody in cases of food allergy (Parish, 1970) and cutaneous vasculitis (Parish, 1971a, b). In contrast to IgE, this reagin-like fraction was able to passively sensitize the skin and isolated tissues of guinea pigs and monkeys for short periods only (four to six hours). It was heat stable resisting heat to 56°C, and was found to be an IgG class. He called it "short-term sensitizing IgG" antibody or S-T S IgG. It apparently belongs to a subclass of IgG, namely IgG_4 (Stanworth & Smith, 1973). S-T S IgG has been found in cases of asthma and rhinitis, and in recent studies of patients with allergic asthma and rhinitis in their family trees (Bruyzeel & Berrens, 1979; Gwynn et al., 1979; Brighton, 1980). However high concentrations of specific IgG_4 have also been reported in asymptomatic beekeepers with chronic antigenic exposure, supporting the alternative explanation that IgG_4 may be a secondary, protective class of antibody in allergic individuals (Aalberse et al., 1983). It has recently been shown that IgD is the antibody involved in cases of sensitivity to Tartrazine. Although this observation is of considerable interest, it is not clear how significant it may be clinically (Weliky & Heiner, 1980).

Blocking Antibodies

In addition to the previously described immunoglobulin properties, IgG also plays a significant role in the form of a "blocking antibody." Blocking activity was first described by Cooke et al. (1935) as a factor in the serum of treated patients with allergic rhinitis which could inhibit the wheal and flare reaction in the skin using the method of passive transfer. The rise of IgG blocking antibody is now almost routinely used as an index of the efficacy of treatment in many such studies (Sobotka et al., 1976). The most consistent results have been found in studies on the effect of pure bee venom immunotherapy due to the fact that the allergen(s) is pure and the degree of protection conferred can be closely related to the increase of IgG blocking antibody (Golden et al., 1980).

IgA also has blocking antibody activity. It is significant that both IgG and IgA blocking antibodies have been demonstrated in nasal secretions, and the levels could be correlated with histamine release from basophils and relief of symptoms (Platts-Mills et al., 1976).

Mast Cells and Basophils

The principal target cell in IgE-mediated atopic diseases is the tissue mast cell and the principal effector agents are the mast-cell–derived mediators. Mast cells are widely distributed throughout various tissues of the body, particularly organs rich in connective tissue, and usually adjacent to blood vessels. Basophil leukocytes have been considered to be circulating mast cells because of the functional and morphological similarities between the two. However, there is mounting evidence that basophils are distinct from mast cells. They differ in histologic properties, granular structure, and biochemical responses to various agents (Wasserman, 1983). The life span of the basophil is in days, whereas that of the mast cell is in months to years. Not only do these cells differ, but differences have been found between mast cells of different locations such as the GI and respiratory tracts (Bienenstock & Befus, 1980; Kaliner, 1980). There is also evidence that two distinct populations of mast cells may exist in the human GI tract (Befus et al., 1979).

Mast cells have been found in the bronchial mucosa (Orange, 1973) and IgE-bearing mast cells have been identified intraepithelially in tonsils, adenoids, and nasal polyps of man (Feltkamp-Vroom et al., 1975). Studies of concentrated dispersed human lung mast cells have shown them to possess granules with a crystalline structure and that IgE-dependent activation leads to transformation of the granule to an amorphous one. As the process continues, further solubilization of the granule occurs which is associated with discharge of the amorphous granular material (Austen, 1980). Most of the initial studies of IgE-mediated processes have been conducted on chopped lung preparations or in vitro observations on basophilic leukocytes (Lichtenstein & Mamburger, 1978), but recent technologic advances have enabled investigators to study purified isolated intestinal mast cells, bone marrow-derived mast cells, and mast cells from enzymatically digested human lung.

CHEMICAL MEDIATORS

The combination of allergen with IgE antibody fixed to tissue mast cells or circulating basophils leads to the release of a variety of chemical mediators which in turn explain many of the resulting changes in the surrounding tissues. As the number and variety of chemical mediators have increased, their classification into one group or another has varied. Thus, some divide them into primary and secondary whereas others prefer to separate them into those which are preformed and are simply released as compared to those which are newly synthesized or generated. A third variety separates those which are rapidly released from those which are released slowly, and finally there are mediators which originate from sources other than mast cells or basophils (Table 8-1).

Primary Mediators

Histamine
Of the primary, those which are known to exist in a preformed state are histamine and eosinophil chemotactic factor of anaphylaxis (ECF-A) (Kay et al., 1971). Histamine accounts for the changes in vascular permeability, vasodilation, stimulation of exocrine glands, contraction of smooth muscle, and the induction of itching. Histamine is also capable of attracting eosinophils or inhibiting eosinophil migration through H_1 and H_2 receptor interactions, respectively. In addition to these many properties, this remarkable amine can stimulate the production of T lymphocytes which bear an H_2 receptor and which in turn suppress the production of IgE-producing B lymphocytes (Beer et al., 1982).

Table 8-1. Mediators of Immediate Hypersensitivity.

MEDIATOR	RELEVANT BIOLOGICAL ACTIVITY
A Preformed—Rapidly released	
*1. Histamine	Increased vascular permeability Smooth muscle contraction
*2. Eosinophil Chemotactic Factor (ECF-A)	Attraction of eosinophils
3. Neutrophil Chemotactic Factor (NCF-A)	Attraction of polymorphs
B Preformed—Slowly released	
1. Arylsulfatase	Inactivates SRS-A
2. Heparin	Anticoagulation
C Newly generated	
*1. Slow-Reacting Substance of Anaphylaxis (SRS-A) Leukotrienes LT C, D, E	Contraction of smooth muscle Increase in vascular permeability
2. Prostaglandins PGD PGE PGF_{2a}	Bronchoconstriction Bronchodilation Bronchoconstriction
*3. Platelet Activating Factor PAF or (AGEPC)	Platelet aggregation Smooth muscle contraction (guinea pig)
D Newly formed from sources other than mast cells or basophils	
1. Acetylcholine	Bronchoconstriction Mucous secretion
2. Serotonin	Increase in vascular permeability
(3. Anaphylatoxins C3a, C4a, C5a)	(Histamine and SRS-A release)

* Primary mediators

Eosinophil Chemotactic Factor (ECF-A)

ECF-A, first described in 1971 (Kay et al., 1971), is a distinct immunologically released factor which selectively attracts eosinophils. It can be extracted from mast cells where it exists in a preformed state. Some of the activity of human ECF-A has been shown to reside in two acidic tetrapeptides (Goetzl & Austen, 1975) and higher molecular weight eosinophil chemotactic factors have also been identified. In addition to ECF-A and histamine, chemotactic activity has been demonstrated in derivatives of arachidonic acid.

Slow Reacting Substance of Anaphylaxis (SRS-A) and Leukotrienes

The third and very important primary mediator group is termed slow reacting substance of anaphylaxis (SRS-A) (Orange & Austen, 1969). In contrast to histamine and ECF-A, it is not present preformed in mast cells but is generated once allergen—IgE combination takes place.

The first description of a substance derived from lung perfusates which produced a slow onset and sustained contraction of guinea pig ileum was that of Feldberg and Kellaway (1938). They called it slow reacting substance. Using human lung in which an immediate hypersensitivity reaction had been induced, Brocklehurst noted that in addition to the release of histamine, a similar slow reacting substance was released in the perfusate and termed it SRS-A (Brocklehurst, 1960). Many subsequent studies have culminated in the definition of the complete structure of these mediators (Goetzl & Austen, 1975; Lewis et al., 1980; Orange et al., 1973; Samuelsson et al., 1980).

As these studies were in progress, exciting advances were being made with reference to mediators derived from arachidonic acid (Murphy et al., 1979; Orange et al., 1980). The products of arachidonic acid stem from two metabolic pathways. One is the cyclooxygenase pathway, which yields various prostaglandins and thromboxanes. More recently, the products of the second, or lipogenase, pathway have been intensively studied. Activity of the 5-lipoxygenase enzyme in mast cells on arachidonic acid produces 5-hydroperoxy 6, 8, 11, 14-eicosatetraenoic acid (HPETE) which may be reduced to 5-hydroxyeicosatetraenoic acid (5-HETE) or alternatively metabolized to the leukotrienes (LT), the active components of SRS-A. Leukotriene A is initially formed (Lewis et al., 1980), but is highly unstable and rapidly converted to LTB_4, a potent chemotactic factor (Goetzl & Pickett, 1980). Addition of a glutathionyl residue to carbon 6 yields LTC_4 (Rouzer et al., 1980) which may be transformed into LTD_4 (Lewis et al., 1980) and on to LTE_4 (Sok et al., 1981), the latter three accounting for the biologic activities of SRS-A.

Whereas the products of the cyclooxygenase pathway, namely the prostaglandins and thromboxanes, can be inhibited by aspirin or indomethacin, those of the lipogenase pathway are not so affected. It has been shown that the leukotrienes are much more potent than histamine in inducing smooth muscle contraction and changes in vascular permeability in both guinea pig and human lung. LTC_4 and LTD_4 are, respectively, approximately 200- and 20,000-fold more potent than histamine in contracting guinea pig lung smooth muscle (Drazen et al., 1980), and a 100-fold greater dose of histamine than LTD_4 or LTE_4 is required to produce a comparable increase in vasopermeability in guinea pig skin (Lewis & Austen, 1981).

It has further been shown that these lipogenase products of arachidonic acid stimulate the migration of human eosinophils and neutrophils as well as increasing the intraneutrophil concentration of cGMP. Thus, they represent a class of chemical mediators which can regulate both cellular and humoral components of human allergic reactions (Goetzl, 1980). It would seem, therefore, that they may also play a significant role in allergic rhinitis.

Platelet Activating Factor (PAF)

The fourth primary mediator is platelet activating factor, or PAF, as it was originally called (Benveniste et al., 1977; Henson & Pinckard, 1977). During IgE-mediated membrane activation, it is newly synthesized and released from basophils, macrophages, neutrophils, and eosinophils, and perhaps tissue mast cells, inducing aggregation of platelets with the release of vasoactive amines. Recently, the chemical structure has been elucidated and shown to be a phospholipid, namely acetyl-alkyl-glyceryl-ether-phosphorylcholine or AGEPC (Demopoulos, Pinckard, & Hanahan, 1979). It has been partially synthesized, providing large quantities of chemically pure material, and shown to possess many potent pharmacologic and inflammatory properties. These include stimulation of human neutrophils (Chignard et al., 1980) and contraction of guinea pig ileum and parenchymal lung strips (Findlay et al., 1981; Stimler et al., 1981a). It is of interest that these properties are independent of H_1 or leukotriene receptors. When administered intravenously, it reproduces IgE-mediated anaphylaxis (Halonen et al., 1980). It seems likely that AGEPC may assume an important role as a major mediator of anaphylaxis.

Secondary Mediators

Prostaglandins

The major group of substances in this category are the prostaglandins, which are a family of unsaturated fatty acids derived from arachidonic acid. They are synthesized in all cells by prostaglandin synthetase. Human lung and rat serosal mast cells generate large amounts of prostaglandin D_2 (PGD$_2$) after challenge with an appropriate secretagogue (Lewis et al., 1982). This product may increase cyclic AMP levels, contract smooth muscle, and increase vascular permeability. There are two other types of prostaglandins which are of potential physiologic significance in terms of allergic disease. These are types of E and F. PGF$_2$ is a powerful constrictor of bronchial smooth muscle. In asthmatic subjects, it requires some 8000 times less to induce bronchial constriction than is required in normals. In contrast, PGE induces bronchodilation in asthmatics. There is evidence that PGE can reduce nasal resistance in some subjects. However, because of irritant properties, it is not suitable as a therapeutic agent.

Kinins

Kinins, which are polypeptides, can contract smooth muscle, dilate blood vessels, and increase vascular permeability. They are derived from kininogens which are found in the alpha$_2$ globulin fraction of the plasma proteins. Bradykinin is formed by the action of kallikrein on bradykininogen. That it may be of some significance in human IgE-dependent inflammatory reactions or anaphylaxis is not clear.

Anaphylatoxins

The complement factors C3a and C5a which are known as anaphylatoxins have long been included as possible mediators of allergic manifestations because of their capacity to release histamine from mast cells and basophils of guinea pig origin, as well as from rabbit platelets (Osler, 1973). More recently it has been shown that C5a releases both histamine and leukotrienes (SRS-A) from pulmonary tissue. C3a also releases histamine and prostaglandins (Glovsky et al., 1979; Hugli, 1981; Stimler et al., 1981). It should be emphasized, however, when considering the possible involvement of anaphylatoxins in allergic manifestations, that they function in quite a different manner from IgE-mediated release of mediators from mast cells and are therefore bracketed in Table 8-1.

IMMUNOPHARMACOLOGY

Cyclic Nucleotides

Cyclic nucleotides are intracellular regulators of mast cell and basophil activity in that the levels which exist in a particular cell influence its ability to release mediators (Austen, 1978b). They consist of cAMP and cGMP, which were originally associated with inhibition and enhancement of the release of mediators, respectively. Considerable controversy has arisen over this rather simplistic explanation, and current evidence suggests a much more complex relationship between cyclic nucleotide levels and mast cell secretion (Holgate et al., 1980). Cyclic nucleotides are modulated by stimulation of the cell receptors α (alpha) and β (beta) which are of adrenergic origin and by a cholinergic receptor site. Cyclic AMP is formed from AMP by the action of the enzyme adenylate cyclase and is inactivated by the enzyme phosphodiesterase. Stimulation of the β-adrenergic receptor by agents such as isoproterenol increases the level of cAMP by activation of adenylate cyclase. Levels of cAMP are also increased by theophylline, which inactivates the enzyme phosphodiesterase or by PGE which also activates adenylate cyclase (Orange et al., 1971; Tauber et al., 1973).

Conversely, the levels of cAMP are decreased by blockade of the β-adrenergic receptor by propanolol. A similar effect is produced when the α-adrenergic receptor is stimulated (Kaliner et al., 1972). PGF also decreases the cAMP levels. Cholinergic agents such as acetylcholine stimulate the cholinergic receptor leading to an increase of cGMP concentrations. It appears that a balance between the two cyclic nucleotides determines the mode in which the cell will react, and in this sense, these two nucleotides display some similarities to the sympathetic and parasympathetic nervous system interactions.

The role of cAMP has been further clarified by the studies of Ishizaka (1981) on rat mast cell preparations activated by the addition of antibody to Fc receptor sites with the subsequent release of mediators. It appears that once the process begins, there is a biphasic change in cAMP consisting of an initial rise followed by a brisk fall. It is during the latter phase that mediator release occurs. In addition, when a histamine liberating agent such as 48/80 or the calcium ionophore A23187 is added instead of the Fc antibody, a rapid release of histamine occurs, but in this case, there is a brisk fall in cAMP without an initial rise. If the level of cAMP is increased by incubating the mast cells with theophylline, or isoproterenol, or if dibutyril cAMP is added, the release of histamine may be inhibited when IgE Fc receptor bridging occurs.

In general, it has been shown that atopic patients with allergic asthma are hyporesponsive to β-adrenergic stimulation and hypersensitive to α-adrenergic and cholinergic stimuli (Henderson et al., 1979). Patients with allergic rhinitis differ slightly, showing similar β-adrenergic hyporesponsiveness and cholinergic hypersensitivity, but their α-adrenergic response is less consistently lowered. It is of interest that similar findings have been shown as well in patients with cystic fibrosis (Davis et al., 1980). It is important to note, however, that the responses investigated were not those pertinent to the disease manifestations in these patient groups and were indirect measurements of drug actions.

These studies have been confirmed indirectly in patients with asthma by the administration of suitable stimulators of either α- or β-adrenergic agents, or specific blocking agents (Patel & Kerr, 1973, 1975; Rose et al., 1978). It is not known to what extent they may be related to the release of mediators from nasal biopsy material. However, it has been shown that β-adrenergic agonists can effectively inhibit the symptoms of rhinitis (Borum & Mygind, 1980; McFadden, 1981; Schumacher, 1980).

Alterations in autonomic responses have been investigated particularly by Kaliner and his group (Shelhamer et al., 1980). Thus, studies of eccrine sweat responses in cases of allergic rhinitis show the same hyperresponsiveness as do cases of allergic asthma who are also more sensitive to inhaled cholinomimetics than normal controls (Kaliner, 1976; Shelhamer et al., 1980).

Recently, the presence of autoantibodies to β_2-adrenergic receptors was demonstrated in the serum of three patients with allergic respiratory disease (Venter, Fraser, & Harrison, 1980). These findings have been further amplified by Fraser, Venter, and Kaliner (1981). They identified autoantibodies to β_2-adrenergic receptors in the plasma of three apparently normal subjects, four patients with allergic asthma, one "preallergic," and one patient with cystic fibrosis. These findings now provide a possible molecular basis to explain β-adrenergic hyporesponsiveness in some patients with allergic disease but, as the antibodies are present in normals and only a small number of asthmatics, no global explanation can be established from this data.

THE EOSINOPHIL

Although the eosinophil has been the object of much investigation ever since it was recognized as a constant but enigmatic component of allergic disease, its precise role is still unclear (Beeson & Bass, 1977; Butterworth & David, 1981; Samter & Wasserman, 1978). It is a highly phagocytic cell and may participate in the preparation of allergen along with the macrophage for the induction of specific IgE antibodies. It is a source of histaminase, the enzyme which is responsible for the inactivation of histamine. As shown more recently and of considerable importance is that it is a source of aryl-sulfatase, an enzyme which binds SRS-A (Wasserman, Goetzl, & Austen, 1975). When allergen is injected into the skin of a sensitive subject, and combines with the Fab portion of the IgE molecule as described above, with the liberation of mediators, it usually takes about 24 hours for eosinophils to accumulate at the site. This may be due primarily to the release of chemotactic factors derived from mast cells. As is well recognized,. eosinophils are present in the nasal smears of patients with both allergic and nonallergic rhinitis, although the count is usually higher in the former. Eosinophil production appears to be dependent on the presence of T lymphocytes as shown originally by Basten and Beeson (1970). Again, the significance of this finding, while highly interesting, is unknown.

There are many features of the eosinophil which lead one to speculate that it may police or in some way modulate the allergic immediate type inflammatory reaction (Samter, 1980). To begin with, there are many factors which attract eosinophils to the site of inflammation. These include ECF-A, histamine (Clark, Gallin, & Kaplan, 1975), HETES (Goetzl, Woods, & Gorman, 1977), the anaphylatoxins C3a and C5a (Kay, Shin, & Austen, 1973), LTB_4, and platelet activating factor (PAF). Once there, the eosinophil is capable of inactivating SRS-A, histamine, heparin, and PAF. It is also capable of releasing PGE, which can inhibit the release of histamine from sensitized basophils. Eosinophils are thought to be a first line of defense against infestation by metazoan parasites in that the eosinophil can kill these in vitro (Bass, 1979; Samter, 1980). There is some evidence that allergens such as house dust, animal danders, and pollen grains share antigenic determinants with metazoan parasites, suggesting that there is a common role for the eosinophil in both metazoan infestation and the common allergies (Kay et al., 1973).

It is well established that many of the agents used in the management of allergic manifestations can produce a substantional reduction in the number of circulating eosinophils. These include those which stimulate the β_2 receptor such as epinephrine and isoproterenol. Corticosteroids also produce a profound reduction but the exact mechanism is not clear. In spite of the mass of information which has accumulated about the eosinophil, its exact role is yet to be determined.

Studies of the eosinophil count, either in the peripheral blood or locally as in nasal smears, must be interpreted with caution. The report of Franklin and Goetzl (1981) in which they describe a patient with a long history of urticaria and rhinitis who had no detectible eosinophils in blood or bone marrow raises questions about the role of the eosinophil in allergic disease. There were no eosinophils in the nasal smears. All other parameters in this thoroughly worked up case, including skin testing and IgE levels, were in keeping with the diagnosis. An explanation for the total absence of eosinophils was found in that the serum contained a complement-dependent IgG-related activity which degranualted eosinophils.

The peripheral blood may show an elevated eosinophil count not only in IgE-dependent asthma, but also in subjects in whom there is no evidence for IgE participation. The count may be higher in the peripheral blood of some patients with nonallergic asthma than in those with atopic asthma. It is also of interest that a local eosinophilia induced by the intradermal injection of an allergen into a sensitive patient is independent of the peripheral eosinophil count. This can be demonstrated by passive transfer of reaginic serum to a nonallergic recipient in whom the count may be quite low or normal. Nevertheless, following the injection of allergen into the sensitized site, but not in a control site, the usual eosinophilia can be demonstrated (Eidenger et al., 1962, 1964).

ROLE OF T AND B CELLS IN THE IGE RESPONSE

The induction of circulating antibodies of all classes are dependent on the presence of a normal T and B cell population (Reinherz & Schlossman, 1980). It appears that of all antibody classes, namely IgG, A, M, D, and E, IgE is the most sensitive to the action of the T suppressor cell (Tada, 1975). In the nonallergic individual, the level of IgE in the serum is apparently maintained by the presence of T suppressor cells in balance with the T helper population (Ishizaka, 1976). As shown in animal studies, the low IgE responder mouse in particular, interference with the T cell production by such means as x-irradiation, or thymectomy results in a marked increase in the IgE level (Chorazzi et al., 1977a). In man, a number of clinical studies support the view that the atopic patient lacks an adequate T suppressor cell population (Buckley & Becker, 1978) and that immunotherapy, in addition to its other effects such as stimulating the production of blocking antibody, also tends to restore the T suppressor cell population (Rocklin et al., 1980b). There is further evidence in support of this contention in the studies on children with very high levels of circulating IgE and who have marked susceptibility to infections (Church et al., 1976). They frequently have eczema and an eosinophilia. As shown by Buckley and her co-workers, a fundamental defect may be a lack of T suppressor cells (Buckley & Becker, 1978).

In a recent study by Beer et al. (1982), further evidence has been provided that supports the view that there is a defect in the ability of the atopic subject to maintain an adequate T suppressor cell population. The study was based on the observation that a subset of T lymphocytes bearing H_2 (type 2) receptors can be triggered by histamine to express their suppressor function (Rocklin et al., 1980a). The percentage of T lymphocytes bearing histamine type 2 receptors was significantly lower in the atopic group as compared to normal controls, and could partly explain the increased levels of IgE.

STUDIES OF NASAL SECRETIONS AND BIOPSIES

There are obvious difficulties in determining the presence of immunoglobulins in nasal biopsy specimens or secretions. However, significant elevations of IgE, IgA, and IgG have been reported in patients with allergic rhinitis (Deuschl, 1976, 1977; Deuschl et al., 1977; Platts-Mills, 1976, 1979). IgA plasma cells have been identified by immunofluorescence in nasal mucosa biopsies from allergic and nonallergic patients.

However, IgE-staining plasma cells were found only in biopsies from allergic patients. An occasional IgG-staining cell but no IgM-staining cells were seen.

Biopsy studies on nasal mucosa directed toward the mast cell population have shown conflicting results. Thus, an overall increase in the numbers present was reported in both atopic and nonatopic individuals (Hastie, Heroy, & Levy, 1979), the latter being patients with nonallergic rhinitis. It has been shown that mast cell degranulation is not necessarily a feature of histamine and other mediator release following the combination of allergen with IgE on sensitized basophils in vitro. Therefore, it is difficult to interpret the electron microscope studies on nasal mucosa from patients taken both before and after challenge with a specific allergen. In these, both intact and degranulated mast cells, primarily the former, have been identified (Okuda & Ohtsuka, 1978). Although indirect, there is strong support for the role of mediators in allergic rhinitis based on the observations of Kaliner et al. (1973). It was shown that when human nasal polyps were passively sensitized in vitro and then challenged with antigen or with anti IgE, there occurred the release of histamine, ECF-A, and SRS-A. As noted previously, the presence of histamine, both in nasal tissue and secretions, strongly suggests its role as well in the increased permeability and vasodilatation of allergic rhinitis.

GENETICS OF ATOPIC DISEASE

Although many fundamental observations have led to a clearer understanding of the allergic state, we still do not know precisely why it is that one individual becomes allergic, in the clinical sense, whereas another may not. As early as 1916, family studies of allergic patients were begun by Cooke and Vander Veer (1916). They noted that positive family histories of allergy tended to be some three times higher in allergic patients than in those without a history of allergy. Although many subsequent studies tended to confirm a familial or inherited tendency, there was still the feeling that the controlling factors were probably a combination of both genetic and environmental. It was not until two important discoveries were made in the late 1960s that the whole approach to this problem was changed. These were first the description of IgE by the Ishizakas (1967) as the major immunoglobulin responsible for atopic allergy in man and, second, the discovery of immune response (Ir) genes linked to H-2, the major histocompatibility complex (MHC) of mammalian species, by McDevitt and his colleagues (1980) (Benacerraf & McDevitt, 1972).

The studies of Vaz and Levine (1970) on inbred pure strain mice demonstrated two fundamental points. These were first that the production of IgE antibody was dependent on the strain of mouse (Levine & Vaz, 1970). Thus, certain strains were unresponsive to the injection of antigen with little or no change in the titer of IgE, whereas others responded with a brisk elevation. The second and equally important finding was that in the responder strains, the level of IgE induced was dose dependent (Vaz & Levine, 1970). Thus, a high dose failed, whereas low levels induced a high IgE antibody response.

This finding is in keeping with the estimated quantities of pollen which may be inhaled during a given pollen season (Marsh et al., 1981).

Investigation of patients and their families was greatly facilitated by two other advances of major importance. The first, resulting from studies on organ transplants, was the definition of the HLA (human lymphocyte antigens) system in man which is the equivalent of the MHC system in mice and other mammalian species (Levine & Vaz, 1970). Although the existence of Ir genes in man has not yet been confirmed, it is very likely that it exists. Stemming from HLA surveys in various diseases, it has been established that susceptibility to certain diseases, of which the autoimmune variety such as SLE is a prime example, are significantly associated with certain HLA antigens. The application of such studies to allergic disease was greatly facilitated by the availability of pure low molecular weight allergens such as those from ragweed, namely Ra 3 and Ra 5 (Lapkoff & Goodfriend, 1974; Mole et al., 1975), and Rye I (Johnson & Marsh, 1966). For a detailed review, see Marsh, Meyers, and Bias (1981).

ALLERGENS

The enigmas of allergic disease are many, not the least of which is why the agents which are involved should be completely innocuous to the rest of the population. They consist of pollens, molds, spores, animal danders, grains, and the like, including foods and certain drugs of which the penicillins are the main examples. In most instances, they are either inhaled through the respiratory tract or are ingested. The nature of an allergen is quite complex in structure and it is only in recent years, with the introduction of more refined methods of analysis, that the major components of a few, ragweed in particular, have been defined. The purification and structural aspects of the major component, namely Antigen E and K by King et al. (1974), provided a major tool for much of the in vitro and in vivo studies in recent years. Similarly, the description of RA 3 and 5 by Lapkoff and Goodfriend (Goodfriend et al., 1981; Mole et al., 1975), because of their purity and low molecular weight, was crucial to the genetic studies by Marsh et al. (1973). In considering allergens, it should be pointed out that all behave as "antigens" but just why they behave as "allergens" with the induction of an IgE antibody response is not clear.

INFECTION

The possible role of infection giving rise to nonallergic rhinitis of chronic form has been debated for many years and controversial forms of treatment such as bacterial vaccines have been employed in the past but now largely abandoned. More convincing evidence had been shown for the association of viral and bacterial respiratory infections with exacerbations of wheezing in young asthmatic children (McIntosh et al., 1973; Minor et al., 1974). In a recent study by Welliver et al. (1981) of nasopharyngeal secretions after infection in a group of 79 children, both respiratory syncytial virus-specific IgE and the release of histamine in nasopharyngeal secretions were found to be higher in children who developed wheezing as compared to those who did not. Although these parameters were correlated with the degree of hypoxia, it seems not improbable that they might also correlate with the onset of rhinitis following viral infections.

CLINICAL DIAGNOSIS AND MANAGEMENT OF RHINITIS

Classification

Because of the lack of knowledge concerning the etiology and pathophysiology of symptoms occurring in a high proportion of patients with rhinitis, a classification is at best difficult and unsatisfactory. A useful and simple classification has recently been proposed by Mullarkey (1981) based on the study by Mullarkey, Hill, and Webb (1980). It consists of allergic rhinitis both seasonal and perennial of known etiology, and nonallergic rhinitis. Mullarkey and colleagues surveyed 142 cases of rhinitis. Of these, 42 were diagnosed allergic on the basis of histories corresponding with skin tests and elevated total serum IgE levels. About 25% of this group may have nasal eosinophilia and in 50% symptoms of asthma. On the basis of the above, this category by definition is a disease of known pathogenesis.

Of the nonallergic cases, in whom there was no evidence for immunologic disease, physical agents as factors, or evidence of respiratory pathology, 52 were classified as vasomotor rhinitis (VMR). A smaller group of 21 patients had symptoms similar to those of VMR but demonstrated nasal eosinophilia and were therefore classified as having eosinophilic nonallergic rhinitis or ENR. They had a high prevalence of nasal polyps and were more responsive to medical therapy than the cases of VMR. The implication is that when there is a known cause such as in rhinitis medicamentosa or the rhinitis of pregnancy, such terms are satisfactory. However, the large group of cases of nonallergic rhinitis which are usually perennial and of no known etiology should be named descriptively without implication concerning etiology. Examples are nonallergic rhinitis with eosinophilia, neutrophilic rhinitis, and nasal polyposis.

As neat and simple as this classification appears, Jacobs, Freedman, and Boswell (1981) have recently described a group of 52 patients with "on and off" perennial sneezing, profuse watery rhinorrhea, itching of the nasopharyngeal mucosa, absence of triggering factors or history of allergy, nasal polyps, or respiratory symptoms. All were characterized by a marked nasal eosinophilia, but the mean total eosinophil count and the total serum IgE were normal. Nasal secretions showed normal values for immunoglobulins, including

IgE, and skin tests were negative. These authors have suggested that they be classified as nonallergic rhinitis with eosinophilia or the eponym NARES syndrome.

The subclassification of this large group of nonallergic rhinitis into VMR and ENR merits consideration from the standpoint of management. Allergic rhinitis, both seasonal and perennial, responds to nonspecific therapy when symptoms are mild and easily controlled with antihistamines alone or in combination with decongestants. When these measures are inadequate, nasal topical steroid sprays are often employed or inhaled cromolyn sodium is administered. If symptomatic control is not achieved or the side effects of the medications are intolerable, immunotherapy is indicated. Of the nonallergic variety, VMR without nasal eosinophilia or evidence of infection is the most difficult and responds mainly to decongestants. On the other hand, when VMR is accompanied with nasal eosinophilia (ENR), steroid therapy would seem to be indicated. Those cases which show mainly neutrophils in nasal smears warrant a trial of antibiotics in addition to decongestants. It would appear that nasal smears are useful in nonallergic rhinitis and its subdivisions but should not be necessary in patients with allergic rhinitis.

ALLERGIC RHINITIS

Allergic rhinitis is a symptom complex consisting of paroxysmal bouts of sneezing, nasal congestion, watery nasal discharge, lacrimation, and itching of the eyes. It may be seasonal, relating to a particular pollen present during a specific season, or perennial usually due to substances present the year around such as dust, molds, or animal danders. The symptoms are related to the inhalation of allergenic substances and are mediated by specific immunological mechanisms. The onset usually occurs prior to age 40 but can occur as early as 6 months of age (Hill, 1961). The condition is quite common. A national survey in 1973 in the United States estimated that 25.6 million suffer from allergic rhinitis, asthma, or both (*Allergy Statistics*, 1974). It occurs primarily in so-called *atopic* individuals, a term originally introduced by Coca and Cooke (1923) to designate allergies of hereditary or familial origin. The word *atopy* means unusual or strange. Depending on the degree of sensitivity and exposure to pollen, the symptoms may vary considerably in intensity, mild and of short duration in some, while in others severe, often accompanied by asthma and associated with irritability, fatigue, asthenia, or depression. The nose commonly becomes sensitive to nonspecific irritants such as odors, pollutants, and changes in atmospheric conditions. Severe symptoms with marked nasal obstruction may interfere with sinus drainage or patency of eustachian tubes, resulting in impairment of hearing and headaches (Connell, 1970; Taylor, 1973).

Although not common, there are patients who develop severe rhinitis on eating a particular food. Usually the skin tests or RAST may be positive. They therefore resemble patients with allergic rhinitis, with the difference that the particular allergen is ingested rather than inhaled. In addition, it is possible to encounter patients who invariably cannot drink beer or certain wines without developing severe rhinitis and who may fall into the category of perennial allergic rhinitis or vasomotor rhinitis. The mechanism is not known.

An accurate and detailed history is essential for proper diagnosis. Symptoms confined to a particular month or season such as the spring, midsummer, or fall are generally related to pollens (trees, grasses, or weeds). However, the assumption that symptoms are due to a particular allergen simply because they are repeated each year during a particular period can lead to errors. For example, on the Eastern seaboard, symptoms beginning sometime in August could be due either to ragweed or to wormwood or molds. In contrast, perennial symptoms which, by definition, occur the year around, are usually related to allergen exposure at home (animal danders, molds, feathers, or dust), or to some occupational factor such as trimellitic anhydride (Sale et al., 1981). It is necessary to go into detail with reference to the time of appearance, location, and other pertinent factors such as air conditioning, or nature of working habits, and always to what medication has been used. Frequently other manifestations of atopy such as asthma associated with either rhinitis or exposure to cold air or exercise, or eczema may have preceded the onset of rhinitis.

On examination, fever is uncommon unless there is a complication such as pharyngitis, otitis, or sinusitis. The nasal mucosa is sometimes pale and usually thickened, and the turbinates markedly swollen. In allergic rhinitis of the seasonal variety, there is generally a thin watery nasal secretion, and in a few patients nasal polyps may be found. Eye symptoms such as itching and lacrimation, or injection of the conjuntivae are common. However, these are much less frequent in cases of perennial allergic rhinitis.

NONALLERGIC RHINITIS

This term has been applied to a large group of patients who have rhinitis of a chronic nature of unknown etiology. The symptoms are related to nonallergic factors such as irritants, emotional factors, and climatic changes, all of which are poorly defined. Nasal secretions are generally watery. A careful history should clarify the diagnosis, because in general, apart from a clearly related factor, there is no history of either personal or familial allergy. It is characteristic to be told that either one side or the other is blocked, particularly at night, depending on which side the patient may sleep. It is common for the patient to complain of loss of taste and smell. On examination, the major finding is a pale, boggy-looking nasal membrane. The nasal smears may show no or many eosinophils and skin tests are negative. IgE levels are usually normal (Knight et al., 1979) but may occasionally be elevated (Jacobs et al., 1981; Mullarkey et al., 1980).

In a large survey of some 1300 biopsies in cases of chronic rhinitis over a period of 10 years, Connell (1976) classified the microscopic findings according to type of infiltrating cell, basement membrane appearance, and the epithelial type. These findings were correlated with the appearance of the nose on examination and clinical history. He concluded that there could be some 12 different types of chronic rhinitis.

Rhinitis Medicamentosa

The excessive use of nasal decongestants, in particular such agents as naphazoline hydrochloride, can lead to chronic nasal congestion, usually accompanied by a watery discharge but absent pruritis and has been referred to as "rhinitis medicamentosa" (Black & Remsen, 1980). It has been ascribed to a "rebound" phenomenon in which the agent is sprayed into the nares with relief, only to be followed by another more severe bout requiring more of the same medication. The exact pharmacology of the reaction is not known, although a down-regulation of local α-adrenergic receptors and resulting hyposensitivity to α-adrenergic agonists is possible. The patient, if carefully questioned, may relate that he was well until he developed a "head cold," occasionally infectious although not necessarily, and began using the preparation for relief. A correct diagnosis with cessation of the offending drug will often lead to complete disappearance of the symptoms. Nasal steroid administration is often a helpful adjunct to therapy of this disorder. Although not as frequent today, it was not uncommon to see patients with marked symptoms of nasal obstruction following the use of reserpine derivatives, with complete relief on stopping the medication. Although the mechanism is not clear, it has been postulated that depletion of norepinephrine from the nasal epithelium may be a cause (Norn & Shore, 1971).

Hormonal Rhinitis

It is not uncommon for either rhinitis or asthma to make its first appearance during pregnancy about the third trimester. Curiously, the opposite may be the case—namely, that a patient with allergic seasonal rhinitis or asthma may remain free of symptoms while pregnant. There are two reasons which could explain the latter. The first is the well-described increase in the production of cortisol during pregnancy, and the second is the marked increase in blood histaminase which continues until parturition, and the source of which is the placenta (Rose, Harkness, & Forbes, 1946). However, it is not clear what the fundamental difference between these two types of response might be. Rhinitis of a chronic nature is sometimes associated with hypothyroidism and may disappear when the thyroid deficiency is corrected.

Rhinitis and Nasal Polyps

Nasal polyps are grapelike structures. They arise from the mucosa of the sphenoidal sinuses and from the posterior nasal mucosa. The etiology of nasal polyps is essentially unknown although they have been the subject of much investigation (Knight et al., 1979; Settipane & Chafee, 1977). They were thought at one time to be "allergic" or "infectious" in origin but this classification is no longer acceptable. They tend, however, to occur most frequently in asthmatics (29.6%) (Settipane & Chafee, 1977; Webb, 1978) and less so in cases of rhinitis, 13.7% in nonallergic rhinitis and 13.2% in allergic rhinitis. Various surveys have more or less agreed with these figures.

Mygind (1979) divides nasal polyps into two varieties according to the histology. These are neutrophil polyps found primarily in about 25% of children with cystic fibrosis and 10% to 15% of polyposis in adults. The adult cases usually are associated with chronic infection or inflammation. Eosinophil polyps usually occur in cases of asthma or perennial rhinitis. It is now thought that the coexistence with allergy could support the etiology of polyps as being allergic, but this is in dispute and it is thought that the situation is coincidental. However, it has been shown that IgE synthesis occurs in nasal polyps and that the concentration of IgE is more elevated in the nasal secretions of these patients than in those with conventional allergic rhinitis (Lichtenstein et al., 1973); Platts-Mills et al., 1976).

The cells most frequently encountered when polyps are sectioned are eosinophils (Baxter & Rose, 1953) and plasma cells, with varying numbers of neutrophils. Degranulated mast cells have been demonstrated, suggesting that the release of histamine also occurs, possibly secondary to denervation.

It is well known that some 25% of children with nasal polyps are prone to develop cystic fibrosis. In this connection, the recent studies of Davis, Shelhamer, and Kaliner (1980) are of particular interest. They examined the responses of patients with cystic fibrosis to the administration of α-adrenergic, β-adrenergic, and cholinergic agents, and found abnormalities in all three components of the autonomic nervous system. There was diminished sensitivity to β-adrenergic stimulation, and increased sensitivity to both α-adrenergic and cholinergic stimulation. As noted above, these investigators found similar changes using the same protocol in patients with asthma and rhinitis.

Aspirin Sensitivity

Some patients use aspirin to control the symptoms of rhinitis. A portion may become sensitive with the production of generalized urticaria, marked rhinitis, moderate to severe asthma, and hypotension (Stenius & Lemola, 1976). Although death due to aspirin sensitivity is relatively rare, reports continue to appear (Aaron & Muttitt, 1982). A useful list of aspirin-containing preparations will be found in this same article. The reported incidence of sensitivity to aspirin in asthmatics varies from 2.8% to 19% depending on the authors (Walton & Randle, 1957; Editorial, 1980) and apparently increases with age. It is important to note that most of the nonsteroidal anti-inflammatory agents such as indomethacin or ibuprofen (Motrin) may induce the same symptomatology. These patients generally have nasal polyps, asthma, and invariably a high circulating eosinophil count (Samter & Beers, 1968; Samter & Wasserman, 1978). An accurate history is essential with reference to drug habits since the patient may be inducing symptoms by taking an aspirin or one of the nonsteroid anti-inflammatory agents for headache or arthralgias.

The mechanism of action of aspirin and the newer nonsteroid anti-inflammatory drugs may be explained on the basis of their ability to suppress prostaglandin synthetase

(Vane, 1971). There are two current theories. The first suggests that interference with the cyclooxygenase pathway of arachidonic acid derivatives prevents the production of prostaglandin E (PGE2), thereby inducing bronchoconstriction and presumably other symptoms such as rhinitis. The second indicates there is a diversion from the normal cyclooygenase pathway to the lipogenase pathway with consequent production of leukotrienes (Burka & Paterson, 1980). Both of these explanations remain speculative. Recently, tolerance to aspirin has been described by administering small quantities orally, and increasing the dose by small increments (Stevenson et al., 1980), but clinical improvement has been demonstrated in a minority of these patients.

Between 10% and 40% of aspirin-sensitive patients have been found sensitive to the food-coloring agent tartrazine. The reactions characteristic of allergy range from systemic anaphylaxis and severe asthma to urticaria and mild rhinitis (Michaelson & Juhlin, 1973; Neuman et al., 1978). It is of interest that in a recent study of patients sensitive to tartrazine, Weliky and Heiner (1980) have shown a correlation of symptoms with serum IgD but not with IgE.

DIAGNOSTIC PROCEDURES

Skin Testing

While a diagnosis can often be made on the basis of history alone, it must always be confirmed by an objective method based on the specific immediate sensitivity conferred by IgE antibodies. This is carried out by direct skin testing with dilute extracts of the suspected allergens. Patients must be cautioned to stop antihistamines at least 24 and preferably 72 hours prior to testing. On the other hand, corticosteroids do not alter the immediate IgE-mediated response in the skin. It is also important to establish whether or not dermographism is present before skin testing in order to obviate false-positive results. In the case of a patient with dermographism, the administration of an antihistamine such as diphenhydramine hydrochloride (Benadryl), mg 50, or chlorpheniramine maleate, (Chlor-Trimeton) mg 4 to 8, one-half hour before testing may allow for significant skin responses providing the control injection site is negative. In marked dermographism, it is advisable to resort to testing by the RAST method.

The first of these is the so-called scratch or prick method. After cleansing the skin surface with alcohol or ether, a series of superficial scratches are made, usually on the forearms, suitably spaced, so that one does not interfere with another at an adjacent site. Extracts for scratch testing are provided in dropper vials containing an allergen in 50% glycerine as preservative, as well as 0.5% NaCl and 0.275 sodium bicarbonate. Drops of the various allergens are then placed over each scratch and the patient is observed. Within 15 to 20 minutes, if the test is positive, a wheal with a surrounding flare varying in size according to the sensitivity of the reaction will appear. A control solution consisting of dilution fluid must always be included. The prick test is done in a similar fashion,

TABLE 8-2.

	GRADING OF SKIN TEST REACTIONS	
Grade	Erythema (mm)	Wheal (mm)
±	5	5
1+	5—10	5—10
2+	11—20	5—10
3+	21—30	5—10
4+	31—40	10—15

but in this instance the drops of allergen extracts are first placed on the skin, and then using a sterile 25-gauge needle, a superficial prick is made into the skin underlying each drop, allowing the extract to enter the superficial layers. When using the prick method, the needle should be cleansed between pricks or separate sterile needles used. The advantage of these tests is that in the case of an individual who may be very sensitive and who may develop constitutional reactions such as urticaria, asthma, or vascular collapse, the solution can be immediately wiped off, thus preventing the absorption of more of the extract, and suitable procedures instituted immediately. Reactions are graded roughly according to the size of the wheal and surrounding erythema (Table 8-2) compared to saline negative controls and histamine or codeine positive controls.

The second method of testing is by the intradermal injection of an allergenic extract, usually more dilute. The volume is usually 0.01 to 0.02 cc, and a separate syringe and needle is required for each solution to be tested. The reaction time is similar to that described for scratch tests. Again the patient is observed carefully. If it appears that the patient is developing a "constitutional" reaction, immediate steps should be taken. A tourniquet must be placed above the site of the reactions to prevent further absorption of the extracts. Usually, the upper arm is used for intradermal testing since it is convenient for this purpose. The subsequent mode of treating a constitutional reaction is described below. As a general rule, it is important to carry out the intradermal tests, since they are often more sensitive and will reveal positive reactions confirming the history and which might have otherwise been missed. In addition, having done the scratch method first, one avoids or minimizes the danger of provoking a constitutional reaction. When interpreting the results, it cannot be too strongly emphasized that a positive skin test does not necessarily mean that the patient is clinically sensitive to that particular allergen. In all cases the tests must coincide with the clinical history.

The number of tests used by either method will depend on the nature of the problem. For a case of seasonal rhinitis, it should not be necessary to do more than 15 to 20 by the scratch method. If a strongly positive reaction is observed to an extract, it should not be repeated by an intradermal test with the same allergen. In the case of a negative reaction to a mixed pollen extract such as the trees or grasses, tests should be repeated with individual allergens, particularly if the history suggests that these may be involved.

In general, the number of intradermal tests should not exceed some 15 to 30 at one sitting. It may be necessary to dilute a test solution for intradermal use although these are generally safe to use. The grading of the reaction is similar to that for scratch tests (Table 8-2).

Late Phase IgE-mediated Reactions (LPR)

The local reaction to the intradermal injection of an allergen into the skin of an allergic patient gives rise to the so-called immediate response consisting of a wheal and flare which appears within 15 to 20 minutes, and has usually subsided within an hour. Although late cutaneous reactions had been noted by early observers, these dual reactions were given little attention until Dolovich and his co-workers began an investigation of the nature of the delayed response to the injection of pollen extracts (Dolovich et al., 1973). The LPR continue to develop, peaking at six to 12 hours, with erythema, edema, pruritis, and tenderness, usually subsiding by 24 to 48 hours. In contrast to the Arthus (type III) reaction which was described by Pepys in the late phase of the dual response on skin testing patients with allergic bronchopulmonary aspergillosis (Pepys, 1968) and which could be explained by the presence of both IgE and IgG antibodies to the fungal antigens, these late phase reactions are dependent on IgE antibody (Dolovich et al., 1973; Solley et al., 1976; Zetterstrom, 1979). The histology of the LPR reveals edema, mast cell degranulation, eosinophilia, and neutrophilia and does not differ essentially from those found in the immediate reaction without LPR (Richerson et al., 1979). Just what the significance of these LPR may be in allergic disease is still unknown, though their appearance may be inhibited by prior administration of corticosteroids.

Nasal and Conjunctival Tests

Provocative tests are thought by some to be the most reliable in that the allergen is placed in direct contact with the target organ, such as the nasal mucous membrane or the conjunctiva (Malmberg et al., 1978; Pepys et al., 1975; Taylor & Shivalkar, 1971). Although proposed many years ago, they have not been generally accepted because of the potential hazards involved such as the precipitation of a severe local reaction (Pepys et al., 1975). In the vast majority of cases, however, one can obtain the necessary confirmation by conventional skin tests and the history. Nasal challenge techniques have had their major application in experimental studies (Guercio et al., 1980). They are time consuming, and may give both false-positive and false-negative results. They require pure allergen, and must be carefully monitored in that one does not wish to use an extract of excessive strength. Therefore, one uses as little allergen as possible. Because of difficulties due to nasal obstruction or severe symptoms, it is best to carry out the test during a symptom-free period.

Normally, 0.1 to 0.2 mL of a standard extract is sprayed into the nose using a suitable nebulizer. The choice of allergen may present difficulties since there is no good correlation between nasal sensitivity and skin test sensitivity to pollens in hay-fever patients. Alternatively, house stock solutions, or powdered allergens, or pollen grains may be used. Stock solutions may be sprayed into the nose. An arbitrary quantity of powder, such as that which can be balanced on the tip of a toothpick, can be sniffed. Some authors prefer the insufflation of pollen grains direct by means of a rubber balloon or capillary tube, but sophisticated methods are only possible with specially designed apparatus for research purposes.

Patients with allergic asthma and rhinitis must be very carefully managed because the dose of pollen used for nasal challenge is much greater than that used in skin testing. Consequently, the hazard of severe asthma or anaphylaxis is constantly present. It is not recommended that nasal challenge techniques be used in these patients unless the facilities for dealing with severe asthma or anaphylaxis are available.

The interpretation of results may not be easy. The number of sneezes, and time of onset may be due either to the allergenic properties, or simply irritation of the nasal mucosa. The amount of nasal secretion may be collected and measured. Some suggest that rhinomanometry be combined with the above, but there is debate as to whether it really adds any further information.

Several recent publications may however alter this point of view. The first is by Berdel, Gast, and Huber (1981) in which they describe a simplified oscillation method for measuring nasal resistance during nasal tests with allergens in children. Apparently, there is no physical difficulty on the part of the patients who wear a mask, and breathe through the nose only. The second paper by Clement, van Dishoeck, and colleagues (1981) utilizes a Heyer nebulizer into which the provocation solution is placed, and which is inserted into the nostrils of different sizes according to the patient physiognomy. The effect of the provocation was measured by means of passive anterior rhinometry (PAR). Prior to testing the patency of the nasal airways was determined twice in each nostril by PAR after which the challenging extract was administered. These were performed at intervals of 24 hours to avoid interference of a possible late reaction. The patients comprised 55 children with chronic lung diease and had bronchial provocation tests as well. The object of this study was not to replace conventional skin testing with nasal provocation, but to verify the significance of a positive skin reaction to an extract of high potency which may or not be significant. As pointed out by Norman (1980), when skin tests are not carefully titrated, and when too strong an extract is used, some 25% of normal subjects react positively. Consequently, one may become committed to an unnecessary course of immunotherapy. If the nasal provocation test is positive using the same allergen, then these authors claim that immunotherapy is justified and it is for this use only that they recommend it. If the skin test is negative, there is no need to perform the nasal provocation test.

Nasal Smears

In the case of a clear-cut history and confirmation by the skin tests, it should not be necessary to do anything further in the way of diagnostic procedures. However, if there should be doubt, nasal smears may be helpful for if they show a significant eosinophilia, it is likely that the symptoms are allergic in origin or that they may respond to intranasal corticosteroids. This is not universal in that the reverse may be found (Mullarkey et al., 1980; Whelan, 1980).

Hemogram

The eosinophil count is usually elevated in allergic asthma, and less so in allergic rhinitis. However, it may also be raised in asthma or rhinitis secondary to infection, and is virtually always elevated in the triad of aspirin sensitivity, nasal polyposis, and asthma. There is also the possibility that a patient may have parasitic disease or some major illness, the presenting symptoms being some nasal obstruction and a watery serosanguinous discharge which could be the early signs of carcinoma of a sinus or Wegener's granulomatosis.

Radioimmunosorbent Test for IgE (RIST)

This test, based on the conventional radioimmunoassay technique, is used for the determination of the level of "total" IgE in the serum (Berg & Johansson, 1969; Ishizaka et al., 1966; Johannsen et al., 1976; Wide et al., 1967). The level, which has been expressed in various denominations, is now expressed in units which vary from 0 to 150 normally, but may vary more according to the standards used (Bazaral et al., 1971). The serum concentrations of IgE are usually but not always elevated in patients with atopic dermatitis, allergic asthma, allergic rhinitis, parasitic infestations, and allergic bronchopulmonary aspergillosis. The level is slightly higher in individuals who have no evidence of allergy, but whose family history is positive for allergy (Bazaral, Orgel, & Hamburger, 1971; Sears et al., 1980). In the case of an individual in whom the diagnosis is questionable, this test may be useful. It is usually, but not invariably, normal or low normal in cases of nonallergic rhinitis. Unfortunately, surveys have shown inconsistent findings. Most cases of allergic rhinitis will have a higher value, but normal and very low values may be found. Conversely, although the majority of cases of nonallergic rhinitis will have low or very low values, some, with negative skin tests, as well as a history which complies may show an elevated IgE level. It is difficult to explain such findings (WHO Memorandum, 1981).

Radioallergosorbent Test (RAST)

In contrast to the RIST test, the radioallergosorbent or RAST test is used for the measurement of specific IgE antibody in serum (Aas & Johanssen, 1971; Wide et al., 1967). Basically, it consists of (1) coupling a known quantity of allergen to a paper disc which is then (2) reacted with a sample of the patient's serum containing an unknown quantity of IgE antibody to the allergen. The next step (3) is the addition of ^{125}I labeled anti-IgE after which the test can be read in a suitable counter, the number of counts indicative of the quantity of labeled anti-IgE and consequently of that of the IgE antibody in the serum sample.

While the RAST test and its newer modifications such as the enzyme-labeled anti-IgE (ELISA) represent a major advance in the field of IgE-mediated disease, its prime use at the moment is in the area of basic and clinical investigation for the following reasons: the test is quite expensive to carry out and in effect tells no more about the patient than does a conventional skin test. The commercial kits commonly used yield results related to a single reference serum. Therefore, comparison with other results is almost impossible and RAST classes for different allergens are not comparable. Furthermore, the test is dependent on the availability of pure allergens since a false positive result may occur with crude preparations.

The number of available pure allergens has increased in recent years and now include antigen E, K, and several components such as RA 3 and 5 ragweed, rye, and timothy grass, birch pollen, horse dander, cat dander, codfish, bovine milk, chicken, egg, and the venoms of several stinging insects. A modified RAST test has become quite useful as a method for determining the potency of allergenic extracts (Foucard et al., 1973). However, the results obtained from skin tests are available within 30 minutes, whereas it presently takes a minimum of 48 hours for the results from RAST testing. As pointed out by Adkinson (1981) "The indiscriminate wholesale replacement of skin testing with RAST in the clinical practice of allergy is fraught with numerous difficulties, not the least of which is obtaining reliable results." Present RAST results from commercial laboratories are affected by the presence of blocking IgG antibodies (Zeiss et al., 1981). Similar results wee reported by Zimmerman, Yungiger and Gleich (1980) when positivity is critical with ragweed (Pharmacia) and honeybee discs. In addition, when the threshold was set at a low level using a modified RAST procedure, 33% false-positive results were obtained among non-IgE–containing controls (Santrach et al., 1981). In contrast, the conventional Phadebas RAST threshold is set so high that half of the RAST negative patients in the group studied by these same authors had positive nasal provocation tests. It seems obvious that until the RAST test can be made more reliable, its use at the moment cannot be recommended when skin tests are available (WHO Memorandum, 1981). It must be noted, however, that there are a number of distinct advantages to the RAST test. It is without risk to the patient, can be performed in patients taking anti-histamines or those with dermographism, and when carried out properly is quite reproducible. As the procedure becomes more useful in terms of the availability of pure allergenic extracts, and less expensive, it may well come into regular use clinically.

TREATMENT

Allergen Elimination

In all cases of allergic nasal disease, the simplest and most certain method of treatment is to eliminate the allergen, common examples being the removal of a pet, including dogs, cats, or birds, or the elimination of feather pillows. It is impossible to completely eliminate house dust, but the patient can be cautioned not to be present when the vacuum is being used or when there is general house cleaning. Obviously this is often not possible in the case of a housewife, but she can be cautioned to keep windows open and to wear a mask during the carrying out of her arduous duties. Special mattress and box springs covers may be purchased to limit dust exposure from these sources. It has been recommended that carpets be removed, old furniture in which there may be dust mite (*Dermatophagoides*), curtains, etc, must all be removed from the bedroom in particular. This can be a very traumatizing experience for many patients and the results are questionable, except in the case of young children where the procedure may be quite simple. One should be quite sure that the carpet is really at fault before insisting that it should now be removed. It is, however, very important to caution patients, particularly those with perennial allergic rhinitis, not to expose themselves to the dust produced during the renovation of an old house. The same precaution pertains to fresh paint, such as veneers of the turpentine variety. Latex paint, on the other hand, seems to be tolerated. In all cases, the rigorousness of such precautions must be balanced with the severity of symptoms. For those whose symptoms are mild and easily controlled with nonspecific therapy such as a suitable antihistamine, they should not be necessary. On the other hand, it is always possible that the patient is a potential asthmatic and if this should be the case, then more rigorous dust control should be undertaken. In the case of an individual whose livelihood depends on caring for animals, such as farmers or veterinarians, a careful trial of immunotherapy is indicated.

SYMPTOMATIC TREATMENT OF ALLERGIC RHINITIS

Antihistamines

Antihistamines, first studied some 35 years ago (Henderson & Rose, 1947), are the most widely used of all the preparations available. They are believed to act as competitive inhibitors of histamine by blocking the histamine receptor sites of the H_1 variety: that is, those sites which, when stimulated, increase vascular permeability and the contraction of smooth muscle. In recent years, a second receptor for histamine called H_2 has been described. It stimulates the secretion of gastric acid. However, the recent H_2 blocking agent, cimetidine hydrochloride, which is used for the treatment of gastric ulcers, has no apparent role in the treatment of rhinitis. In addition to their primary action, antihistamines that are used in the treatment of rhinitis have anticholinergic, sedative, and antiemetic properties. Consequently, their side effects may include sedation, dryness of the mouth, and blurred vision. One should always caution a patient about the sedative effects when driving or in particular those engaged in a hazardous occupation. There are four groups according to their chemical structure (see Table 8-3). They consist of a heterocyclic or benzene structure linked to a basic ethylamine by (1) a nitrogen (ethylenediamine derivative) or (2) oxygen (aminoalkyl ether derivative), or (3) carbon

TABLE 8-3. Classes of H_1 Blocking Antihistamines.

Class	Trade Name	Dose (Adult)	Sedation
Ethanolamines			
Diphenhydramine hydrochloride	Benadryl	25 or 50 mg	marked
Carbinoxamine maleate	Clistin	4 mg	moderate
Ethylenediamines			
Tripelennamine hydrochloride	Pyrabenzamine	50 mg	moderate
Tripelennamine citrate	Pyrabenzamine	Elixir 37.5 mg per 5 mL	
Antazolin phosphate	Vasocon-A Ophthalmic solution 0.5% (with 0.05% naphazoline)		
Alkylamines			
Chlorpheniramine maleate	Chlor-Trimeton (US) Chlortripolon (Canada)	4 mg	moderate
Brompheniramine maleate	Dimetane	4–8 mg	moderate to marked
Phenothiazines			
Promethazine hydrochloride	Phenergan	25–50 mg	marked

(alkylamine). A fourth group, although not chemically related, are the cyclizines, of which hydroxizine is an example. Finally, there is a miscellaneous group which includes cyproheptadine (Periactin) and dimethendine.

There is considerable variation in the effectiveness of the antihistamines and it is useful to prescribe several for a patient to try before ordering a large quantity. In general, the ethanolamines tend to be the most effective but may cause the most sedation, although this is not invariable. Several new nonsedating antihistamines are currently undergoing clinical trials and may be available for patient use in the very near future.

TABLE 8-4. Sympathomimetic Drugs.

Nonproprietary name	Trade name	Form	Dose
Propylhexedrene	Benzedrex	NI	250 mg
Tuaminoheptane sulfate	Tuamine	NI	325 mg
Naphazoline hydrochloride	Privine	NS	0.1%
		OS	0.02 - 0.1%
Oxymetazoline hydrochloride	Afrin	NS	0.025 - 0.05%
Xylometazoline hydrochloride	Otrivin	NS	0.05 - 0.1%
Phenylpropanolamine	Propadrine	C	25 50 mg
		E	4 mg/ml
Pseudoephedrine	Sudafed	T	60 mg
	Sudafed SA	C	120 mg
		E	30 mg/5 ml
	Afrinol	RT	120 mg

Legend: NI—nasal inhaler; NB—nebulizer; NS—nasal spray; OS—ophthalmic solution; C—capsules; E—elixir; T—tablets; RT—repetabs.

Combination of Antihistamines with Pseudoepinephrine or Norepinephrine

A variety of such preparations, usually in capsule form, are often quite effective and have the advantage of prolonged action requiring a morning and nightime dose only. In general, nasal sprays, such as xylometazoline hydrochloride and in particular, naphazoline hydrochloride are to be discouraged because of the possibility of a rebound phenomenon (see rhinitis medicamentosa).

Sympathomimetic Amines

These agents, which are listed in Table 8-4 act primarily by stimulating the α-adrenergic receptor sites. They have been employed for many years either alone as nasal sprays or in combination with antihistamines for the management of all forms of rhinitis. They are most effective in shrinking the nasal mucosa and reducing nasal secretions in the allergic forms of rhinitis. They may be the cause of so-called rhinitis medicamentosa when used to excess. It should be noted that they also stimulate β receptors and should not be administered to patients with heart disease or hyperthyroidism with the production of untoward side effects such as nervousness and palpitations with a tachycardia (Weiner, 1980). Preparations such as albuterol (Ventolin and Proventi) and fenoterol (Berotec) are not generally used for relief of rhinitis although there are reports that they may be effective (Schumacher, 1980).

Cromolyn Sodium (Intal)

Although cromolyn sodium has been in use for the treatment of allergic asthma for some years, its performance raises some questions in clinical practice (Knight & Underdown, 1975; Manners & Ezeoke, 1973). It seems to be effective in some patients but not in others for reasons that are not clear (Craig et al., 1977; Frostad, 1977). It is said to act by stabilizing the mast cell and thereby preventing the release of mediators. It has recently been introduced in the form of a nasal aerosol for the treatment of allergic rhinitis and appears to be superior to placebo in this regard. One drawback of cromolyn nasal spray is its short duration of action, requiring up to six administrations per day for optimal results. Cromolyn has also been effective as a solution in cases of laboratory workers who have developed an allergy to laboratory animals such as mice and rabbits (Posey & Nelson, 1977). Some newer compounds with properties similar to that of cromolyn sodium have been introduced and show promise of being useful in allergic rhinitis (Blair, 1977; Vilsvik & Jenssen, 1976).

Corticosteroids

Although corticosteroids are the most highly effective form of therapy, their use in the oral or injectible forms has been largely supplanted by the newer topical spray preparations (Harding & Heath, 1976; Okuda & Mygind, 1980). The first topical preparation for rhinitis was dexamethasone sodium phosphate (Decadron Turbinaire) which is propelled by freon from a container, each puff delivering 0.08 mg of dexamethasone. The average starting dose is two puffs in each nostril three times daily which is equivalent to about 1.0 mg of prednisone per day. It is absorbed systemically in amounts equivalent to 2.5 to 4 mg of prednisone, which is not an insignificant quantity and can cause adrenal suppression, sometimes weight gain, and hyperglycemia. However, this is usually reversible if the preparation is discontinued. It has been supplanted by two newer topical steroid preparations. These are beclomethasone dipropionate (Beconase or Vancenase) and flunisolide (Nasalide). Beclomethasone has been in clinical use in Britain and Canada for some ten years (Brompton Hospital, 1980; Sahay et al., 1980a,b; Schulz et al., 1978).

These two preparations have several major advantages. They are much more potent and, when used in clinically effective doses, there is no evidence of systemic absorption.

The usual dose for beclomethasone dipropionate is one puff in each nostril, four times daily. Each puff delivers 50 μg for a total dose of 400 μg daily. The dose for flunisolide is two puffs into each nostril twice a day for a total of 200 μg since each actuation delivers 25 μg. The amount required per patient on a daily basis is an individual assessment. In a recent large survey by Munch, Gomez et al. (1981), an open comparison of dosage frequencies of beclomethasone was made on 123 adult patients with seasonal allergic rhinitis. They were divided into three groups and each received a total daily dose of 400 μg as (1) one puff in each nostril four times daily, (2) two puffs in each nostril twice daily, and (3) four puffs in each nostril once daily. It was concluded that the twice daily dose of two puffs was as effective as that given four times a day. In allergic rhinitis marked improvement was reported by Mygind (1973) in 85% of subjects receiving a daily dose of 400 μg of beclomethasone dipropionate and similar results were observed by Cockroft et al. (1976). The results of similar schedules for patients with perennial rhinitis are somewhat less, varying from 54% to 89% (Cockroft et al., 1980). It is of interest that in the studies of Mullarkey et al. (1980), in the group of nonallergic cases of rhinitis with nasal eosinophilia (ENR), the response to intranasal steroids was particularly effective.

Prior to the advent of these newer preparations, the management of patients with nasal polyposis was mostly unsatisfactory, consisting primarily of polypectomy, or oral steroids with their attendant side effects. There are now a number of reports which are encouraging for the management of this vexing problem (Deuschl & Drettner, 1977; Mygind, 1975; Webb, 1978), with response rates of 68%.

Untoward effects are rare when these preparations are used intranasally. The small incidence of candidiasis which has been reported when beclomethasone is inhaled orally for cases of asthma has not been noted in cases of rhinitis. In a long term study of flunisolide treatment in perennial rhinitis, nasal biopsies taken before and after treatment showed no significant change in the histological appearance or morphological characteristics (Sahay et al., 1980b). However, in a combined trial comparing two dosage schedules of beclomethasone dipropionate over a period of 12 months, 12 out of 40 patients developed epistaxis necessitating a reduction in dosage (Brompton Hospital, 1980), although the use of saline nasal lavage may help to alleviate this reaction.

Immunotherapy

The basic principle of immunotherapy is to treat the patient with an extract containing allergen(s) which are of clinical significance. This infers that the extract contains only those allergens which, on the basis of careful history and corresponding skin tests, coincide with the production of symptoms. For example, if, on performing the skin tests, positive reactions are obtained to the trees, grasses, ragweed, and several animal danders, but the symptoms occur only during the months of June and July, the extract should contain only the grass pollens. It is useless to send a copy of skin test results to a commercial company and have them make up an extract without any further information or indeed

TABLE 8-5. Standard Equivalent Values of Extracts.

Weight by volume	1 mL of 1:50
Pollen units	20,000
Freeman-Noon units	20,000
Protein nitrogen units	10,000
Total nitrogen units	26,000
Total nitrogen	0.26 mg

Note: These values are only approximate.

any direct contact with the patient and such practice is only to be condemned. Although treatment with food allergens has been tried in the past, it is not used for the chief reason that no therapeutic effect has been obtained.

A second principle concerns the number of allergens which may be included in a single extract. These should be limited to three or four at the most. Thus in general for a patient who has both seasonal and perennial allergic rhinitis with symptoms occurring during the three seasonal periods and whose reactions on skin testing include the tree, grass, and ragweed pollens as well as dust and mite (*D. farinea*), two separate extracts should be used: one containing the pollens and the other dust and mite (Aas, 1971).

Standardization of Allergens

Because of the complexity of allergens, the problem of standardization has been difficult and has as yet not been completely solved. The initial Noon unit was based on weight by volume, which is the ratio of crude pollen to the volume of extracting fluid. The protein nitrogen unit (PNU) which is still widely used was introduced by Cooke and Stull (1933). A PNU was defined as 0.00001 mg of protein nitrogen. However, neither of these are a true index of biological activity and the potency of commercial extracts labeled in these terms may vary considerably (see Table 8-5). More recently, it has become possible to estimate the biological potency of some pollen extracts by a modification of the radioallergosorbent (RAST) method (Foucard et al., 1973). With pure allergens, of which the venoms of stinging insects are the best examples, standardization can be quite accurately measured on a weight basis.

Extracts of pollen and other inhalants generally are provided in two forms. These are first the aqueous preparation using Coca's solution as the vehicle, and second preparations in phosphate-buffered saline with 50% glycerol. The glycerinated variety has the advantage of remaining stable for long periods at all temperatures up to 35 °C. The major disadvantage is that injections may be quite irritating or painful. Aqueous preparations, on the other hand, are generally well tolerated, but may lose their potency quite rapidly if not kept at 4 °C (Anderson & Baer, 1982).

In general, treatment extracts are available in strengths based on the two methods of calibration referred to above. The first, weight by volume, is expressed in dilutions of a given quantity diluted to 1/10,000, 1/1,000, 1/100, and 1/10. The second is expressed in protein nitrogen units or PNU. These are generally 100, 1,000, and 10,000 PNU. Treatment schedules provided by the various companies are only a guide and have to be carefully monitored for each patient to avoid any undesirable and often serious reactions (see below). In the case of a patient who on skin testing responds with a very large reaction, it may be necessary to start with a lower concentration such as 10 PNU, or 1/100,000 wt/vol.

Forms of Treatment

The basic principle of immunotherapy consists of beginning with a low dose which can be tolerated and which is increased slowly according to the tolerance of the patient, usually at intervals of seven days, until the highest tolerated dose is reached. In the case of ragweed, as an example, this would be a final maintenance dose of 0.5 mL or more of 1:10 wt/vol or 10,000 PNU. Twenty-five or more injections may be required to reach the final dose using aqueous extracts, but it may be necessary to make adjustments downward to avoid too large local or constitutional reactions. Many studies have shown that the effectiveness of such treatment is specific and dose related (Lichtenstein et al., 1973; Lowell & Franklin, 1965; Norman et al., 1979).

In general, there are three types of treatment schedules. *Coseasonal therapy* consists of the administration of injections during the particular pollen season, such as when the patient is seen for the first time when symptoms are present. It is not recommended for long-term therapy and is not commonly used. *Preseasonal therapy* is that form which is begun some 3 to 6 months prior to the onset of the pollen season, the highest dose being attained before the usual onset of symptoms at which time the injections are stopped. These are resumed again in the following year in the same manner.

The treatment of choice is *perennial therapy* because it appears to provide the greatest degree of clinical improvement (Franklin & Lowell, 1967; Johnstone et al., 1968). In this form, one begins with the same schedule as that used in preseasonal therapy, but once the maintenance dose is reached, the interval between each injection is increased to every 2 weeks or up to a maximum of an injection every 3 to 4 weeks. There are, however, some patients who may report that symptoms may recur at this interval between injections and that they require one every 2 weeks, but this is not common. It is important to note that when starting with a new supply of extract, usually at the end of a year, the starting dose must be reduced by at least one third and built up at weekly intervals again to the top maintenance dose. Recently, a "clustered" schedule for Hymenoptera venom immunotherapy consisting of three injections the first day, followed by a single injection given every 2 weeks with rapid increase in the dosage was suggested (Golden et al., 1980). It was found to have no advantage over the preseasonal schedule (Van Metre, Jr et al., 1982).

Precautions

There are certain precautions which must be taken when administering extracts for treatment. The injections are given subcutaneously using a sterile tuberculin syringe and 25-gauge needle. Before injection, the skin site must be cleaned with alcohol. After inserting the needle, the plunger must first be drawn back to make certain that it is not in a blood vessel in order to avoid injection intravenously, which could precipitate a severe anaphylactic reaction. If blood is withdrawn, the needle should be withdrawn and a second site used with the same precautions. Patients should be advised not to come for treatment after a heavy meal, or after strenuous exertion such as a game of squash. In the case where two extracts are administered on the same day, a separate needle and syringe is used for each extract.

Tolerance or Ceiling

A small proportion of patients, usually quite sensitive both clinically and on skin testing, may develop what has been called a "ceiling" beyond which the dose cannot be increased without inducing both large local and general reactions. In this circumstance, the dose must be reduced to a level which is tolerated. Sometimes changing the type of extract, usually aqueous, to an alum-precipitated variety may eliminate the problem. The administration of an antihistamine such as 4 mg of chlorpheniramine one hour prior to the injection, may be useful in preventing such reactions.

COMPLICATIONS

Untoward reactions may occur both on skin testing and treatment procedures. Therefore, certain precautions are essential (see Table 8-6). At all times (1) a physician must be present, (2) a syringe containing adrenalin 1:1000 freshly prepared, must be available, (3) antihistamines such as Benadryl available for intramuscular (IM) injection, (4) oxygen with a suitable mask for administration, (5) patients must remain where they can be observed by a nurse or the physician for a period of at least 20 minutes before leaving.

Pollen extracts, when administered subcutaneously, may give rise to three types of allergic reactions. With the first few injections, it is usual for a wheal and flare to appear at the site resembling a positive reaction to a skin test. It usually subsides within an hour or so. A second type which appears within two to four hours after the injection consists of local itching and an erythematous swelling with wheal formation. These may reach a maximum of 16 to 24 hours and then subside within another 24 hours. There is no

TABLE 8-6. Management of Reactions to Immunotherapy or Skin Testing.

A. Local reactions

    1. Oral antihistamine
    2. Review of dosage schedule

B. Systemic reactions (including generalized erythema, urticaria, angioedema, bronchospasm, laryngeal edema, shock and cardiac arrest)

    1. 0.01 mL/kg up to 0.2 mL of aqueous epinephrine 1:1000 subcutaneously at site of immunotherapy injection
    2. 0.01 mL/kg up to 0.3 mL of epinephrine 1:1000 subcutaneously at another site
    3. Diphenhydramine intravenously or intramuscularly 1.25 mg/kg up to 50 mg
    4. Tourniquet above the site of injection of allergen
    5. Specific reactions
       a. Bronchospasm: Intravenous aminophylline 4 mg/kg up to 500 mg given *slowly* over 10–15 minutes, aqueous hydrocortisone (Solucortef) up to 200 mg, oxygen
       b. Laryngeal edema: oxygen, intubation, tracheostomy
       c. Hypotension: vasopressors, steroids
       d. Cardiac arrest: resuscitation, sodium bicarbonate, defibrillation, antiarrythmia medications

    6. Review of dosage schedule

Adapted from Immunotherapy by Patterson et al in Allergy, Principles and Practice Edited by Middleton, Reed and Ellis, 1978 C.V. Mosby Company, St. Louis, Missouri.

necrosis. In both of these types of reaction, there is participation of IgE. Both are of minor significance.

The third type is the so-called *constitutional reaction*. Although relatively rare, it nevertheless constitutes a potentially serious hazard of therapy and requires prompt treatment, because it is a form of anaphylaxis. Symptoms consist of a feeling of uneasiness, often associated with generalized urticaria. Asthma, varying from mild to severe, can occur, accompanied by tachycardia, hypotension, and syncope. A tourniquet should be placed around the arm *above* the site of injection and epeniphrine administered promptly. However, IM antihistamines and oxygen may be necessary. In general, it may be said that the sooner symptoms begin, following the injection of the extract, the more severe is the reaction. It is well established that the administration of corticosteroids have no immediate effect either on the local reaction or the occurrence of a constitutional reaction. It is sometimes useful to instruct the patient to take an antihistamine one-half hour before the administration of the extract. Detailed procedures are outlined in Table 8-6. Finally, there are some patients who develop a feeling of uneasiness, followed by syncope, pallor, sweatiness, drop in BP, and a bradycardia. These are usually vasovagal in origin. The patient usually recovers quickly when the head is lowered, and is helped by the subcutaneous injection of epinephrine or a small dose of atropine.

Intranasal Immunotherapy

The use of intranasal sprays of pollen extracts for the treatment of allergic rhinitis is not new and was first suggested by Herxheimer (1951). Although early trials reported alleviation of symptoms (Deuschl & Johanssen, 1977), the induction of local adverse symptoms counteracted the later beneficial effects as emphasized by Welsh, Zimmerman et al. (1981) in a recent trial. They used short ragweed extract sprayed six times daily intranasally for a 12-week period preseasonally. A control group received a similar treatment using histamine solutions as the placebo. The treatment did not alter serum antibody levels to crude short ragweed or a number of pure fractions including AgE, Ra3, and Ra5 in either group.

Effect of Immunotherapy

With the widespread use of immunotherapy in the early stages following its introduction in 1911 by Noon, most of the evidence supporting its efficacy was anecdotal. The first well carried out studies were those of Frankland and Augustin (1954) and later those of Lowell and Franklin (1965). The latter were done with adequate controls and double blind. In that study of 154 patients, 80% of the treated were improved whereas only 43% of the placebo treated group were similarly improved. These studies were done with conventional aqueous extracts. With the advent of antigen E, the purified and most active fraction of ragweed, a number of well-designed and carefully controlled investigations were carried out by Norman (Norman et al., 1968), and Lichtenstein et al. (1973). These were correlated with the pollen count, symptom scores, technique of in vitro histamine release, specific IgE levels by the RAST method, and the blocking (IgG) antibody. They showed that either conventional ragweed aqueous extract or Antigen E administered in gradually increasing doses over a period of 5 years resulted in amelioration of the symptoms of ragweed hay fever, whereas the placebo had no effect. Similarly, that of Lichtenstein showed that an average of 80% of treated patients improved as compared to only 30% of the placebo group. In general, most of the effective results were dependent on the ultimate dose achieved, in that low doses were generally ineffective. It seems clear that each case is an individual problem and that the objective would seem to be to achieve as high a dose as possible. Obviously, there are hazards to this approach with these types of extract because of the possibility of untoward reactions. It should also be noted that few so-called cures are achieved, and that most cases relapse with cessation of treatment after a period of 5 years of therapy.

The Mode of Action of Immunotherapy

A clear understanding of the mode of action of immunotherapy is not yet available in terms of crude pollen extracts. However, the availability of more sophisticated techniques have clarified this considerably (Evans et al., 1976; Lichtenstein et al., 1973). These consist of the accurate measurement of specific IgE antibody, the measurement of blocking IgG antibody, the studies on histamine release from circulating basophils and the availability of pure allergens (Lichtenstein et al., 1966). Thus, it seems clear that immunotherapy induces a definite rise in IgG blocking antibody which in turn inhibits the combination of allergen with IgE. Unfortunately, in many of the studies performed, there is no consistent trend. The one exception would seem to be the recent studies on the treatment of patients sensitive to stinging insects using pure venom. Studies on histamine release in vitro also demonstrate two important points (Platts-Mills et al., 1976). These are that when pretreatment serum is tested, it can be shown that it takes a given amount of allergen to deplete these cells of 50% of their histamine content. Following an adequate course of immunotherapy, it now takes considerably more allergen to induce the release of the same quantity of histamine (50%) presumably because of the increase in blocking antibody. An additional point of interest is the finding that in some cases post treatment basophils are much more resistant to histamine release, in that any amount of antigen will not release all of the histamine. Studies of the serum IgE levels in untreated hay-fever patients have shown that with the advent of a pollen season the level of IgE antibody rises and again falls when the season is over (Lichtenstein et al., 1973). In similar studies on patients undergoing treatment, the rise of IgE is inhibited in most cases, but again there is no consistent correlation. Although IgE, IgA, and IgG have been demonstrated in nasal secretions (Dolovich et al., 1970, 1973; Pepys, 1968), it is difficult to correlate these with severity of symptoms, clinical course, or serum IgG or IgE levels (Deuschl, 1976; Deuschl & Johanssen, 1977; Deuschl et al., 1977). A better correlation between IgG and IgA antibodies and immunotherapy was obtained by Platts-Mills et al. (1976). They found that IgG- and IgA-blocking antibodies in nasal secretions increased in the treated patients and these could be correlated with the inhibition of histamine release from basophils and relief of symptoms.

It seems evident from the foregoing brief discussion that a major stumbling block in many of these studies has been the lack of purified antigens. With the recent availability of pure venom extracts, much more concrete evidence has been obtained not only in diagnosis on skin testing, therapeutic result with complete immunity, but, of major interest, mode of action. The study of Golden et al. (1980) shows that treatment with the venom of insects of the order Hymenoptera can specifically protect insect-allergic patients against anaphylactic reactions to the stings of these insects. Although there was no change in

IgE antibody levels, protection could be clearly related to the level of IgG-blocking antibody induced.

As noted in the section on basic mechanisms, further evidence for the effectiveness of immunotherapy is the increase of type 2 (H_2)-bearing T suppressor lymphocytes which suppress the number of IgE-producing B cells (B lymphocytes) with a consequent decrease in circulating IgE (Rocklin et al., 1980).

Some Controversial Tests and Procedures for Diagnosis and Treatment for Allergic Diseases

Over the years, procedures for diagnosis and treatment have come and gone in the practice of medicine, and the allergic diseases are certainly no exception. Many of these were nevertheless adhered to tenaciously by their proponents, unfortunately without adequate controls. Either to substantiate these claims or to clarify their possible use, a number of carefully organized studies have been carried out and the results presented in the *Journal of Allergy and Clinical Immunology* at the request of the Federal Register, the National Center for Health Care Technology (American Academy of Allergy, 1981). These include cytotoxicity testing, urine autoinjection, provocative and neutralization testing, and the Rinkel method.

Cytotoxicity Testing (Bryan's Test). The test is based on the claim that the addition of a specific allergen in vitro to either whole bood or to serum leukocyte suspensions results in a reduction of the leukocyte count or death of the leukocytes, and is consequently useful in diagnosis. A number of well-controlled studies, on the other hand, have clearly shown that the results are inconsistent, often showing no difference between controls to which saline was added instead of allergen. The conclusions were that there is no proof that leukocytotoxic testing is effective for the diagnosis of food or inhalant allergy.

Urine autoinjection (autogenous urine immunization). This very controversial procedure consists of collecting urine from the patient in sterile containers, either filtering or boiling it, and then injecting it back into the same patient intramuscularly. Suffice it to say that there is no evidence for its effectiveness. In addition, the procedure is potentially dangerous, in that injections of kidney protein (glomerular basement membrane) could induce nephritis.

Provocative and Neutralization Testing (subcutaneous) and Provocative Testing (sublingual). When examined under controlled conditions, it was concluded that subcutaneous provocation and neutralization as a method for the treatment and diagnosis of allergic disease has no plausible rationale or immunologic basic. Similarly, in the case of provocative testing, no adequate control studies appear to have been done by the proponents. Since the results by others using adequate controls indicate that the method is ineffective, demonstration of the effectiveness of this method should be the responsibility of the proponents.

The Rinkel Method. Finally, in this group of contentious methods is the question of the rationale and/or effectiveness of the so-called Rinkel method of treatment. This method of treatment, which is still widely used for allergic rhinitis (Williams, 1971; Willoughby, 1974), stems from the original observations of Vaughan (1923). He noted that a proper low dose of ragweed extract was promptly followed by good relief of symptoms in 80% of previously unimmunized patients and emphasized that the dose must be low and that when higher doses were used, they were less effective. These observations were followed by those of Hansel (1941) and Rinkel (1949). The latter devised a method of calculating the optimum dose for treatment based on end-point skin testing using serial dilutions to determine sensitivity. He found the end-point dilution to be closely related to the optimal dose for treatment. Essentially, using serial dilutions of extract, the weakest extract which just produces a positive reaction is the end-point dilution. The optimal treatment dose is then arrived at by subcutaneous injections once weekly starting with 0.1 mL of the end-point dilution. The optimal dose is usually 1 to 5 times the size of the starting dose and is usually close to the end-point dilution. The problem lies in the fact that although it is said to be effective by its proponents, this does not appear to be the case when properly controlled double-blind studies are carried out.

The first of these was that of Van Metre, Adkinson et al. (1980) who studied 24 patients with ragweed hay fever. They were divided into two groups based on in vitro histamine release tests and skin test reaction to antigen E (AgE). A battery of immunological parameters were measured. One group of 12 was treated by the Rinkel method, and the control group was treated with placebo given in an immitation of the Rinkel method. There was no difference in the symptom scores or immunological parameters of either group in this double-blind study. The second, sponsored by the American Academy of Allergy and conducted by Hirsch, Kalbfleish et al. (1981) was a 2-year double-blind multicenter study of the effect of Rinkel injection therapy compared with a histamine placebo in 155 subjects with atopic rhinitis. These were divided into two groups—81 treated and 74 placebo. With one exception, none of the centers reported a consistent significant difference between the pollen extract treated and placebo treated groups in any of the weekly mean scores or the RAST before, during, and after the pollen seasons. It was concluded that the Rinkel method of treatment is no more effective than a histamine-placebo in influencing the weekly mean symptom, medication, and physical examination scores or IgE levels.

NEWER APPROACHES TO IMMUNOTHERAPY

It seems clear from the foregoing section on immunotherapy that, although we have a better understanding of its effects and mode of action, the current form of treatment leaves much to be desired (Norman, 1980; Patterson, 1981). The most effective treatment at the moment is that for the management of insect allergy. However, the nature of the allergens involved is quite different from that of the pollens, and the availability of pure venoms makes for more precise evaluation.

TABLE 8-7. Newer Preparations for Immunotherapy.

1. Alum precipitated
2. Pyridine treated
3. Formaldehyde treated (allergoids)
4. Gluteraldehyde polymers
5. Gluteraldehyde modified pollen-tyrosine adsorbates
6. Synthetic polymer D-Glutamic D-lysine (D-GL) fraction A of SRW (A: D-Gl)
7. Conjugates of allergens to polyethylene glycol

A number of newer modified extract methods have been tried in recent years. The objectives are (*a*) attempts to increase the antigenicity and decrease the allergenicity (*b*) to stimulate the production of T suppressor cells, (*c*) to increase the levels of IgG-blocking antibody, and (*d*) to suppress the production of IgE antibody. It would also be desirable to achieve such objectives with fewer injections than the present schedules require (Table 8-7). These modifications have been reviewed by Patterson (1981).

Alum-Precipitated Extracts

Alum-precipitated extracts of pollens provide an advantage as a long-acting depot, because the injected material is released slowly in one or two hours' time. The number of injections required is reduced by about one half, and the incidence of systemic reactions such as urticaria, rhinitis, or asthma is usually less than with aqueous extracts. Depot preparations such as oil emulsions, which were in vogue for a short period some years ago, are no longer used, because they have carcinogenic properties when injected into mice (Potter & Boyce, 1962).

Pyridine-Treated Extracts

The modification of allergenic extracts by chemical manipulation is another means of reducing allergenicity while maintaining immunogenicity. One such preparation using pyridine, which is an organic solvent, followed by alum precipitation, has been available for many years (Fuchs & Strauss, 1959). The final product of this treatment is a suspension of water-insoluble whole pollen complex. However, in the case of ragweed, it has been shown that treatment with pyridine virtually denatures antigen E, which is the major allergen in ragweed. Nevertheless, some IgG antibody to ragweed has been demonstrated in patients treated with this preparation.

Chemically Modified Extracts

Formaldehyde treated

Two agents, formaldehyde and glutaraldehyde, have been used to modify allergenic extracts. The formaldehyde extract has been referred to as an "allergoid," analogous to the treatment of tetanus antitoxin with formaldehyde to produce tetanus "toxoid" (Marsh et al., 1970; Norman et al., 1979). Preliminary studies have shown that allergenicity is reduced with maintenance of immunogenicity. This preparation has been studied thoroughly since 1972 with the following results. On the basis of antigen E content, it has about one-fiftieth the ability of unaltered whole ragweed extract to induce local delayed and systemic reactions when administered subcutaneously; in other words, allergenicity is greatly reduced. Its antigenicity is increased in that it stimulates a more rapid increase in IgG-blocking antibody. It has a longer shelf life than conventional allergen extracts and has shown no evidence of any ill effects in patients on perennial treatment since 1972 (Norman et al., 1981).

Ragweed allergoid has also been used in preliminary trials of intranasal therapy for allergic rhinitis. Apparently, it is effective in this form of treatment with results similar to those obtained by injection. As compared to ragweed pollen extracts, which induce the symptoms of sneezing and nasal discharge, the allergoid ragweed preparation was free of these side effects and provided relief of symptoms during the ragweed season with accompanying rise in IgG-blocking antibody.

Glutaraldehyde Treated

A promising modification using glutaraldehyde has been intensively studied by Patterson and his group (Hendrix et al., 1980; Kelly et al., 1980). Glutaraldehyde produces complexing so that large polymers of the allergen result. In this case, utilizing whole ragweed, it has been shown that complexes less than 200,000 mol wt still retained allergenicity as defined by the ability to elicit IgE-mediated skin reactivity. A second fraction with molecular weights ranging from 200,000 to 20,000,000 was shown to retain immunogenicity defined as the ability to induce an IgG antibody response but in marked contrast little allergenicity. As a consequence, the latter high molecular weight polymerized ragweed product can be administered with higher dose schedules requiring fewer injections (Hendrix et al., 1981). It is, however, not yet generally available.

A number of trials using chemically modified extracts administered intranasally, in particular glutaraldehyde polymers, have been carried out (Deuschl & Johannsen, 1977; Johannsen et al., 1979; Nickelsen et al., 1981; Welsh et al., 1981). From the results obtained on these double-blind studies, with one exception (Mathews et al., 1980), it appears that these chemically modified extracts are effective for the treatment of allergic pollen induced rhinitis. Although freer of adverse reactions, they are less effective clinically than unmodified pollen extracts. In the study by Nickelsen, Goldstein et al. (1981), both the systemic and the local (nasal secretions) immunologic parameters were followed. Three groups of patients which consisted of a control, an unmodified ragweed treated, and a glutaraldehyde polymer of ragweed treated were studied. A significant rise in serum IgE was found only in the ragweed treated group. There was a significant increase in the nasal secretion of IgA in both treatment groups. Nasal secretion of IgE and IgG were increased in the glutaraldehyde group. There was, however, no consistent correlation between nasal secretion antibodies and symptoms. Ragweed specific serum IgG was not affected by any of the treatments. From these and other studies, it is quite probable that intranasal treatment may be useful when a suitable modified allergen becomes available, in that this form of treatment has many obvious advantages for the patient.

Glutaraldehyde Pollen-Tyrosine Adsorbate (Pollinex)

Recently, another variant of pollen extract, the Pollinex variety, has been in clinical use in Britain for a number of years and is now available in Canada (Johannsen et al., 1974; Miller, 1976; Symington et al., 1977; Verstraeten & Wheeler, 1978). It is a glutaraldehyde-modified pollen-tyrosine adsorbate. The addition of the tyrosine is said to increase its depot property. Like the previous glutaraldehyde-treated pollen extracts, allergenicity is said to be decreased while immunogenicity is retained. Consequently, fewer injections are necessary to achieve a sufficiently high total dose. In the case of the ragweed preparation, four or five injections are given at weekly intervals, the last one just prior to the onset of the ragweed pollen season (Metzger et al., 1981). With the grass preparation, only three injections are given at the same time intervals ending just prior to the advent of the grass season. As with glutaraldehyde-treated pollen preparations, reactions are only occasionally produced, and these are generally mild.

Tolerogens

Another approach to the treatment of allergic manifestations is the use of agents which are capable of suppressing the production of IgE by inducing a state of tolerance (Katz, 1974, 1979; Sehon & Lee, 1979). Such agents have been called "tolerogens." These are synthetic compounds consisting of allergenic determinants linked to carriers. The carrier provides special properties which result in the induction of specific immunological tolerance to the allergenic component. The first of these to be described were (1) the synthetic copolymer D-glutamic, D-lysine (D-GL) (Katz, 1974), and (2) isologous gamma globulin. In the initial studies, haptenic derivatives were used such as the benzylpenicilloyl hapten of penicillin (BPO) which when linked to D-GL induced hapten-specific tolerance upon injection to mice. The tolerance induced to the haptens was irreversible and included not only the abrogation of IgE but also of IgG antibodies. To apply this principle to clinical problems it was desirable to synthesize protein D-GL conjugates such as pollens-D-GL and this has now been achieved using the primary antigen of ragweed, namely antigen E (AgE), to produce AgE-D-GL. When this conjugate was injected into mice which had been sensitized to AgE with the production of high IgE antibodies, it was possible to suppress the IgE antibody response, with little change in the IgG titer. It was further shown that mice so treated were unresponsive to further challenge with AgE. Clearly, this form of immunologic control may have great significance for the management of clinical allergy in that it would seem now possible to treat a specific allergy such as ragweed hay-fever resulting in a marked lowering of the IgE antibody titer, without interfering with the desired IgG-blocking antibody response, and presumably in an irreversible manner.

The first clinical study of this type of tolerogen was recently carried out by Butterfield, Gleich et al. (1981). They employed the nonimmunogenic carrier D-glutamic acid: D-lysine linked to short ragweed (SWR) fraction A (fraction A: D-GL). Three groups of 12 short ragweed sensitive patients were studied. The first, which consisted of 12 with seasonal symptoms, positive skin tests, and who had never received immunotherapy were given a 2-month course of fraction A: D-GL. The control group consisted of 14 patients sensitive to SWR with seasonal hay fever on no immunotherapy, and a third group of 13 SWR-sensitive patients with seasonal symptoms on their 4th year of standard immunotherapy with aqueous SWR. Although the mean symptom scores of the A: D-GL treated group did not differ from those on conventional therapy, and showed a significant decrease in skin test activity to both SWR and antigen E, the expected decrease in IgE did not occur. In contrast, fraction A: D-GL stimulated increases in both IgE and IgG responses, which were significantly greater than in the control groups. In addition mild urticaria and large local reactions were observed. It is, of course, possible that the particular preparation which was used may not have had quite the same characteristics as those used in previous animal studies.

Using a different method, namely the conjugation of an allergen with polyethylene glycol, Sehon and Lee (1978, 1979; Tse et al., 1978) have shown in a series of experiments in animals that these conjugates seem to fulfill the criteria of a tolerogen, since they appear to be nonantigenic, nonallergenic, and nonimmunogenic while still able to suppress the capacity of animals to mount primary as well as secondary IgE responses to diphenylated ovalbumin or of ragweed in an immunologically specific manner. Their most recent preparations, using a variety of antigens, include timothy grass and ragweed conjugated with monomethoxy polyethylene glycol are immunosuppressive and devoid of the antigenic properties of unmodified extracts. These findings have recently been confirmed (King et al., 1979).

As to their respective modes of action, it is interesting that one mechanism of D-GL is to suppress T_h or T helper cells, which induce the production of IgE. On the other hand, results of experiments with monomethoxy polyethylene glycol conjugates indicate that the prime mechanism is the stimulation of T_s or T suppressor cells, thereby preventing the production of IgE. It is also of interest from the standpoint of clinical application for these tolerogens that they do not seem to interfere with the existing levels of the other classes of immunoglobulins.

A number of novel approaches to immunotherapy have been intensively studied in animal experiments and show promise of clinical application. They are extremely interesting and are based on the proposition that atopic disease may represent a deficiency in the regulation of the production of IgE. This deficiency seems to be in the T suppressor lymphocyte of IgE (Chorazzi et al., 1977). In a series of somewhat complicated but highly interesting experiments, Katz (1979) and his co-workers have demonstrated the presence of a normal inhibitor of IgE production in low-responder mice, which is either present in low quantities or absent in high-responder mice. He has termed this the "suppressive factor of allergy" (SFA). It is important to emphasize that SFA is produced by living animals and is biologically active when passively transferred to living recipients. Although the basic reason why an individual should suddenly become allergic to a given allergen is not known, Katz has proposed a concept of what he terms "allergic breakthrough," which concerns the possible pathogenesis of the allergic phenotype (Katz, 1980).

REFERENCES

Aalberse RC, van der Gaag R, van Leeuwen J: Serologic aspects of IgG$_4$ antibodies. I. Prolonged immunization results in an IgG$_4$-restricted response. *J Immunol* 1983; 130:722.

Aaron TH, Muttitt ELC: Reactions to acetylsalicylic acid. *Can Med Assoc J* 1982; 126:609.

Aas K: Hyposensitization in house dust allergy asthma. *Acta Paediatr Scand* 1971; 60:264.

Aas K, Johansson SGO: The radioallergosorbent test (RAST) in the in vitro diagnosis of multiple reaginic allergy. *J Allergy Clin Immunol* 1971; 48:134.

Adkinson NF JR: The radioallergosorbent test in 1981—Limitations and refinements, editorial. *J Allergy Clin Immunol* 1981; 67:87.

Alexander HL: The history of allergy in immunological diseases in Samter M (ed): *Immunological Diseases*. Boston, Little, Brown & Co, 1965.

Allergy Statistics: NIAID, DHEW Publication No. (NIH) 75-757, 1974.

American Academy of Allergy: Position statements—Controversial techniques. *J Allergy Clin Immunol* 1981; 67:333.

Anderson CL, Spiegelberg HL: Macrophage receptors for IgE: Binding of IgE to specific IgE Fc receptors on human macrophage cell line, U937. *J Immunol* 1981; 126(6):2470.

Anderson Mc, Baer H: Antigenic and allergenic changes during storage of a pollen extract. *J Allergy Clin Immunol* 1982; 69:3.

Aspirin sensitivity in asthmatics, Editorial: *Br Med J* 1980; 281:958.

Austen KF: The Atopic Diseases: Definition and Comments, in Samter M (ed): *Immunological Diseases* ed 3. Boston, Little, Brown & Co, 1978a p 781.

Austen KF: The chemical mediators of immediate hypersensitivity reactions, in Samter M (ed): *Immunological Diseases*, ed 3. Boston, Little, Brown & Co, 1978b, p 183.

Austen KF: Chemical mediators originating from human mast cells: A commentary. *Clinical Allergy* 1980; 10 (Suppl):477.

Bach MK, Brashler JR: Ionophore A 23187-induced production of slow reacting substance of anaphylaxis (SRS-A) by rat peritoneal cells in vitro: Evidence for production by mononuclear cells. *J Immunol* 1978; 120:998.

Bass DA: The functions of eosinophils. *Ann Int Med* 1979; 91:120.

Basten A, Beeson PB: Mechanism of eosinophils: II. Role of the leucocyte. *J Exp Med* 1970; 131:1288.

Baxter JD, Rose B: The histamine content of allergic and non-allergic human nasal mucous membrane with simultaneous observations on the eosinophils. *J Allergy* 1953; 24:1.

Bazaral M, Orgel HA, Hamburger RN: IgE levels in normal infants and mothers and an inheritance hypothesis. *J Immunol* 1971; 107:794.

Beer DJ, Osband ME, McCaffrey RP, et al: Abnormal histamine-induced suppressor cell function in atopic subjects. *N Engl J Med* 1982; 306:454.

Beeson PB, Bass DA: *The Eosinophil.* Philadelphia, WB Saunders Co, 1977.

Befus AD, Pearce FL, Gauldie J, et al: Isolating and characteristics of mast cells from the lamina propria of the small bowel, in Pepys J, Edwards AM (ed): *The Mast Cell.* Kent, England, Pitman Medical Publishing Co, 1979. (pp 3)

Benacerraf B, McDevitt HO: Histocompatibility-linked immune response genes. *Science* 1972; 175:273.

Benveniste J, Camussi J, Polonsky J: Platelet-activating factor. *Monogr Allergy* 1977; 12:138.

Berdel D, Gast R, Huber B: The simplified oscillation method for measuring nasal resistance during provocation with allergens. *Clinical Allergy* 1981; 11:385.

Berg T, Johanssen SGO: Immunoglobulin levels in childhood with special regard to IgE. *Acta Paed Scand* 1969; 58:513.

Bienenstock J, Befus AD: Mucosal Immunology. *Immunology* 1980; 41:249.

Black MJ, Remsen KA: Rhinitis medicamentosa. *Can Med Assoc J* 1980; 122:881.

Blair H: A trial of ICI 74,917 in seasonal allergic rhinitis. *Clin Allergy* 1977; 7:397.

Boltz-Nitulescu G, Bazin H, Spiegelberg HL: Specifity of Fc receptors for IgG2a, IgG/IgG2b and IgE on rat macrophages. *J Exp Med* 1981; 154:374.

Boltz-Nitulescu G, Spiegelberg HL: Receptors specific for IgE on rat alveolar and peritoneal macrophages. *Cell Immunol* 1981; 59:1–6.

Borum P, Mygind N: Inhibition of the immediate allergic reaction in the nose by the beta-2 adrenostimulant fenoterol. *J Allergy Clin Immunol* 1980; 66:25.

Bostock J: Case of periodical affection of the eyes and chest. *Med Chir Trans* 1918; 10:161.

Brighton WD: Frequency of occurrence of IgG (ST-S). *Clinical Allergy* 1980; 10:97.

Brocklehurst WE: The release of histamine and formation of slow reacting substance (SRS-A) during anaphylactic shock. *J Physiol* 1960; 151:416.

Bromptom Hospital/MRC: Double blind trial comparing two dosage schedules of beclomethasone dipropionate aerosol with a placebo in the treatment of perennial rhinitis for 12 months. *Clinical Allergy* 1980; 10:239.

Bruyzeel PLB, Berrens L: IgE and IgG4 antibodies in specific human allergies. *Int Arch Allergy Appl Immunol* 1979; 58:344.

Buckley RH, Becker WG: Abnormalties in the regulating of human IgE synthesis. *Immunological Reviews* 1978; 41:288.

Burka JF, Paterson NA: Evidence for lipoxygenase pathway involvement in allergic tracheal contraction. *Prostaglandins* 1980; 19:499.

Butterfield JH, Gleich GJ, Yungiger JW, et al: Immunotherapy with short ragweed fraction A: D-glutamic acid: D-lysine polymer in ragweed hay fever. *J Allergy Clin Immunol* 1981; 67:272.

Butterworth AE, David JR: Eosinophile function. *N Eng J Med* 1981; 304:154.

Chignard M, LeCouedic JP, Vargaftig BB, et al: Platelet activating factor (PAF-acether) secretion from platelets: Effect of aggregating agents. *Brit J Haematol* 1980; 46:455.

Chorazzi N, Tung AS, Katz DH: Induction of a ragweed-specific allergic state in Ir gene-restricted non-responder mice. *J Exp Med* 1977; 146:302.

Chorazzi N, Fox DA, Katz DH: Hapten-specific IgE antibody responses in mice: VII. Conversion of IgE "responders" by elimination of suppressor T cell activity. *J Immunol* 1977; 118:48.

Church JA, Frenkel LD, Wright DG, et al: T-lymphocyte dysfunction, hyperimmunoglobulinemia E, recurrent bacterial infections and defective neutrophile chemotaxis in a Negro child. *J Pediatrics* 1976; 88:982.

Clark RAF, Gallin JS, Kaplan AP: The selective eosinophile chemotactic activity of histamine. *J Exp Med* 1975; 142:1462.

Clement PAR, Van Dishoeck A, Van de Wal J, et al: Nasal provocation and passive anterior rhinomanometry (PAR). *Clinical Allergy* 1981; 11:293.

Coca AF, Cooke RA: On the classification of the phenomenon of hypersensitiveness. *J Immunol* 1923; 8:163.

Cockroft DW, Hargreave FE, Dolovich J: Intranasal beclomethasone dipropionate in rhinitis, in Mygind N, Clark TJH (eds): *Topical Steroid Treatment for Asthma and Rhinitis.* London, Bailliere, Tindall, 1980.

Cockroft DW, MacCormack Newhouse MT: Beclomethasone dipropionate in allergic rhinitis. *Can Med Assoc J* 1976; 115:523.

Connell JT: Allergic rhinitis. Human experimental model. *NY St J Med* 1970; 70:1751.

Connell JT: Asthmatic deaths – Role of the mast cell. *JAMA* 1971; 215:769.

Connell JT: Histological classification of non-infectious and non-surgical nasal disease, in *Proceedings of the International Symposium, Infection and Allergy of the nose and Paranasal Sinuses.* Tokyo, SCIMED Publication, Inc, 1976, p 1.

Conrad DH, Froese A: Characterization of the target cell receptor for IgE: II. Polyacrilamide gell analysis of the surface IgE receptor from normal rat mast cells and from rat basophilic leucocytes. *J Immunol* 1976; 116:319.

Cooke RA, Barnard JH, Hebald S, Stull A: Serological evidence of immunity with co-existing sensitization in a type of human allergy (hay fever). *J Exp Med* 1935; 62:733.

Cooke RA, Stull A: Preparation and standardization of pollen extracts for the treatment of hay fever. *J Allergy* 1933; 4:87.

Cooke RA, Vander Veer A: Human sensitization. *J Immunol* 1916; 1:201.

Corey EJ, Clark DA, Goto G, et al: Stereospecific total synthesis of a "slow reacting substance of anaphylaxis," leukotriene C-1. *J Am Chem Soc* 1980; 102:1436.

Craig S, Rubinstein E, Reisman RE, et al: Treatment of ragweed hay fever with intranasally administered disodium cromoglycate. *Clin Allergy* 1977; 7:569.

Davis PB, Shelhamer JR, Kaliner M: Abnormal adrenergic and cholinergic sensitivity in cystic fibrosis. *N Eng J Med* 1980; 302:1453.

Demopoulos CA, Pinckard RN, Hanahan DJ: Platelet-activating factor. Evidence for 1-0-alkyl-2-acetyl-sn-glyceryl-3-phorylcholine as the active component (a new class of lipid chemical mediators). *J Biol Chem* 1979; 254:9355.

Deuschl H: Immunoglobulins in nasal secretion with special reference to IgE II. Seasonal studies of timothy-specific IgE antibody in patients with allergic rhinitis. *Internat Arch Allergy* 1976; 52:376.

Deuschl H, Drettner B: Nasal polyps treated by beclomethasone nasal aerosol. *Rhinology* 1977; 15:17.

Deuschl H, Johannsen SGO: Hyposensitization of patients with allergic rhinitis by intranasal administration of chemically modified grass pollen allergen. *Acta Allergol* 1977; 32:248.

Deuschl H, Johannsen SGO: Specific IgE antibodies in nasal secretion from patients with allergic rhinitis and with negative or weakly positive RAST on the serum. *Clin Allergy* 1977; 7:195.

Deuschl H, Johannsen SGO, Fagerberg E: IgE, IgG and IgA antibodies in serum and nasal secretion during parenteral hyposensitization. *Clin Allergy* 1977; 7:315.

De Weck AL, Schneider CH, Spengler H, et al: Inhibition of allergic reactions by monovalent haptens, in Goodfriend AH, Sehon AH, Orange RP (eds): *Mechanisms in Allergy (Reagin Mediated Hypersensitivity Immunology Series* vol 1. p 323. New York, Marcel Dekker, 1973.

Dolovich J, Hargreave FE, Chalmers R, et al: Late cutaneous allergic reactions in isolated IgE-dependent reactions. *J Allergy Clin Immunol* 1973; 52:38.

Dolovich J, Tomasi TB, Arbesman CE: Antibodies of nasal and parotid secretions of ragweed allergic subjects. *J Allergy* 1970; 45:286.

Drazen JM, Austen KF, Lewis RA, et al: Comparative airway and vascular activities of leukotrienes C-1 and D in vivo and in vitro. *Proc Natl Acad Sci USA* 1980; 77:4354.

Eidenger D, Raff M, Rose B: Tissue eosinophilia in hypersensitivity reactions as revealed by the human skin window. *Nature (London)* 1962; 196:683.

Eidenger D, Wilkinson R, Rose B: A study of cellular responses in immune reaction utilizing the skin window technique. *J Allergy* 1964; 35:77.

Evans R, Pence H, Kaplan H, et al: The effect of immunotherapy on humoral and cellular responses in ragweed hay fever. *J Clin Invest* 1976; 57:735.

Feldberg W, Kellaway CH: Liberation of histamine and formation of lysolecithin-like substances from cobra venom. *J Physiol* 1938; 94:187.

Feltkamp-Vroom TM, Stallman PJ, Aalberse RC, et al: Immunofluorescence studies on renal tissue, tonsils, adenoids, nasal polyps and skin of atopic and non-atopic patients, with specific reference to IgE. *Clin Immunol Immunopathol* 1975; 4:392.

Findlay SR, Lichtenstein LM, Hanahan DJ, Pinckard RN: Contraction of guinea pig ileal smooth muscle by acetyl glyceryl ether phosphorylcholine. *Am J Physiol* 1981; 241:C130.

Foucard T, Johanssen SGO, Bennicu H, et al: In vitro estimation of allergens by a radioimmune antiglobulin technique using human IgE antibodies. *Int Arch Allergy Appl Immunol* 1973; 43:360.

Frankland AW, Augustin R: Prophylaxis of summer hay fever and asthma. Controlled trial comparing crude grass pollen extracts with isolated main protein component. *Lancet* 1954; 1:1055.

Franklin W, Goetzl EJ: Total absence of eosinophiles in a patient with an allergic disorder. *Ann Int Med* 1981; 94:352.

Franklin W, Lowell FC: Comparison of two dosages of ragweed extract in the treatment of pollenosis. *JAMA* 1967; 201:915.

Fraser CM, Venter JC, Kaliner M: Autonomic abnormalities and autoantibodies to beta-adrenergic receptors. *N Eng J Med* 1981; 305:1165.

Frostad AB: The treatment of seasonal allergic rhinitis with a 2% aqueous solution of sodium cromoglycate delivered by a metered dose nasal spray. *Clin Allergy* 1977; 7:347.

Fuchs AM, Strauss MB: The clinical evaluation and preparation and standardization of suspensions of new water insoluble whole ragweed pollen complex. *J Allergy* 1959; 30:66.

Geha RS, Reinherz E, Leung D, McKee KJ, Jr., Schlossman S, Rosen FS: Deficiency of suppressor T cells in the hyperimmunoglobulin E syndrome. *J Clin Invest* 1981, 68:783.

Glovsky MM, Hugli TE, Ishizaka T, et al: Anaphylatoxin-induced histamine release with human leucocytes: Studies of C3a leucocyte binding and histamine release. *J Clin Invest* 1979; 64:804.

Goetzl EJ: Mediators of immediate hypersensitivity derived from arachidonic acid. *N Eng J Med* 1980; 303:822.

Goetzl EJ, Austen KF: Purification and synthesis of eosinophilotactic tetrapeptides of human lung tissue: Identification as eosinophil chemotactic factor of anaphylaxis. *Proc Natl Acad Sci (USA)* 1975; 72:4123.

Goetzl EJ, Woods JM, Gorman RR: Stimulation of human eosinophile and neutrofil polymorphonuclear leucocyte chemotaxis and random migration by 12-L-hydroxy-5, 8, 10, 14-eicosatetraenoic acid. *J Clin Inv* 1977; 59:179.

Goetzl EJ, Pickett WC: The human PMN leukocyte chemotactic activity of complex hydroxy-eicosatetraenoic acids (HETEs). *J Immunol* 1980; 125:1789.

Golden DBK, Valentine MD, Kagey-Sobotka A, et al: Regimens of Hymenoptera venom immunotherapy. *Ann Int Med* 1980; 92:620.

Gonzales-Molina A, Spielgelberg HL: A subpopulation of normal human peripheral B lymphocytes that bind IgE. *J Clin Invest* 1977; 59:616.

Goodfriend L, Roebber M, Lundkvist U, et al: Two variants of ragweed allergen Ra3. *J Allergy Clin Immunol* 1981; 67:299.

Guercio JP, Birch S, Fernandez RJ, et al: Deposition of ragweed pollen and extract on nasal mucosa of patients with allergic rhinitis: Effect of nasal airflow resistance and nasal mucus velocity. *J Allergy Clin Immunol* 1980; 66:61.

Gwynn CM, Morrison Smith J, Leon Leon G, et al: IgE and IgG4 subclass in atopic families. *Clin Allergy* 1979; 9:119.

Halonen M, Palmer JD, Lohman IC, et al: Respiratory and circulatory alterations induced by acetyl glyceryl ether phosphorylcholine (AGEPC), a mediator of IgE anaphylaxis in the rabbit. *Amer Rev Resp Dis* 1980; 122:915.

Hansel FK: Coseasonal intracutaneous treatment of hay-fever. *J Allergy* 1941; 12:457.

Harding SM, Heath S: Intranasal steriod aerosol in perennial rhinitis: comparison with an antihistamine compound. *Clin Allergy* 1976; 6:369.

Harper TB, Gaumer HR, Waring W, et al: A comparison of cell mediated immunity and suppressor T cell function in asthmatic and normal children. *Clin Allergy* 1980; 10:555.

Hastie R, Heroy JH, Levy DA: Basophil leucocytes and mast cells in human nasal secretions and scrapings studies by light microscopy. *Lab Invest* 1979; 40:554.

Henderson AT, Rose B: Pyribenzamine (n-Pyridl, N-Benzyl, Dimenthyl-Ethylenediamine Hydrochloride) in the treatment of allergy. *Cdn Med Ass J* 1947; 57:136.

Henderson WR, Shelhamer JH, Reingold DB, et al: Alpha-adrenergic hyper-responsiveness in asthma. *N Eng J Med* 1979; 300:642.

Hendrix SG, Patterson R, Zeiss CR, et al: Further studies on the safety of polymerized antigens for immunotherapy. *J Allergy Clin Immunol* 1981; 67:124.

Hendrix SG, Zeiss R, Levitz D, et al: Polymerized whole ragweed: A two year follow-up of patients treated with an improved method of immunotherapy. *J Allergy Clin Immunol* 1980; 65:57.

Henson PM, Pinckard RN: Platelet activating factor (PAF). A possible direct mediator of anaphylaxis in the rabbit and a trigger for the vasculator deposition of circulating immune complexes. *Monogr Allergy* 1977; 12:13.

Herxheimer H: Bronchial hypersensitization and hyposensitization in man. *Int Arch Allergy Appl Immunol* 1951; 2:40.

Hiley CR, Wilson H, Yates MS: Identification of beta-adreno receptors and histamine receptors in the cat nasal vasculature. *Acta Otolaryngol (Stocjh)* 1978; 85:444.

Hill LW: Certain aspects of allergy in children. *N Eng J Med* 1961; 265:1194.

Hirsch SR, Kalbfleisch JH, Golbert TM, et al: Rinkel injection therapy: A multicenter controlled study. *J Allergy Clin Immunol* 1981; 68:113.

Holgate ST, Lewis RA, Maguire JF, Roberts LJ II, Oates JA, Austen KF: Effects of prostaglandin D_2 on rat serosal mast cells: Discordance between immunologic mediator release and cyclic AMP levels. *J Immunol* 1980; 125:1367.

Hugli TE: The complement anaphylatoxin, in Hofstaetter T, Schorlemmer HU (eds): *Topics of Allergology.* Behring Institute Mittellungen (BIM), 1981; 68:68.

Ishizaka K: Cellular events in the IgE antibody response. *Advances in Immunol* 1976; 23:1.

Ishizaka K, Ishizaka T: Identification of IgE as carrier of reaginic activity. *J Immunol* 1967; 99:1187.

Ishizaka K, Ishizaka T, Hornbrook MM: Physico-chemical properties of reaginic antibody V. Correlation of reaginic activity with gamma E-globulin antibody (for gamma-type Y). *J Immunol* 1966; 97:840.

Ishizaka T: Analysis of triggering events in mast cells for immunoglobulin E-mediated histamine release. *J Allergy Clin Immunol* 1981; 67:90.

Ishizaka T, Ishizaka K, Conrad DH, et al: A new concept of IgE histamine release. *J Allergy Clin Immunol* 1978; 61:320.

Jacobs RL, Freedman PM, Boswell RN: Nonallergic rhinitis with eosinophilia (NARES syndrome). *J Allergy Clin Immunol* 1981; 67:253.

Johannsen SGO, Berglund A, Kjellman N-IM: Comparison of IgE values as determined by different solid phase radioimmunoassay methods. *Clin Immunol* 1976; 6:91.

Johannsen SGO, Deuschl H, Zeterstrom O: The use of glutaraldehyde modified timothy grass pollen extract in nasal hyposensitization treatment of hay fever. *Int Arch Allergy Appl Immunol* 1979; 60:477.

Johanssen SGO, Miller ACML, Overell BG, et al: Changes in serum antibody levels during treatment with grass pollen-tyrosine adsorbate. *Clin Allergy* 1974; 4:57.

Johnson P, Marsh DG: Allergens from common rye grass pollen *(Lolium perenne)*: I. Chemical composition and structure. *Immunochemistry* 1966; 3:91.

Johnstone DE, Dutton A: The value of hyposensitization therapy for bronchial asthma in children—a 14 year old study. *Pediatrics* 1968; 43:793.

Kaliner MA: The cholinergic nervous system and immediate hypersensitivity: I. Eccrine sweat responses in allergic patients. *J Allergy Clin Immunol* 1976; 58:308.

Kaliner MA: Is a mast cell a mast cell a mast cell? *J Allergy Clin Immunol* 1980; 66:1.

Kaliner M, Orange RP, Austen KF: Immunologic release of histamine and slow reacting substance of anaphylaxis from human lung: IV. Enhancement by cholinergic and alpha adrenergic stimulation. *J Exp Med* 1972; 136:556.

Kaliner MA, Wasserman SI, Austen KF: Immunologic release of chemical mediators from human nasal polyps. *N Eng J Med* 1973; 289:277.

Katz DH: Hapten-specific tolerance induced by the DNP derivative of D-Glutamic acid and D-Lysine (D-GL) copolymer, in Katz DH, Benacerra FB (eds): *Immunological Tolerance: Mechanisms and Potential Therapeutic Applications,* New York, Academic Press, 1974, p 189.

Katz DH: New concepts concerning the clinical control of IgE synthesis. *Clin Allergy* 1979; 9:609.

Katz DH: Recent studies on the regulation of IgE antibody synthesis in experimental animals and man. *Immunology* 1980; 41:1.

Kay AB, Shin HS, Austen KF: Selection of eosinophiles, and synergism between eosinophile chemotactic factor of anaphylaxis (ECF-A) and a fragment cleaved from the fifth component of complement (C5a). *Immunol* 1973; 24:969.

Kay AB, Stechschulte DJ, Austen KF: An eosinophile leukocyte chemotactic factor of anaphylaxis. *J Exp Med* 1971; 133:602.

Kelly JF, Zeiss CR, Patterson R, et al: Polymerized whole ragweed: Human safety and immune response. *J Allergy Clin Immunol* 1980; 65:50.

King TP, Kochoumian, Chorazzi N: Immunological properties of conjugates of ragweed pollen antigen E with methoxypolyethylene glycol or a copolymer of D-glutamic acid and D-lysine. *J Exper Med* 1979; 149:424.

King TP, Norman PS, Tao N: Chemical modifications of the major allergen of ragweed pollen: Antigen E. *Immunochemistry* 1974; 11:83.

Knight A, Underdown BJ: Disodium cromoglycate in ragweed allergic rhinitis. *J Allergy Clin Immunol* 1975; 55:(abstracted) 116.

Knight A, Underdown BJ, Connell JT, et al: Immunological parameters in perennial rhinitis. *Clin Allergy* 1979; 9:159.

Lapkoff CB, Goodfriend L: Isolation of a low molecular weight ragweed pollen antigen: Ra-5. *Int Arch Allergy Clin Immunol* 1974; 46:215.

Lee TH, Brown MJ, Nagy L, Causon R, Walport MJ, Kay AB: Exercise-induced release at histamine and neutrophil chemotactic factor in atopic asthmatics. *J Allergy Clin Immunol* 1982; 70:73.

Levine BB, Vaz NM: Effect of combinations of inbred strain, antigen and antigen dose on immune responsiveness and regin production in the mouse. *Int Arch Allergy Appl Immunol* 1970; 39:156.

Lewis RA, Austen KF: Mediation of local homeostasis and inflammation by leukotrienes and other mast cell-dependent compounds. *Nature* 1981; 293:103.

Lewis RA, Austen KF, Drazen JM, Clark DA, Marfat A, Corey EJ: Slow reacting substances of anaphylaxis: Identification of leukotrienes C1 and D from human and rat sources. *Proc Natl Acad Sci USA* 1980a; 77:3710.

Lewis RA, Drazen JM, Austen KF, et al: Identification of the C(6)-S-conjugate of leukotriene A with cysteine as a naturally occurring slow reactive substance of anaphylaxis (SRS-A). Importance of the 11-*cis*-geometry for biological activity. *Biochem Biophys Res Commun* 1980; 96:271.

Lewis RA, Soter NA, Diamond PT, Austen KF, Oates JA, Roberts LJ II: Prostaglandin D^2 generation after activation of rat and human mast cells with anti-IgE. *J Immunol* 1982; 129:1627.

Lichtenstein LM, Ishizaka K, Norman PS, et al: IgE antibody measurements in ragweed hay fever: Relationship to clinical severity and the results of immunotherapy. *J Clin Invest* 1973; 52:472.

Lichtenstein LM, Mamburger RN: IgE and atopic disease, in Samter M (ed): *Immunological Diseases* Boston, Little, Brown & Company, 1978, p 804.

Lichtenstein LM, Norman PS, Winkenwerder WL, et al: "In vitro" studies of human ragweed allergy: Changes in cellular and humoral activity associated with specific desentization. *J Clin Invest* 1966; 45:1126.

Lowell FC, Franklin W: A "double blind" study of the effectiveness and specifity of injection therapy in ragweed hay fever. *N Eng J Med* 1965; 273:675.

Malmberg CHO, Holopainen EEA, Stenius-Aarniala BSM: Relationship between nasal and conjunctival tests in patients with allergic rhinitis. *Clin Allergy* 1978; 8:397.

Manners B, Ezeoke A: Serum IgE levels and the use of sodium cromoglycate in hay fever: A study of 46 patients from a single general practice. *Clin Allergy* 1973; 3:311.

Marsh DG, Bias WB, Hsu, SH, et al: Associations between major histocompatibility (HK-A) antigens and specific reaginic antibody responses in allergic men. In Goodfriend L, Sehan AH, Orange RP (eds): Mechanisms in Allergy: Reagin-Mediated Hypersensitivity. New York, Marcel Decker, Inc., 1973.

Marsh DG, Hsu SH, Hussain R, et al: Genetics of human response to allergens. *J Allergy Clin Immunol* 1980; 65:322.

Marsh DG, Lichtenstein LM, Campbell DH: Studies on "allergoids" prepared from naturally occurring allergens: I. Assay of allergenicity and antigenicity of formalized rye group I component. *Immunol* 1970; 18:705.

Mathews KP, Bayne NK, Banas JM: A controlled study of intranasal immunotherapy with polymerized ragweed antigen. *J Allergy Clin Immunol* 1980; 65:191.

Melewicz FM, Spiegelberg HL: Fc receptors for IgE on a subpopulation of human peripheral blood monocytes. *J Immunol* 1980; 125:1026.

Melewicz FM, Zeiger RS, Mellon MH, et al: Increased peripheral blood monocytes with Fc receptors for IgE in patients with severe allergic disorders. *J Immunol* 1981; 126:1592.

Metzger WJ, Dorminey HC, Richerson HB, et al: Clinical and immunologic evaluation of glutaraldehyde-modified tyrosine-absorbed short ragweed extract: A double-blind placebo-controlled study. *J Allergy Clin Immunol* 1981; 68:442.

Michaelson G. Juhlin L: Urticaria induced by preservatives and dye additives in food and drugs. *Br J Derm* 1973; 88:525.

Miller ACML: A comparative trial of hyposensitization in 1973 in the treatment of hay fever using Pollinex and Alavac -P. *Clin Allergy* 1976; 6:551.

Minor T, Dick E, De Meo AN, et al: Viruses as precipitants of asthmatic attacks in children. *JAMA* 1974; 227:292.

Mole LE, Goodfriend L, Lapkoff CB, et al: The aminoacid sequence of ragweed pollen Ra 5. *Biochemistry* 1981; 14:1216.

Mullarkey MF: The classification of nasal disease: An opinion, editorial. *J Allergy Clin Immunol* 1981; 67:251.

Mullarkey MF, Hill JS Webb DR: Allergic and non allergic rhinitis: Their characterization with attention to the meaning of nasal eosinophilia. *J Allergy Clin Immunol* 1980; 65:122.

Munch E, Gomez G, Harris C, et al: An open comparison of dosage frequencies of beclomethasone dipropionate in seasonal allergic rhinitis. *Clin Allergy* 1981; 11:303.

Murphy RC, Hammarstrom S, Samuelsson B: Leukotriene C: A slow-reacting substance from murine mastocytoma cells. *Proc Natl Acad Sci* 1979; 76:4275.

Mygind N: Local effect of intranasal beclomethasone dipropionate aerosol in hay fever. *Br Med J* 1973; 4:464.

Mygind N: *Nasal Allergy,* ed 2. Oxgord, Blackwell Scientific Publications, 1979.

Mygind N, Pederson CB, Prytz S: Treatment of nasal polyps with intranasal beclomethasone dipropionate aerosol. *Clin Allergy* 1975; 5:159.

McDevitt HO: Current concepts: Regulation of the immune response by the major histocompatibility system. *N Eng J Med* 1980; 303:1514.

McFadden ER Jr: Beta[2] receptor agonist, metabolism and pharmacology. *J Allergy Clin Immunol* 1981; 68:91.

McIntosh K, Ellis EF, Hoffman LS, et al: The association of viral and bacterial respiratory infections with exacerbations of wheezing in young asthmatic children. *J Pediatr* 1973; 82:578.

Neuman I, Elian R, Nahum H, et al: The danger of "yellow" dyes (tartrazine) to allergic subjects. *Clin Allergy* 1978; 8:65.

Nickelsen JA, Goldstein S, Mueller U, et al: Local intranasal immunotherapy for ragweed allergic rhinitis: I. Clinical response. *J Allergy Clin Immunol* 1981; 68:33.

Nickelsen JA, Goldstein S, Mueller U, et al: Local intranasal immunotherapy for ragweed allergic rhinitis: II. Immunologic response. *J Allergy Clin Immunol* 1981; 68:41.

Noon L: Prophylactic inoculation for hay fever. *Lancet* 1911; 1:1572.

Norman PS: An overview of immunotherapy: Implications for the future. *J Allergy Clin Immunol* 1980; 65:87.

Norman PS, Lichtenstein LM: Comparisons of alum-precipitated and unprecipitated aqueous ragweed pollen extracts in the treatment of hay fever. *J Allergy Clin Immunol* 1978; 61:384.

Norman PS, Lichtenstein LM, Marsh DG: Studies on allergoids from naturally occurring allergens: IV. Efficacy and safety of long-term allergoid treatment of ragweed hay-fever. *J Allergy Clin Immunol* 1981; 68:460.

Norman PS, Marsh DG, Lichtenstein LM: Long-term immunotherapy with ragweed allergen and allergoid. *J Allergy Clin Immunol* 1979; 63:167.

Norman PS, Winkenwerder W, Lichtenstein LM: Immunotherapy of hay fever with ragweed antigen E: Comparisons with whole pollen extract and placebo. *J Allergy* 1968; 42:93.

Norn S, Shore PA: Failure to affect tissue reserpine concentrations by alteration of adrenergic nerve activity. *Biochem Pharmacol* 1971; 20:2133.

Okuda M, Mygind N: Pathophysiological basis for topical steroid treatment in the nose, in Mygind N, Clark TJH, (eds): *Topical Steroid Treatment for Asthma and Rhinitis*. London, Bailliere & Tindall, 1980.

Okuda M, Ohtsuka H: Electron microscopy study of basophilic cells in allergic nasal secretions. *Arch Otorhinolaryngol* 1978; 221:215.

Orange RP: Immunopharmacological aspects of bronchial asthma. *Clin Immunol* 1973; 3(suppl):521.

Orange RP, Austen KF: Slow reacting substance of anaphylaxis. *Adv Immunol* 1969; 10:105.

Orange RP, Austen WG, Austen KF: Immunological release of histamine and slow reacting substance of anaphylaxis from human lung: I. Modulation by agents influencing cellular levels of cyclic 3'5' adenosine monophosphate. *J Exp Med* 1971; 134:136.

Orange RP, Moore EG, Gelfand EW: The formation and release of slow reacting substance of anaphylaxis (SRS-A) by rat and mouse peritoneal mononuclear cells induced by ionophore A23187. *J Immunol* 1980; 124:2264.

Orange RP, Murphy RC, Karnofsky ML, et al: The physicochemical characteristics and purification of slow reacting substance of anaphylaxis. *J Immunol* 1973; 110:760.

Osler AG: The C3 shunt participation in allergic tissue injury, in Goodfriend, Sehon A, Orange RP (eds): *Mechanisms in Allergy; Reagin-Mediated Hypersensitivity*. New York, Marcel Dekker, Inc, 1973.

Parish WE: Short term anaphylactic IgG antibodies in human serum. *Lancet* 1970; 2:591.

Parish WE: Detection of reaginic and short-term sensitizing anaphylactic or anaphylactoid antibodies to mild in sera of allergic and normal persons. *Clin Allergy* 1971; 1:369.

Parish WE: Studies on vasculitis: IV. The low incidence of antibacterial anaphylactic antibodies in the sera of persons with cutaneous casculitis following bacterial infection. *Clin Allergy* 1971; 1:433.

Patel KR, Kerr JW: The airways response to phenylephrine after blockade of alpha and beta receptors in extrinsic bronchial asthma. *Clin Allergy* 1973; 3:439.

Patel KR, Kerr JW: Effect of alpha receptor blocking drug thymoxamine on allergen induced bronchoconstriction in extrinsic asthma. *Clin Allergy* 1975; 5:311.

Patterson R: Allergen immunotherapy with modified allergens. *J Allergy Clin Immunol* 1981; 68:85.

Pepys J, Turner-Warwick M, Dawson PL, et al: Arthus (type III) reactions in man. Clinical and immunopathological features. *Allergology Excerpta Med Inter Cong Ser* 1968; 162:221.

Pepys J, Roth A, Carroll KB: RAST, skin and nasal tests and the history in grass pollen allergy. *Clin Allergy* 1975; 5:431.

Platts-Mills TAE: Local production of IgG, IgA and IgE antibodies in grass pollen hay fever. *J Immunol* 1979; 122:2218.

Platts-Mills TAE, Von Maur RK, Ishizaka K, et al: IgA and IgG anti-ragweed antibodies in nasal secretions: Quantitative measurements of antibodies and correlation with inhibition of histamine release. *J Clin Invest* 1976; 57:1041.

Posey WC, Nelson HS: Controlled trials with 4% cromolyn spray in seasonal allergic rhinitis. *Clin Allergy* 1977; 7:485.

Potter M, Boyce CR: Induction of plasma-cell neoplasms in strain BALB/C mice with mineral oil and mineral oil adjuvants. *Nature (London)* 1962; 193:1087.

Prausnitz C, Kustner H: Studien uber die Uberempfindlichkeit. *Z Bakt* 1921; 86:160.

Reinherz EL, Schlossman SF: The differentiation and function of human T Lymphocytes. *Cell* 1980; 19:8.

Richerson HB, Rajtova DW, Perrick GD, et al: Cutaneous and nasal responses in ragweed hay fever: Lack of clinical and histopathologic correlations with late phase responses. *J Allergy Clin Immunol* 1979; 64:67.

Richter M, Harter JG, Sehon AH, et al: Studies on ragweed pollen: III. Estimation of the minimum number of allergens in the water soluble extract of ragweed pollen and a critical evaluation of the neutralization technique. The demonstration of two different reagins in sera of ragweed sensitive individuals. *J Immunol* 1957; 79:13.

Rinkel HJ: Inhalant allergy: III. The coseasonal application of serial dilution testing (titration). *Ann Allergy* 1949; 7:639.

Rinkel HJ: Inhalation allergy: I. The whealing response of the skin to serial dilution testing.*Ann Allergy* 1949; 7:625.

Rocklin RE, Breard J, Gupta S, et al: Characterization of the human blood lymphocytes that produce a histamine-induced suppressor factor (HSF). *Cell Immunol* 1980; 51:226.

Rocklin RE, Sheffer AL, Greineder DK, et al: Generation of antigen-specific suppressor cells during allergy desensitization. *N Eng J Med* 1980; 302:1213.

Rose B: Studies on the role of histamine in hypersensitivity to cold. *J Clin Invest* 1948; 27:553.

Rose B, Harkness EV, Forbes RP: Plasma histaminase in pregnancy. *Annual Report of the John and Mary Markle Foundation,* 1946; p 69.

Rose B. Hogg JC, Macklem P: The pathogenesis of bronchial asthma, in Samter M (ed): *Immunological Diseases.* Boston, Little, Brown & Co, 1978, p 852.

Rose B, Rusted I, Fownes JA: Intravascular catheterization studies on bronchial asthma: I. Histamine levels in arterial and mixed venous blood of asthmatic patients before and during induced attacks. *J Clin Inv* 1950; 29:1113.

Rouzer CA, Scott WA, Cohn ZA, et al: Mouse peritoneal macrophages release leukotriene C in response to a phagocytic stimulus. *Proc Natl Acad Sci USA* 1980; 77:4928.

Rouzer CA, Scott WA, Hamill AL, et al: Dynamics of leukotriene C production by macrophages. *J Exper Med* 1980; 125:1236.

Sahay JN, Chatterjee SS, Engler C: A comparative trial of flunisolide and beclomethasone dipropionate in the treatment of perennial allergic rhinitis. *Clin Allergy* 1980; 10:65.

Sahay JN, Ibrahim NBN, Chatterjee SS, et al: Long term study of flunisolide treatment in perennial rhinitis with special reference to nasal mucosal histology and morphology. *Clin Allergy* 1980; 10:451.

Sale SR, Roach DE, Zeiss CR, et al: Clinical and immunologic correlations in trimellitic anhydride airway syndromes. *J Allergy Clin Immunol* 1981; 68:188.

Samter M: Eosinophils—Nominated but not elected, editorial. *N Eng J Med* 1980; 303:1175.

Samter M, Beers RF Jr: Intolerance to aspirin. *Ann Int Med* 1968; 68:975.

Samter M, Wasserman SI: Eosinophils, in Samter M (ed): *Immunological Diseases,* ed 2. Boston, Little, Brown & Co, 1978, p 230.

Samuelsson B. Hammarstrom S, Murphy RC, et al: Leukotrienes and slow reacting substance of anaphylaxis (SRS-A). *Allergy*1980; 34:375.

Santrach PJ, Parker, JL, Jones RT, Yunginger JW: Diagnostic and therapeutic applications of a modified radio allergosorbent test and comparison with the conventional radioallergosorbent test. *J Allergy Clin Immunol* 1981; 67:97.

Schultz JI, Johnson JD, Freedman SO: Double-blind trial comparing flunisolide and placebo for the treatment of perennial rhinitis. *Clin Allergy* 1978; 8:313.

Schumacher MJ: Effect of a beta-adrenergic agonist, fenoterol, on nasal sensitivity of allergen. *J Allergy Clin Immunol* 1980; 66:33.

Sears MR, Chow CM, Morseth DJ: Serum total IgE in normal subjects and the influence of a family history of allergy. *Clin Allergy* 1980; 10:423.

Sehon AH, Lee WY: Tolerance induction in immediate hypersensitivity. *Clin Allergy* 1979; 9:625.

Settipane GA, Chaffee GH: Nasal polyps in asthma and rhinitis. *J Allergy Clin Immunol* 1977; 59:17.

Shelhamer JH, Metcalfe DD, Smith LJ, et al: Abnormal beta adrenergic responses in allergic subjects: Analysis of isoproterenol-induced cardiovascular and cyclic adenosine monophosphate responses. *J Allergy Clin Immunol* 1980; 66:52.

Sobotka AK, Valentine MD, Lichtenstein LM: Measurement of IgG antibodies: Development and application of a radioimmunoassay. *J Immunol* 1976; 117:84.

Sok DE, Pai JK, Atrache V, Kang VC, Sih CJ: *Biochem Biophys Res Commun* 1981; 101:222.

Solley GE, Gleich GJ, Jordon RE, et al: The late phase of the immediate wheal-and-flare reaction: Its dependence on IgE antibodies. *J Clin Invest* 1976; 58:408.

Stanworth DR, Smith AK: Inhibition of reagin-mediated PCA reactions in baboons by the human IgG4 subclass. *Clin Allergy* 1973; 3:37.

Stenius RSM, Lemola M: Hypersensitivity to acetylsalicylic acid (ASA) and tartrazine in patients with asthma. *Clin Allergy* 1976; 6:119.

Stevenson DD, Simon RA, Mathison DA: Aspirin-sensitive asthma: Tolerance to aspirin after positive oral aspirin challenges. *J Allergy Clin Immunol* 1980; 66:82.

Stimler NP, Brocklehurst WE, Bloor CM, et al: Anaphylatoxin mediated contraction of Guinea pig lung strips: A non-histamine tissue response. *J Immunol* 1981; 126:2258.

Symington IS, O'Neill D, Kerr JW: Comparison of a glutaraldehyde-modified pollen-tyrosine adsorbate with an alum-precipitated pollen vaccine in the treatment of hay fever. *Clin Allergy* 1977; 7:103.

Tada T: Regulation of reaginic antibody in animals. *Progress in Allergy* 1975; 19:122.

Tauber AI, Kaliner M, Stechschulte DJ, et al: Immunological release of histamine and slow reacting substance of anaphylaxis from human lung: V. Effects of prostaglandins on release of histamine. *J Immunol* 1973; 111:27.

Taylor G: Allergic diseases of the upper respiratory tract. *Clin Allergy* 1973; 3(Supp):639.

Taylor G, Shivalkor PR: Changes in nasal airways resistance on antigenic challenge in allergic rhinitis. *Clin Allergy* 1971; 1:63.

Tomasi TB Jr, Larson L, Challacombe S, et al: Mucosal immunity: The origin and migration patterns of cells in the secretory system. *J Allergy Clin Immunol* 1980; 65:12.

Tse KS, Kepron W, Sehon AH: Effects of tolerogenic conjugates in a canine model for reaginic hypersensitivity. *J Allergy Clin Immunol* 1978; 61:303.

Tse KS, Wicher K, Arbesman CE: Effect of immunotherapy on appearance of antibodies to ragweed in external secretions. *J Allergy* 1973; 51:208.

Unkeless JC, Eisen HN: Binding of monomeric immunoglobulins to Fc receptors of mouse macrophages. *J Exp Med* 1975; 142:1520.

Unkeless JC, Kaplan G, Plutner H, et al: Fc-receptor variants of a mouse macrophage cell line. *Proc Natl Acad Sci USA* 1979; 76:1400.

Vane JR: Inhibition of prostaglandin synthetase as a mechanism of action for aspirin-like drugs. *Nature New Biol* 1971; 231:232.

Van Metre TE Jr, Adkinson NF, Amadio FJ, et al: A comparison of immunotherapy schedules for injection treatment of ragweed pollen hay fever. *J Allergy Clin Immunol* 1982; 69:181.

Van Metre TE Jr, Adkinson NF, Lichtenstein LM, et al: A controlled study of the effectiveness of the Rinkel method of immunotherapy for ragweed pollen hay fever. *J Allergy Clin Immunol* 1980; 65:288.

Vaughan WT: Specific treatment of hay-fever during the attack. *JAMA* 1923; 80:245.

Vaz NM, Levine BB: Immune responses of inbred mice to repeated low doses of antigen. Relationship to histocompatibility (H-2) type. *Science* 1970; 168:852.

Venter JC, Fraser CM, Harrison LC: Autoantibodies to B^2-adrenergic receptors: a possible cause of adrenergic hyporesponsiveness in allergic rhinitis and asthma. *Science* 1980; 207:1361.

Verstraeten JM, Wheeler AW: A comparative study of an aqueous grass pollen extract and glutaraldehyde-treated grass pollen-tyrosine adsorbate in the treatment of pollenosis. *Clin Allergy* 1978; 8:435.

Vilsvik JS, Jenssen AO: The effect of a new anti-allergic drug ICI 74, 917 given by aerosol, on nasal stenosis induced by allergen. *Clin Allergy* 1976; 6:487.

Walker WS: Separate Fc receptors for immunoglobulins IgG2a and IgG2b on an established cell line of mouse macrophages. *J Immunol* 1976; 116:911.

Walton CH, Randle DL: Aspirin allergy. *Can Med Assoc J* 1957; 76:1016.

Wasserman SI: Mediators of immediate hypersensitivity. *J Allergy Clin Immunol* 1983; 72:101.

Wasserman SI, Goetzl EJ, Austen KF: Inactivation of slow reacting substance of anaphylaxis by human eosinophile arylsulfatase. *J Immunol* 1975; 114:645.

Webb DR: Clinical characteristics and therapy of nasal polyps. *J Allergy Clin Immunol* 1978; 59:85.

Webb DR: Clinical characteristics and therapy of nasal polyps. *J Allergy Clin Immunol* 1978; 61:185.

Weiner N: Norepinephrine, epinephrine and the sympathomimetic amine, in Goodman, Gilman (eds): *The Pharmacological Basis of Therapeutics.* New York, MacMillan Publishing Co, Inc, 1980, p 138.

Weliky N, Heiner DC: Hypersensitivity to chemicals. Correlation of tartrazine hypersensitivity with characteristic serum IgD and IgE immune response patterns. *Clin Allergy* 1980; 10:375.

Welliver RC, Wong DT, Sun M, et al: The development of respiratory syncytial virus-specific IgE and the release of histamine in nasopharyngeal secretions after infection. *N Eng J Med* 1981; 305:841.

Welsh PW, Zimmermann EM, Yunginger JW, et al: Preseasonal intranasal immunotherapy with nebulized short ragweed extract. *J Allergy Clin Immunol* 1981; 67:237.

Whelan CJ: Problems in the examination of nasal smears in allergic rhinitis. *J Laryngol Otol* 1980; 94:399.

WHO Memorandum: Use and abuse of eight widely-used diagnostic procedures in clinical immunology. *Bulletin of the World Health Organization* 1981; 59:717.

Wide L, Bennich H, Johanssen SGO: Diagnosis of allergy by an in vitro test for allergen antibodies. *Lancet* 1967; 2:1105.

Williams RI: Skin titration: Testing and treatment. *Otolaryngol Clin N Am* 1971; 4:507.

Willoughby JW: Serial dilution titration skin tests in inhalant allergy. *Otolaryngol Clin N A* 1974; 7:579.

Wraith DG, Cunnington AM, Seymour WM: The role and allergenic importance of storage mites in house dust and other environments. *Clin Allergy* 1979; 9:545.

Yodoi J, Ishizaka K: Induction of Fc receptor bearing cells "in vitro" in human peripheral lymphocytes. *J Immunol* 1980; 124:934.

Zeiss CR, Grammer LC, Levitz D: Comparison of the radioallergosorbent test and a quantitative solid-phase radioimmunoassay for the detection of ragweed specific immunoglobulin E antibody in patients undergoing immunotherapy. *J Allergy Clin Immunol* 1981; 67:105.

Zetterstrom O: Dual skin reactions and serum antibodies to subtilisin and aspergillus fumigatus extracts. *Clin Allergy* 1979; 8:77.

Zimmerman EM, Yunginger JW, Gleich GJ: Interference in ragweed pollen and honeybee venom radioallergosorbent tests. *J Allergy Clin Immunol* 1980; 66:386.

Chapter 9

Hyperimmune and Autoimmune Diseases

David A. Mathison
Robert C. Bone

OUTLINE

CLASSIFICATIONS OF IMMUNOPATHOLOGY

IgE AND NON-IgE MEDIATED RHINOSINUSITIS

ANGIOEDEMA-URTICARIA

BLISTERING MUCOCUTANEOUS DISEASES

VASCULITIDES

AUTOIMMUNE EXOCRINOPATHIES

AMYLOIDOSES

DISEASES OF OBSCURE ORIGIN WITH IMMUNOLOGIC FEATURES

CLASSIFICATIONS OF IMMUNOPATHOLOGY

Immunologic responses to exogenous or autologous substances sometimes initiate chemical mediator and effector cell responses that go beyond protection of the host from the antigen to injury of the host. Diseases which can be attributed to immunopathologic injury are termed "allergic, immunological, hyperimmune," or "autoimmune" when autologous antigens initiate the immune response. Two decades ago Coombs and Gell (1962) conveniently classified these disorders by the nature of the immunologic component to include anaphylactic or immediate hypersensitivity reactions (type I), tissue or cell lytic reactions (type II), immune complex reactions (type III), and reactions mediated by specifically sensitized lymphocytes (type IV); (see also chapter 1). Although knowledge of the nature of antigens, antibodies, and the dynamics of cellular and molecular interactions that account for the immunologic-inflammatory response has greatly expanded in the intervening years, the Gell and Coombs classification remains a useful reference point. For the purpose of this review antibody dependent and independent lymphocytotoxic reactions are included in type IV.

In addition to immune responses, selective immunodeficiencies (see chapters 7, 8, 10) and neoplastic proliferations, either benign or malignant, of lymphocyte-plasma cell lines may account for disease.

The spectrum of immunopathologic disorders which affect the mucous membranes and blood vessels of the head and neck are listed in Table 9-1. These range from the transient inflammation of acute IgE-mediated immediate hypersensitivity conjunctivitis-rhinopharyngitis to the relentless and progressive destruction of midline granuloma. Allergic rhinitis is the prototype disorder for which there is reasonably precise understanding of the immunologic events which lead to mediator release, tissue change, symptoms and signs, and for which specific prevention and treatment are available. Midline granuloma lies at the other end of the spectrum in that there is but a speculation as to an immunologic basis, and lack of understanding allows for but ablative radiotherapy for treatment.

The IgE-mediated allergic disorders have been discussed in the previous chapter. This chapter reviews the clinical and immunologic features of the remaining disorders listed in Table 9-1, especially as applicable to the head and neck; for each disorder the nature of the known antigen and putative immunologic response(s) which account for the pathophysiologic events and histologic findings are also listed.

IgE AND NON-IgE-MEDIATED RHINOSINUSITIS

Perennial tendency to nasal and paranasal congestion accompanied by eosinophilic nasal discharge in the absence of immediate hypersensitivity reaction to aeroallergen may occur in children or adults (Mullarkey et al., 1980).

The presence of a greater than 25% eosinophilia in the nasal secretions sets this syndrome apart from ordinary vasomotor rhinitis. In both syndromes there is enhanced nasal reactivity to irritant, thermal, atmospheric, and postural stimuli. Unlike vasomotor rhinitis, in nonallergic eosinophilic rhinitis there is propensity to polyp formation and this syndrome blends into that of rhinosinusitis-nasal polyps-asthma without or with aspirin sensitivity (Mathison & Stevenson, 1979).

In a typical patient with rhinosinusitis-asthma and aspirin sensitivity there are consecutive stages of disease covering years or decades. These include an initial eosinophilic

TABLE 9-1. Disorders with Immunopathologic Features Which Affect the Head and Neck

Disease	Antigen(s)	Putative immunopathologic response(s)
IgE mediated allergic rhinitis	Aeroallergens	Type I — IgE
Eosinophilic non IgE rhinosinusitis		None demonstrated
Angioedema-urticaria	Foods; drugs; viruses; autogenous—nuclear	Type I — IgE, ± Type III
Pemphigus	Autogenous—epidermal intercellular substance	Type II — IgG
Pemphigoid	Autogenous—basement membrane	Type II — IgG
Erythema multiforme		None demonstrated
Vasculitides		Types III and IV
Polyarteritis	Hepatitis B virus; metamphatamine; unknown	Type III
Allergic granulomatosis (Churg and Strauss)	Unknown	Types III and IV
Wegener's granulomatosis	Unknown	Types III and IV
Hypersensitivity vasculitides	See text	Type III
Systemic lupus erythematosus	Autogenous—nuclear, DNA and others	Types II and III
Giant cell arteritis		None demonstrated
Mucocutaneous lymph node syndrome		None demonstrated
Cogan's syndrome		None demonstrated
Behçet's syndrome	See text	Types II and III
Autoimmune exocrinopathies	Autoimmune—cytoplasmic (SS-A and SS-B), ? exocrine	Types III and IV ± neoplastic
Amyloidosis		Neoplastic (primary forms)
Relapsing polychrondritis		? Type IV
Eosinophilic granuloma-histiocytosis X		? Suppressor T lymphocyte deficiency
Midline granuloma		Neoplastic (except Wegener's)

rhinosinusitis complicated by polyp formation, asthma which usually requires corticosteroid treatment for adequate control, and a unique sensitivity response to aspirin characterized by acute flush, rhinitis, and severe asthma attack within an hour or so of ingesting ordinary doses of aspirin or other nonsteroidal antiinflammatory drug. Although aspirin exacerbates the disease, the rhinosinusitis-asthma occurs and continues without ingestion of aspirin or aspirin-like drugs. Approximately 35% of patients with rhinosinusitis, nasal polyps, and asthma are sensitive to aspirin.

The pathophysiologic mechanisms which underlie the eosinophilic infiltrate in the mucosa lining of the respiratory tract are not fully understood. Of the known eosinophil chemotactic factors of inflammation, eosinophil chemotactic factor of anaphylaxis (ECFA) and the C5 anaphylatoxin might be incriminated. Alteration of releasability of mediators from peripheral blood basophils (and presumably from tissue mast cells), as has been observed in patients with asthma (Findlay & Lichtenstein, 1980), might allow release of a histamine or ECFA from upper respiratory mast cell stores in response to stimuli that are without similar effect in most individuals. Absence of immunoglobulins and complement components in the respiratory tissues of individuals with eosinophilic rhinitis-polyps suggest that the C5 anaphylatoxin is not involved unless there is a fluid phase activation without tissue deposition of complement proteins.

Positive evidence for immunologic reaction to aspirin in apsirin-sensitive patients has not been found. Aspirin and other nonsteroidal antiinflammatory drugs are known to inhibit the cyclooxygenase pathway of arachidonic acid metabolism and generation of prostaglandins and thromboxanes; however, as yet there is no link between this inhibition and the aspirin-sensitivity phenomenon, including the eosinophilic inflammation. Perhaps products of the lipoxygenation of arachidonic acid, the hydroxyeicosatetraenoic acids (HETEs) and leukotrienes, are of importance to this type of inflammatory disorder (Goetzl, 1980).

A diagnosis of eosinophilic non-IgE-mediated rhinosinusitis depends upon the presence of eosinophils in the nasal secretions and negative tests for IgE antibodies. Patients with mild forms of this syndrome ordinarily respond to antihistamine-decongestant medication. More severe inflammation without obstructing polyp formation responds to topical corticosteroid, such as the poorly absorbed beclomethasone dipropionate (Cockcroft et al., 1980; Drettner & Deuschl, 1980).

For individuals with such severe disease as to occlude the nasal passages by swelling and polyp formation, or when there is associated sinusitis with retained bacterial infection, a short course of oral cortisone in therapeutic dose (ie, prednisone 20 to 40 mg daily for ten to 20 days if not contraindicated) combined, if indicated, with antibiotic treatment can ordinarily be expected to clear the nasal passages and allow institution of topical corticosteroid treatment. Surgical removal of a polypoid tissue from the nose and paranasal sinuses is indicated for those patients who have failed on systemic corticosteroid treatment, those for whom such treatment is contraindicated, and in those instances where there is inadequate drainage of infected sinus, roentgenographic evidence of bony erosion, or uncertainty of diagnosis.

ANGIOEDEMA-URTICARIA

Angioedema or urticaria or both are common conditions that afflict 20% of the United States population at sometime during their lives.

Angioedema of the face and neck ordinarily is manifest as giant asymmetric swelling affecting the eyelids, lips, tongue, pharynx, or larynx. Swelling appears over several hours and subsides over several days.

Acute cases of urticaria with or without angioedema can often be attributed to a food substance, pharmacological agent, microbe, or physical stimulus that has provoked immunologic or nonimmunologic release of histamine or other mediators from cutaneous mast cells. Immediate reactions (ie, within minutes of exposure) following ingestion of nuts, crustaceans, fish, or injection of penicillin are examples of IgE-mediated mast cell degranulation. Urticaria appearing in the prodrome of serum sickness, hepatitis, or systemic lupus erythematosus, probably reflect a combination of type I and type III reactions on blood vessels. The morphine-codeine family of drugs and dermographism are examples of nonimmunologic triggers of mast cell mediator release that lead to urticaria.

The diagnosis of chronic urticaria is applied to those patients with daily recurrence of urticaria of more than 6 weeks' duration. In the majority of these patients, precise pathophysiologic mechanisms are not recognized; approximately 10% of these patients may have hypocomplementemia associated with circulating immune complexes and a classical and/or alternative pathway of complement activation (Mathison, Arroyave, & Bhat, 1977).

A syndrome of transient attacks of fever with urticaria, progressive perceptive deafness, and amyloidosis affecting nine members of four successive families was reported by Muckle and Wells (1962). Subsequently, there has been report of a sporadic case with chromasomal aberration and response to corticosteroid (Anderson et al., 1967).

Hereditary angioedema is an uncommon variety of acute angioedema associated with deficiency or dysfunction of plasma C1 inhibitor; uninhibited activation of the contact (Hageman factor) system (Schapira et al., 1983) and/or the classical pathway of complement activation with generation of anaphylatoxins C3a and C5a may account for the angioedema in these patients (Prograis et al., unpublished data, 1982).

The progression of acute angioedema and urticaria ordinarily is halted by subcutaneous administration of epinephrine and oral or parenteral antihistamine. Tracheostomy is indicated for angioedema which compromises airway or threatens to compromise the airway by progressing despite treatment. Purified C1 inhibitor concentrate has been used successfully to treat acute episodes of hereditary angioedema (Gadek et al., 1980). Regular prophylactic treatment with an attenuated androgen such as stanozolol or danazol stimulates production of increased amount of C1 inhibitor sufficient to prevent serious angioedema attacks in patients with hereditary angioedema (Sheffer, Fearon, & Austen, 1981).

BLISTERING MUCOCUTANEOUS DISEASES

Pemphigus, pemphigoid, and erythema multiforme are the major immunologic diseases which damage the mucous membranes of the mouth and pharynx (Pearson, 1977).

In *pemphigus*, there is intraepidermal acantholysis attributable to circulating and tissue-fixed IgG autoantibodies to an epidermal intercellular substance antigen. Complement components are also found in the epidermis, and anticomplementary activity resides in the suprabasal intraepidermal bullae which mark the disease. Oral lesions are usually present; if there is extension into the pharynx and larynx hoarseness occurs; such extension carries relatively poor prognosis. Disease activity correlates with titer of serum antibody as determined by indirect immunofluorescent technique. Therapy includes corticosteroids, gold, and immunosuppressives according to activity and extent of disease.

Pemphigoid reflects subepidermal bullae attributable to complement-fixing IgG autonantibody to the basement membrane of skin. Compared to pemphigus, pemphigoid is more chronic, benign, and oral and mucosal lesions are small but may heal with fibrosis and scarring. Failure to transmit the disease to monkeys via serum, even though antibodies can be shown to fix to basement membrane, probably means that immunopathologic mechanisms alone do not account for the disease.

Erythema multiforme is a pattern of reaction in the mucous membranes and skin manifested by angiitis in the upper corium leading to erythematous and bullous lesions that darken with age and leave concentric rings of a "target" lesion. Erythema multiforme may consist of but a few scattered lesions of the mouth and extremities to life-threatening eruptive fever associated with stomatitis and ophthalmia (Stevens-Johnson syndrome). Acute appearances and relapses have been associated with infection, particularly herpes simplex and *Mycoplasma pneumoniae*, immunizations, malignancy, drugs, particularly the sulfas, and thermal or radiation stimuli. These associations have raised a suggestion that immunologic factors may contribute to the pathophysiology; however, immune reactants ordinarily have not been found in the lesions or serum. Systemic corticosteroids are usually used in severe cases but the response is not as prompt as that seen in pemphigus.

VASCULITIS

Inflammation and necrosis of blood vessels constitute vasculitis. Within the spectrum of vasculitis any size or type of blood vessel in any organ system can be involved. Most vasculitides can be associated with immunopathologic mechanisms, particularly immune complex mediation. Classification, clinical, pathologic, immunologic, and therapeutic considerations for the vasculitic disorders are summarized by Cupps and Fauci (1981); their classification is used in Table 9-1.

The necrotizing vasculitides are either caused by or closely associated with deposition of immune complexes (type III reaction) (Cochrane & Dixon, 1978). Circulating foreign (particularly viral or other microbial) or an usually cloistered autogenous antigen gains access to the circulation and forms soluble complexes in antigen excess with antibody as it is synthesized. Complexes not cleared by the reticuloendothelial system are deposited in blood vessel walls. Immune complexes localize in vessels whose permeability has been increased by vasoactive amines released from aggregated platelets (serotonin) or activated basophils (histamine). Complexes tend to lodge along the basement membrane of the vessel wall where they serve as a nidus for complement activation. Complement activation in turn amplifies the inflammation via the anaphylatoxins (C4a, C3a, C5a) which further increase vascular permeability and chemotactic factors (C3a, C5a, C567) which attract neutrophils and eosinophils. Neutrophils and eosinophils in turn intensify the damage by release of protease enzymes including collagenases and elastases. The end result is a damaged and necrotic vessel wall subject to hemorrhage and occlusion. Fortunately, showers of vasculitic injury triggered by soluble antigen-antibody complexes are usually short-lived as continued antibody production results in clearing of complexes in antibody excess by the reticuloendothelial system.

Cell-mediated immunity (type IV reaction) (Miller, 1978) may also be involved in vascular damage. This is not as common or well studied a mechanism as is immune complex reaction. It is assumed that sensitized T lymphocytes are triggered by circulating antigen to release chemical mediators (David & Rocklin, 1978) such as macrophage migration inhibitory factor or to interact directly with monocytes and macrophages, causing these latter cells to influx and accumulate at the site of vessel damage. Macrophages release enzymes causing effects similar to polymorphonuclear leukocytes and, when the antigen is complex and not readily cleared, transform to the epithelioid cells and multinucleated giant cells that constitute classic granuloma (Unanue, 1978).

Systemic necrotizing vasculitides include polyarteritis nodosa, allergic granulomatosis of Churg and Strauss (1951), and that syndrome which does not have the distinguishing charactericstics of either of these syndromes but shares a feature with both and is thus an "overlap syndrome."

Polyarteritis nodosa affects small and medium-size muscular arteries producing aneurysmal dilatations, particularly in the renal, hepatic, and intestinal vasculature. Eosinophilia, granulomata, lung, and spleen involvement ordinarily are absent. Apart from case reports of onset of polyarteritis nodosa following acute serous otitis (Sergent & Christian, 1974) and during hyposensitization treatment for allergic rhinitis (Phanuphak & Kohler, 1980), polyarteritis nodosa ordinarily has not been associated with head or neck disorder. Classic polyarteritis has been associated with hepatitis B virus infection (Duffy et al., 1976) and intravenous metamphetamine abuse (Citron et al., 1970).

Allergic granulomatosis with angiitis is distinguished by high peripheral blood eosinophilia, eosinophilic tissue infiltration with granulomatous reactivity, and lung involvement in addition to the fibrinoid necrosis of muscular arteries as in classic polyarteritis nodosa.

Untreated systemic necrotizing vasculitides have a progressive course with a 5-year survival of less than 15%. Corticosteroid treatment may control mild or limited disease. Severe systemic vasculitis responds favorably to treatment with cytotoxic agents, particularly cyclophosphamide (Fauci et al., 1979).

Wegener's granulomatosis is a distinct syndrome of necrotizing granulomatous vasculitis of the upper and lower respiratory tracts, glomerulonephritis, and variable degrees of disseminated small-vessel vasculitis. Paranasal sinusitis with necrotizing granuloma and secondary bacteria infection are found in 90% of patients. Nasopharynx involvement by granuloma with mucosal ulceration and/or cartilage involvement leading to saddle nose deformity are found in 75% of patients. Keratoconjunctivitis or granulomatosus sclerouveitis are found in 60% and serous otitis media in 35% of patients. Lung involvement with multiple nodular cavitary infiltrates is found in 95%; focal and segmental glomerulitis followed by necrotizing glomerulonephritis is found in 85% of patients.

The etiology of the disease is unclear. A combination of hypersensitivity reactions including immune complex and delayed hypersensitivity probably are involved.

The combination of involvement of upper and lower respiratory tracts with granulomatous vasculitis and necrotizing glomerulonephritis helps to distinguish Wegener's from allergic granulomatosis in which the respiratory involvement is ordinarily limited to the lung and associated with eosinophilic infiltrate and eosinophilia; from midline granuloma in which destructive inflammation is limited to the upper respiratory tract, orbit, and face and which may or may not include granuloma; and from lymphoid granulomatosis in which the granulomatous reaction is characterized by angiotrophic and angiodestructive infiltration of various tissues, particularly lung, with atypical lymphocytoid and plasmacytoid cells (Israel et al., 1977).

Within the past decade, the finding of dramatic response of Wegener's granulomatosis to cyclophosphamide therapy has altered the prognosis from almost uniform fatality to curability.

Hypersensitivity vasculitides are characterized by immune complex deposition in postcapillary venules predominantly in the skin. Palpable purpura, reflecting vessel infiltration by polymorphonuclear leukocytes and their nuclear debris (leukocytoclastic vasculitis), fibrinoid necrosis, and extravasation of erythrocytes, appear in crops with predilection for the lower extremities. Vasculitic lesions of the palate are not uncommon.

Distinct syndromes within this group of vasculitides reflect immune responses to distinct antigens. Serum sickness and serum sickness-like reactions occur following exposure to heterologous antisera and to nonprotein drugs (pencillin, sulfa). In Henoch-Schonlein purpura, attacks follow infection and are associated with IgA antibody in the immune complexes. In essential mixed cryoglobulinemia, there is IgM rheumatoid factor against IgG. Lymphoid malignancies including chronic lymphocytic leukemia, lymphoma, Hodgkins' disease, and multiple myeloma are sometimes accompanied by typical leukocytoclastic vasculitis.

Severe erosive and nodular rheumatoid arthritis and lupus erythematosus are vascular disorders in which circulating complexes of autoantibody and autoantigen account for the vasculitis. In discoid lupus erythematosis, raised erythematous lesions with irregular margins of active inflammation with telangiectasia, follicular scales and plugging, and central healing with atrophy, hypo- or hyperpigmentation appear on the malar face, ears, and scalp. Avoidance of sun exposure and intralesional corticosteroid infiltration may control the skin lesions; antimalarial and corticosteroid treatment are sometimes required. Less than 5% of patients with discoid lupus erythematosis go on to develop progressive systemic lupus erythematosis.

Systemic lupus erythematosus is a disease of unknown cause and protean manifestations and course. Autoantibodies to nuclear antigens including DNA are associated with the disease and evidence for immune complex vasculitis is found in affected organs and even unaffected skin. Approximately 40% of patients have the typical butterfly rash, 30% alopecia, and 12% mucous membrane lesions. The clinical course may be discordant from the serologic activity. Recent evolutions in the understanding and treatment of systemic lupus erythematosis including use of corticosteroid and cytotoxic drugs are reviewed by Decker and colleagues (1979).

Giant cell arteritis is characterized by panarteritic inflammation of medium and large-sized arteries. There are two major varieties, Takayasu's arteritis of the aortic arch and its branches and cranial arteritis with involvement of branches of the carotid artery, particularly the temporal artery, thus the term "temporal arteritis."

The classic clinical picture of cranial arteritis includes headache, fever, markedly elevated erythrocyte sedimentation rate, and anemia in a person over 50 years of age. Often there are associated symptoms of polymyalgia rheumatica, including stiffness and aching in the muscles of the neck, back, shoulder, and pelvic girdles. Occular involvement may lead to sudden blindness. Cranial arteritis and its associated manifestations are promptly responsive to corticosteroid treatment. Prednisone treatment is begun at a dose of 60 mg per day, and tapered downward to a maintenance dose in the range of 7.5 to 20 mg per day according to symptoms and erythrocyte sedimentation rate, and continued for at least 1 year to reduce risk of a relapse.

Although immunologic mechanisms have been implicated in giant cell arteritis, immune reactants specific to these disorders have not been identified (Hamilton, Shelley, & Tumultz, 1971).

Mucocutaneous lymph node syndrome (Kawasaki, 1967) is an unusual and distinct symptom complex including self-limited febrile illness, dryness and erythema of the lips, mouth, and pharynx with "strawberry tongue," indurative edema of the hands and feet with erythema of palms and soles followed by desquamation from the fingertips, and polymorphous exanthema of the trunk. Associated features have included cervical or other lymphopathia, pyorrhea, aseptic meningitis, diarrhea, arthritis, arthralgia, and in several cases, coronary arteritis with aneurysmal dilatation and thrombosis. Early reports were of disease in infants and young children of Oriental origins; more recent reports have come from the United States and included older children and young adults (Everett, 1979; Bell et al., 1981).

Quantitative immunoglobulins in these children are normal, tests for antinuclear antibodies and rheumatoid factor are negative, and searches for microbial infection have not yielded positive result. Biopsies of lymph nodes show only nonspecific hyperplasia.

Because of severe morbidity and several percent mortality in this syndrome, corticosteroid therapy has been advocated even though efficacy in modifying the course or preventing fatal termination has not been documented by controlled trials.

Cogan's syndrome is nonsyphilitic interstitial keratitis with photophobia and vestibuloauditory dysfunction including vertigo and hearing loss (Cheson, Bluming, & Alroy, 1976). This is a rare clinical syndrome affecting primarily young adults and associated with systemic illness such as fever, abdominal pain, myalgias, arthralgias, lymphadenopathy, cerebral artery occlusion, or aortic valvulitis. Infiltration of large veins and muscular artery walls and aortic leaflets with mononuclear and polymorphonuclear cells has been reported. The course is variable from death within months of onset to an acute phase lasting months or years followed by chronic residual damage 15 years after diagnosis. High dosage prednisone treatment may be of benefit in the acute and active phase. Successful aortic valve replacements have been reported for several patients.

Behçet's syndrome is the triad of recurrent oral and genital ulcerations and relapsing iridocyclitis (Lehner 1979). Oral ulceration occurs in 98% of patients and is accompanied by genital ulceration and occular disease in about 80% of patients. Ulcerative hemorrhagic lesions involve the mouth, lips, gums, tongue, palate, or posterior pharynx. In addition, relapsing multisystem disease including seronegative inflammatory polyarteritis of knees, ankles, or wrists, erythema nodosum, thrombophlebitis, neurologic involvement, or intestinal disease occurs in one-third of patients. The multisystem patterns that constitute Behçet's syndrome reflect an obliterative necrotizing vasculitis of arteries and veins.

Immune complexes and complement have been identified in the involved tissues and serum of affected patients. Autoantibodies reactive with oral mucosa have also been found. HLA-B5 is associated with occular disease, B12 with mucocutaneous involvement, and B27 with arthritis.

Corticosteroid therapy is used to treat all manifestations. Recurrences are commonplace and additional treatment with azathioprine, chlorumbucil, and levamisole have been reported to be of benefit.

AUTOIMMUNE EXOCRINOPATHIES

Sjögren (1933) described 19 patients with keratoconjunctivitis sicca and xerostomia and noted that two-thirds of the patients also had arthritic disorder. In the intervening years, a broad spectrum of clinical disorders (Martinez-Lavin, Vaughan, & Tan, 1979), genetic, (Moutsopoulous et al., 1979), and autoimmune markers (Alspaugh, Talal, & Tan, 1976) have been associated with sicca-Sjögren syndromes.

Sicca syndrome reflects a dysfunction of exocrine glands caused by lymphocytic and plasma cell infiltration, hence the term "autoimmune exocrinopathy." The cardinal manifestations are dryness of the eyes and mouth reflecting decrease in lacrimal secretion associated with devitalization and denuding of the corneal and bulbar conjunctival epithelium (keratoconjunctivitis sicca) and decreased saliva with dryness of the mouth (xerostomia). In addition, widespread involvement of mucosal glands may result in dryness of the nares, pharynx, trachea, bronchi, and in severe cases, skin and vagina.

Postmenopausal women comprise 90% of patients with autoimmune exocrinopathies (Kassen & Grady, 1978).

Autoimmune exocrinopathy is termed primary when it occurs alone and secondary when it is associated with another autoimmune disease. In the primary form, a high percentage of patients have autoantibodies to antigens (SS-A, SS-B) extracted from human lymphoblastoid cell line; the frequency of the lymphocyte defined antigens HLA-B8 and HLA-Dw3 also are increased. Diagnosis is confirmed by Schirmer's test for tearing and biopsy of minor salivary glands. Displacement of the acini and hypertrophy of ductal epithelium occur as lymphocyte aggregates enlarge. Both B and T lymphocytes are involved and focal immunoglobulin synthesis occurs.

Approximately 30% to 50% of patients have enlargement of one or more of major salivary glands. The term "pseudolymphoma" has been used to describe extra glandular tumor-like aggregates of lymphoid tissue that do not meet criteria for malignancy. Ordinarily these swellings are asymptomatic and self-limited; however, patients with Sjögren syndrome have died from malignant lymphomas including histiocytic lymphoma, immunoblastic sarcoma, and Waldenstrom's macroglobulinemia. Progression in the lymphoproliferative lesions from a polyclonal infiltrate to a monoclonal B-cell neoplasm accounts for the malignant lymphomas (Zulman, Jaffe, & Talal, 1978).

Additional extraglandular involvements in primary autoimmune exocrinopathy may include Raynaud's phenomenon, lymphocytic interstitial pneumonitis, and distal renal tubular involvement with acidosis and hyposthenuria. More than half of patients have hyperimmunoglobulinemia including rheumatoid factor and circulating immune complexes; however, only occasional patients have active vasculitis.

Autoimmune exocrinopathy is considered to be secondary when associated with rheumatoid arthritis, systemic lupus erythematosus, or other autoimmune-connective tissue disorder. Approximately 50% of patients with sicca syndromes have arthritis, and up to 20% of patients with rheumatoid arthritis and as many as 30% of patients with systemic lupus erythematosus have sicca syndromes. In the secondary form HLA-DRw4 has increased frequency and the serum more often contains precipitating autoantibody to rheumatoid arthritis nuclear antigen. The remaining clinical, histologic, and immunologic features are similar to those with the primary form save that aggressive lymphocytic behavior and extraglandular involvements occur less frequently.

Treatment of autoimmune exocrinopathy is aimed at limiting the damaging effects of xerophthalmia and xerostomia. Artificial tears containing methylcellulose and sour sugar-free candies given as sialogogues are helpful. Topical corticosteroids should be avoided. Staphylococcal blepharitis occurs in the majority of patients and requires antibiotic treatment. Progressive dental caries can be prevented in part by vigorous plaque control and fluoride applications.

Individuals with severe functional disability or life-threatening complications require corticosteroid or immunosuppressive therapy. Prednisone therapy ordinarily will suppress salivary gland swelling and may improve pulmonary disease. Severe renal and pulmonary involvement may warrant cytotoxic immunosuppressive therapy.

AMYLOIDOSES

The amyloidoses are a group of diseases characterized by the deposition of proteinaceous infiltrate in a variety of tissues. Amyloid consists of fibrils 10 nm in diameter composed of longitudinal filaments separated by a clear space. The amyloid protein is a portion of immunoglobulin light chain in the primary forms and other proteins in the secondary (to chronic inflammation), familial, endocrine, senile, and cutaneous forms. Amyloid fibrils are nonimmunogenic, resist phagocytosis and proteolysis, and thus normal host defense mechanisms are ineffective in preventing/removing the tissue deposits.

The primary form includes amyloid associated with myeloma and macroglobulinemia and is encountered most commonly. In this form amyloid infiltrates are found mainly in the tongue, heart, gastrointestinal tract, including liver and spleen, skin, and muscu-loligamentous structures. The presenting complaint may be a difficulty with swallowing or speaking due to macroglossia.

Secondary amyloidosis ordinarily is manifest only after many years of underlying infection (osteomylitis, tuberculosis, bronchiectasis, pyelonephritis, leprosy) or in association with rheumatoid arthritis or regional ileitis. In this form, amyloid infiltration occurs in organs beneath the diaphragm, primarily in the kidney, spleen, liver, and adrenals. Macroglossia is rarely found in secondary amyloidoses.

The most prevalent hereditary forms are familial Mediterranean fever and the Portuguese type of lower limb neuropathy. Localized amyloid may occur in isolated organs including the larynx.

Presence of degradation products of homogeneous light chain (Bence Jones proteins) are found in 90% of patients with primary amyloidosis; such a finding is unusual in the secondary, familial, and localized forms. Diagnosis of amyloidosis requires confirmation by Congo red dye of metachromatic staining. Gingival or rectal biopsy provides histologic evidence of amyloidosis in over 90% of the patients with the systemic forms of the disease.

The current knowledge regarding the varieties of proteins found in different forms of amyloid and speculations as to the immune system involvement in the amyloidosis is reviewed by Franklin (1980). Apart from colchicine treatment to prevent febrile attacks of familial Mediterranean fever and progression of amyloidosis in that condition, there is no proven treatment for the amyloidoses.

DISEASES OF OBSCURE ORIGIN WITH IMMUNOLOGIC FEATURES

In addition to non-IgE rhinosinusitis and several of the vasculitic disorders for which immunopathologic mechanisms have not been demonstrated, several syndromes are herein reported for which an immunologic stimulus response has not been fully demonstrated.

Relapsing polychondritis is a rare disease characterized by a loss of mucopolysaccharide matrix, inflammation, and degeneration of cartilaginous structures. Stages of inflammation include acute neutrophil infiltration of the superficial portions of cartilage, followed later by a granulomatous and then fibrotic change.

The most common site of cartilage inflammation is the pinna which becomes acutely red or violescent, tender, and swollen. Other sites include cartilage of the nasal septum, larynx, trachea, and bronchi sometimes resulting in a life-threatening respiratory obstruction. Involvement of inner ear structures or eustachian tubes may cause deafness, tinnitus, or vertigo. Other sites of damage may include joints, aortic valve ring, and media of the aorta with aortic incompetence or aneurysm.

Immunologic phenomena associated with the disorder have included evidence of lymphocyte transformation and monocyte migration inhibition by the cells of affected patients in reactions with purified cartilage matrix. Approximately one-third of patients have associated autoimmune or vasculitic disorders. Elevation of erythrocyte sedimentation rate and anemia are found in the majority of patients.

Cortiscosteroid therapy dampens the intensity of the inflammatory manifestations and needs to be continued over long periods of time on a daily basis because the natural course of this disorder is for continued and progressive involvement. Surgical intervention for respiratory or cardiovascular disease is sometimes required (McAdam, 1976).

Eosinophilic granuloma is characterized by granulomatous formation by mononuclear cells of phagocytic origin, multinucleated giant cells, foamy histiocytes, and eosinophils. Eosinophilic granuloma occurs most frequently as isolated bone lesions but soft tissue involvement including isolated granuloma of the salivary glands, gingiva, lung, skin, and vulva have also been reported. Multifocal forms involve bone and soft tissue sites and may be accompanied by recurrent bouts of otitis media or mastoiditis. Hand-Schuller-Christian syndrome—exophthalmus, diabetes insipidus, and bone destruction—is one variety of multifocal eosinophilic granuloma.

"Histiocytosis X" links the eosinophilic granulomas with Letterer-Siwe disease of infants in which granuloma formation with proliferation of histiocytes also occurs.

Osband and colleagues (1981) found a majority of patients with histiocytosis X to have circulating lymphocytes cytotoxic to cultured human fibroblasts, antibody to autologous erythrocytes, or lack of histamine H2 surface receptors on T-lymphocytes suggestive of suppressor-cell deficiency. Lymphocyte abnormalities responded to crude extract of calf thymus gland and several patients treated with this extract had clinical response with normalization of their immunologic abnormalities. Prior to this report, treatment ordinarily has included topical corticosteroid to oral and respiratory lesions, radiation therapy to localize bone lesions, surgical decompression of mastoid involvement, and chemotherapy for multifocal lesions inaccessible to these other modalities.

Midline granuloma is a clinical entity now generally recognized as a grouping of diverse pathologic entities all having as a common basis a rapidly developing necrotic process of the midface, nose, and/or the palate. The term itself should be thought of in much the same sense that head and neck clinicians employ "leukoplakia." Neither designation implies a histologic diagnosis or a prognosis—only a clinical picture and set of circumstances. In fact, Burston (1959) has listed over 20 specific disease entities to be included in the differential diagnosis of this syndrome including syphilis, leprosy, tularemia, and rhinoscleroma.

Typically, however, the great majority of cases may be thought of as falling into one of three categories: a recognized histiopathologic type of malignant lymphoma that initially presents in the midface; Wegener's granulomatosis in either its classical or a more limited form; and, finally, (malignant) midline reticulosis, a separate lymphoproliferative disorder capable of rapid infiltration into adjacent paranasal tissues and characterized by vasculitic necrosis with secondary infection.

The differentiation among these three entities is based to a large extent on histological study, although in rare instances even the biopsy is nondiagnostic and one must diagnose on the basis of overall clinical findings. This situation seems to occur most frequently in Wegener's disease where the pathognomic picture of perivascular infiltrate may be obscured. The diagnosis of Wegener's disease requires a careful search for evidence of involvement of the lower respiratory system and kidneys as mentioned above. Lymphoma having its primary site of origin in the midface may present a histological picture of any of the recognized subgroupings of this tumor and is therefore staged and treated accordingly.

Midline reticulosis (MR) is a unique disease entity that comprises a large subgroup of midline granulomas and is characterized by some experts as a lymphoreticular neoplasm containing a peculiar mixture of neoplastic reticular and lymphocytic cells with a normal inflammatory response (Kassel, Echevarria, & Guzzo, 1969). A key factor in the diagnosis of MR is a wide range of pleomorphism in the lymphoreticular elements. Because perivascular grouping of cellular infiltrates can occur, a superficial resemblance to Wegener's granulomatosis is sometimes seen. Fechner and Lamppin (1972) note, however, that the perivascular infiltrate in this case is neoplastic and not inflammatory. These authors also mention the fact that inflammatory reaction and necrosis can exist over a large area so that multiple biopsies are occasionally necessary to include all likely diagnostic foci of lymphoreticular neoplasm.

REFERENCES

Alspaugh MA, Talal M, Tan EM: Differentiation and characterization of autoantibodies and their antigens in Sjögren's syndrome. *Arthritis Rheum* 1976; 19:216–222.

Anderson V, Buck NH, Jensen MK, et al: Deafness, urticaria and amyloidosis. *Ann Intern Med* 1967; 42:449–456.

Bell DM, Brink EW, Nitzkin JL, et al: Kawasaki syndrome: Description of two outbreaks in the United States. *N Engl J Med* 1981; 304:1568–1575.

Burston H: Lethal midline granuloma: Is it a pathological entity? *Laryngoscope* 1959; 69:1–43.

Cheson BD, Bluming AZ, Alroy J: Cogan's syndrome: A systemic vasculitis. *Amer J Med* 1976; 609:549–555.

Churg J, Strauss L: Allergic granulomatosis, allergic angiitis and periarteritis nodosa. *Am J Pathol* 1951; 27:277-301.

Citron BP, Halpern M, McCarron, et al: Necrotizing angiitis associated with drug abuse. *N Engl J Med* 1970; 283:1003-1011.

Cochrane CG, Dixon FJ: Immune complex injury, in Samter M (ed): *Immunological Diseases*. Boston, Little, Brown Co, 1978, pp 210-229.

Cockcroft DW, Hargreave FE, Dolovich J: Intranasal beclomethasone dipropionate in rhinitis, in Mygind M, Clark TJH (eds): *Topical Steroid Treatment for Asthma and Rhinitis*. London, Cassell Ltd, 1980, pp. 155-161.

Coombs, RRA, Gell PGH: The classification of allergic reactions underlying diseases, in Gell PGH, Coombs RRA (eds): *Clinical Aspects of Immunology*. Philadelphia, FA Davis Co, 1962, pp 317-337.

Cupps TR, Fauci AS: The vasculitides, in Smith LH (ed): *Major Problems In Internal Medicine*. Philadelphia, WB Saunders, 1981, vol 21, pp 1-211.

David JR, Rocklin RE: Lymphocyte Mediators: The "Lymphokines", in Samter M (ed): *Immunological Diseases*. Little, Brown & Co, 1978, pp 307-324.

Decker JL, Steinberg AD, Reinertsen JL, et al: Systemic lupus erythematosus: Evolving concepts. *Ann Intern Med* 1979; 91:587-604.

Drettner B, Deuschl H: Intranasal beclomethasone dipropionate in nasal polyposis, in Mygind M, Clark TJH (eds): *Topical Steroid Treatment for Asthma and Rhinitis*. London, Cassell Ltd, 1980, pp 155-161.

Duffy J, Lidskyt MD, Sharp JT, et al: Polyarthritis, polyarteritis and hepatitis B. *Medicine (Baltimore)* 1976; 55:19-37.

Everett ED: Mucocutaneous lymph node syndrome (Kawasaki disease) in adults. *JAMA* 1979; 242:542-543.

Fauci AS, Katz P, Hayes BF, et al: Cyclophosphamide therapy of severe systemic necrotizing vasculitis. *N Engl J Med* 1979; 301:235-238.

Fechner RE, Lamppin DW: Midline malignant reticulosis, a clinicopathologic entity. *Arch Otol* 1972; 95:467-476.

Findlay SR, Lichtenstein LM: Basophil "releasibility" in patients with asthma. *Am Rev Resp Dis* 1980; 122:53-59.

Franklin EC: Immunopathology of the amyloid diseases. *Hospital Practice* 1980; Sept, 70-77.

Gadek JE, Hosea SW, Gelfand JA, et al: Replacement therapy in hereditary angioedema. *N Engl J Med* 1980; 302:542-546.

Goetzl EJ: Mediators of immediate hypersensitivity derived from arachidonic acid. *N Engl J Med* 1980; 303:822.

Hamilton CR, Shelley WM, Tumultz PA: Giant cell arteritis: Including temporal arteritis and polymyalgia rheumatica. *Medicine* 1971; 50:1-27.

Israel HL, Patchefsky AA, Soldana MJ: Wegener's granulomatosis, lymphoid granulomatosis and benign lymphocytic angiitis and granulomatosis of lung: Recognition and treatment. *Ann Intern Med* 1977; 87:691-699.

Kassan SS, Grady M: Sjogren's syndrome: An update and overview. *Amer J Med* 1978; 64:1037-1046.

Kassel JH, Echevarria, Guzzo FP: Midline malignant reticulosis (so called lethal midline granuloma). *Cancer* 1969; 23:920-935.

Kawasaki T: Acute febrile mucocutaneous syndrome with lymph node involvement with specific disquaniation of the fingers and toes in children. *Jpn J Allergy* 1967; 16:178-222.

Lehner N (ed): *Behçet's syndrome: Clinical and Immunological Features.* New York, Academic Press, 1979, pp 1-323.

Martinez-Lavin M, Vaughan JH, Tan EM: Autoantibodies and the spectrum of Sjogren's syndrome. *Amer J Med* 1979; 91:185-190.

Mathison DA, Arroyave CM, Bhat KN, et al: Hypocomplementenia in chronic idiopathic urticaria. *Ann Intern Med* 1977; 86:534-538.

Mathison DA, Stevenson DD: Hypersensitivity to nonsteroidal anti-inflammatory drugs. *J Allergy Clin Immunol* 1979; 64:669-674.

McAdam LP: Relapsing polychrondritis: Prospective study of 23 patients and a review of the literature. *Medicine* 1976; 55:193-215.

Miller JFAP: The cellular basis of immune response, in Samter M (ed): *Immunological Diseases.* Boston, Little, Brown & Co, 1978, pp 35-48.

Moutsopoulos HM, Mann DL, Johnson AH, et al: Genetic differences between primary and secondary sicca syndrome. *N Engl J Med* 1979; 301:761-763.

Muckle TJ, Wells M: Urticaria, deafness and amyloidosis: A new heredo-familial syndrome. *Quart J Med* 1962; 31:235.

Mullarkey F, Hill JS, Webb DR: Allergic and non-allergic rhinitis: Their characterization with attention to the meaning of nasal eosinophilia. *J Allergy Clin Immunol* 1980; 65:122-126.

Osband ME, Lipton JM, Lavin P, et al: Histiocytosis X: Demonstration of abnormal immunity, T-cell histamine H-2 receptor deficiency, and successful treatment with thymic extract. *N Engl J Med* 1981; 304:146-153.

Pearson RW: Advances in the diagnosis and treatment of blistering diseases: A selective review, in Malkinson FD, Pearson R (eds): *The Year Book of Dermatology.* Chicago, Year Book Medical Publishers, 1977, pp 7-52.

Phanuphak P, Kohler PF: Onset of polyarteritis nodosa during allergic hyposensitization treatment. *Amer J Med* 1980; 68:479-485.

Sergent JS, Christian CC: Necrotizing vasculitis after acute serous otitis. *Ann Intern Med* 1974; 81:195-199.

Schapira M, Silver LD, Scott CF, et al: Prekallikrein activation and high molecular-weight kininogen consumption in hereditary angioedema. *N Engl J Med* 1983; 308:1050-1053.

Sheffer AL, Fearon DT, Austen KF: Clinical and biochemical effects of stanazolol therapy for hereditary angioedema. *J Allergy Clin Immunol* 1981; 68:181-187.

Sjögren H: Zur Kenntnis der Keratoconjunctivitis sicca (Keratitis filiformis bein Hypofunktion der Tranendriissen). *Acta Opthal Mol (Kbh)* 1933; 11:1-151.

Unanue ER: The immune granulomas, in Samter M (ed): *Immunological Diseases.* Boston, Little, Brown & Co, 1978, pp 297-306.

Zulman J, Jaffe R, Talal N: Evidence that the malignant lymphoma of Sjögren syndrome is a monoclonal B-cell neoplasm. *N Engl J Med* 1978; 299:1215-1220.

Chapter 10

Immunodeficiency Diseases: Head and Neck Manifestations

Jeffrey P. Harris
Mary Ann South

OUTLINE

INTRODUCTION

IMMUNODEFICIENCY INVOLVING THE B-CELL SYSTEM
X-Linked Infantile Agammaglobulinemia (Bruton's disease)
Common Variable Immunodeficiency
X-Linked Immunodeficiency with Hyper-IgM
Selective IgA Deficiency

IMMUNODEFICIENCY INVOLVING THE T-CELL SYSTEM
Thymic Hypoplasia/DiGeorge Syndrome
Chronic Mucocutaneous Candidiasis (CMC)

IMMUNODEFICIENCY INVOLVING BOTH T-CELL AND B-CELL SYSTEMS
Severe Combined Immunodeficiency Diseases (SCID)
Wiskott-Aldrich Syndrome
Ataxia-Telangiectasia

DISORDERS OF PHAGOCYTOSIS
Neutropenia
Chronic Granulomatous Disease of Childhood (CGD)

DISORDERS OF THE COMPLEMENT SYSTEM
C1 Inhibitor Deficiency: Hereditary Angioneurotic Edema (HANE)
Other Complement Disorders

SUMMARY

INTRODUCTION

Upper respiratory infections represent the most prevalent illness to affect normal children during their development. Similarly, immunodeficient children exhibit upper respiratory infections as the major manifestation of their altered immunologic state. Head and neck surgeons are often confronted with children who historically appear to have an increased susceptibility to infections. How, then, can one distinguish between the "normal" child and one who is immunodeficient? An accurate history of the nature of the infections is of great help. Do the infections truly occur more frequently than would be expected? Are they more severe or do they last longer than expected? Do unexpected complications occur, especially from organisms with low pathogenicity? Positive responses to these questions could indicate that the patient is immunodeficient.

The head and neck manifestations of immunodeficiency disorders commonly present as recurrent suppurative otitis media, tonsillitis, sinusitis, rhinitis, and nasopharyngitis. Complications may develop, ultimately leading to mastoiditis with chronic otorrhea, osteomyelitis, or abscessed cervical lymph nodes. Despite appropriate antibiotic therapy, recurrences of these infections often occur from the same organism; that is, one of the common respiratory pathogens such as *Pneumococcus, Hemophilus influenzae,* and *Streptococcus* (Table 10-1). The immunodeficient individual may also have non-head-and-neck manifestations, which include pneumonia, bronchiectasis, chronic diarrhea, failure to thrive, malabsorption, skin lesions (such as rash, pyoderma or eczema), thrush, hepatosplenomegaly, chronic conjunctivitis, and hematologic abnormalities.

The incidence of immunodeficiency disorders is difficult to determine because many of these individuals go undiagnosed. An extrapolation of one study places the incidence of humoral immune deficiency at 0.002% of the new births in the general population (Medical Research Council Working Party, 1969). When one examines the hospitalized patient population, the incidence of primary humoral immunodeficiency rises to an estimated 0.3% of admissions (Hobbs, 1966). In addition, cellular immune deficiencies are at least as frequent, since severe combined immunodeficiency disease (SCID) occurs at a rate of about 1 in 30,000 or 0.03%.

The age distribution at the time of diagnosis of an immunodeficiency disorder is as follows: 17% in infants less than 1 year old, 41% in children between 1 and 15 years old, and 42% in adults (Medical Research Council Working Party, 1969). These data

From the Division of Otolaryngology (Head and Neck Surgery), University of California, San Diego Medical Center, San Diego, CA (Dr. Harris); and NINCDS-Infectious Disease Branch. Bethesda. MD (Dr. South). From Head and Neck Surgery. 5:114-124. 1982, with permission of John Wiley & Sons Publishing Company. This work was supported in part by Teacher-Investigator Development Award. NIH-NINCDS No. 1 KOH NS00606 (Dr. Harris). The authors acknowledge the assistance of Mary E. Bartoo in the preparation of this work.

TABLE 10-1. Special susceptibility to infection with specific classes of organisms*

	Humoral immune deficiency	Cellular immune deficiency	Combined immune deficiency	Phagocytic defects	Complement defects
Bacteria					
High-grade pathogens encapsulated (*Pneumococcus, B. strep, H. influenzae, Meningococcus*)	++++	-	++++	++	+
Low-grade pathogens enteric organisms	+	+	+	++++	+
Intracellular bacteria (mycobacteria, listeria)	-	+++	+++	-	-
Viruses					
High-grade pathogens	-	++++	++++	-	-
Low-grade pathogens (warts, fever blisters)	++	++++	++++	-	-
Fungi	+	++++	++++	++	+
Protozoa (*Pneumocystis carinii*)	++	++++	++++	-	-

*Coded for degree of susceptibility to infection: + + + +, most susceptible: +, least susceptible: −, equal to the susceptibility of the general population.

primarily reflect a population of hypogammaglobulinemics; however, other primary immunodeficiencies seem to show the same incidence.

The sex distribution shows a male predominance (62%), which is especially pronounced among children less than 15 years of age (83%) (Medical Research Council Working Party, 1969). This male predominance is in part due to the X-linked inheritance pattern of certain of the immunodeficiency diseases.

The heterogeneous nature of primary immunodeficiency disorders is probably the best evidence of their multiple etiologies. It is recognized that most of these disorders are congenital and that inheritance plays a major role in many of them. Investigation often has led to the identification of a defect in the structure or development of the immune system. With the increasing sophistication of immunologic tests, new and more subtle defects of the immune system are rapidly being uncovered (Table 10-2). Thus, it would be difficult and confusing to cover each and every immunodeficiency state that is now recognized in a review of this type. Instead, this paper examines the prototype for immunodeficiency disorders involving the B cell, T cell, phagocytic, and complement systems, illustrating the major defects involved and their common head and neck manifestations.

IMMUNODEFICIENCY INVOLVING THE B-CELL SYSTEM

B lymphocytes (B cells) are recognized as having the capacity to respond to antigenic stimulation by proliferating and giving rise to antibody-producing mature plasma cells. B cells can be found distributed throughout the body in lymph nodes, spleen, tonsils, appendix, Peyer's patches, and the peripheral blood.

T cells, on the other hand, are responsible for cell-mediated immunity and are the effector cells in delayed hypersensitivity reactions. While this division of labor exists within the immune system, the operation of B-cell functions requires the cooperation of T cells. For example, antibody response to an antigen as well as amplification of that response, immunologic memory, and transition from IgM to IgG production, all require T lymphocytes to provide a helper function. Not only is this cellular cooperation responsible for the production of antibody, it is also responsible for its ultimate regulation and control, leading in some instances to abnormal suppression of the antibody response (T suppressor cells).

X-Linked Infantile Agammaglobulinemia (Bruton's Disease)

Case History

The patient, a Caucasian boy, was the first child in his family. He had pneumonia at 2 years of age, and at 4 he contracted meningitis due to *Hemophilus influenzae.* The physician who treated his meningitis noted that he had no visible tonsils, and that his lymph nodes were very small. The mother's only brother had died at age 20 from chronic

TABLE 10-2. Laboratory examination of a patient with too many infections.

	Humoral immune deficiency, B Cell	Cellular immune deficiency, T Cell	Combined immune deficiency	Phagocytic defects	Complement defects
Screening tests (all patients)					
CBC	Normal (rarely neutropenia associated)	Lymphopenia	Lymphopenia Eosinophilia	Neutropenia Neutrophilia Monocytosis Eosinophilia	Normal
Immunoglobulins IgG, -M, -A, -E	*Absent, disproportional	Normal, absent IgA paraproteins	*Absent; low	Normal or high	Normal
Isohemagglutinins	*Absent	Normal, low, or absent	Absent	Normal	Normal
Skin tests for delayed hypersensitivity	Normal	Negative	Negative	Normal; induration without erythema	Normal
CH_{50}, C_3	Normal	Normal	Normal	Normal	Low, rarely normal
Nitroblue tetrazolium (NBT)	Normal (if opsonins furnished)	Normal	Normal (if opsonins furnished)	*Negative in CGD	Normal
Follow-up tests (selected patients)					
T-cell and B-cell enumeration by rosettes; surface immunoglobulins	Absent B cells; normal in common variable	Absent T cells; normal	Absent T and B cells; normal	Normal	Normal
Mutagenic response of lymphocytes in culture	Normal	*PHA, Con A negative	*PHA, Con A negative, MLC negative or low	Normal	Normal

*Most important and diagnostic for the condition listed. CGD, chronic granulomatous disease of childhood; PHA, phytohemagglutinin; Con A, concanavalin-A; MLC, mixed leukocyte culture.

(Continued next page)

TABLE 10-2. Laboratory examination of a patient with too many infections. (continued)

	Humoral immune deficiency, B Cell	Cellular immune deficiency, T Cell	Combined immune deficiency	Phagocytic defects	Complement defects
Bone marrow aspiration	Absent plasma cells	Normal; lymphocytes low	Normal; lymphocytes low	*Neutropenia	Normal
Lymph node biopsy	Absent germinal follicles and plasma cells	Absent T-dependent areas	Absence of both T-cell and B-cell areas	Normal	Normal
Skin graft rejection	Normal	Absent	Absent	Normal	Normal
Rebuck skin window	Normal	Normal	Normal	Normal; abnormal in some chemotactic defects	Normal; rarely abnormal in C_3 deficiency
Chemotaxis and random mobility of phagocytes	Normal	Normal	Normal	Abnormal in chemotactic defects	*Abnormal chemotactic defect
Phagocytic killing test, intracellular metabolism phagocytic index	Normal	Normal	Normal	Abnormal in CGD	Normal if phagocytosis occurs
Characterization of T-cell subsets by monoclonal antibody technique	Normal	Abnormal	Abnormal	Normal	Normal
Complement components by chemical or functional assay	Normal	Normal	Low C_{1q}	Normal	*Abnormal according to specific defects

*Most important and diagnostic for the condition listed. CGD, chronic granulomatous disease of childhood; PHA, phytohemagglutinin; Con A, concanavalin-A; MLC, mixed leukocyte culture.

lung infection, thought to be secondary to paralytic polio which he had as a young child. This family history and the physical findings were suggestive of an immune defect, and immunoglobulin levels were obtained. All immunoglobulins were undetectable except IgM, which was low at 4 mg/dL. Isohemagglutinins were negative. The delayed hypersensitivity response was positive for *Candida*. Meanwhile, he had recovered normally after antibiotic therapy for meningitis. He was started on intramuscular immune serum globulin, 1.2 cc/kg as a loading dose and then 0.6 cc/kg every month. A year later the mother reported that he was a different child while on treatment. She stated that although she had denied that he had frequent infections in the initial history, he always had a "runny nose" beginning at 6 months of age, which she thought was normal. On therapy he had no more serious infections; he continued to have purulent nasal discharge but it was a very small amount, and his general well-being was greatly improved.

Etiology

The X-linked inheritance of this disorder is considered highly likely; however, there has been no definitive proof for the X-linked transmission of the disease. Most suggestive, however, is the observation that 80% of congenital antibody-deficient children are male (Squire, 1962).

The primary defect in X-linked agammaglobulinemia is the lack of B lymphocytes. The search for a structural or anatomic defect in this condition stems from animal experiments in which bursectomized chicks were found to be completely devoid of antibody production, indicating that in chickens, at least, the bursa of Fabricius is the anatomic site responsible for the differentiation of stem cells or precursor cells into B-committed cells (Cooper et al., 1966). However, even though in mammals the bursal equivalent appears to reside in the fetal liver and bone marrow, no specific anatomic defect has been identified as yet (Owen et al., 1974). What has been reported is the absence of B lymphocytes with surface immunoglobulins (Cooper & Lawton, 1972). Additionally, it has been reported that populations of suppressor cells exist in the peripheral blood of these patients which, when cultured along with normal patients' peripheral blood lymphocytes, can prevent differentiation of B lymphocytes into plasma cells (Siegal et al., 1976). It is not clear, however, if the genetic defect results in the presence of suppressor cells which prevent B-cell function or whether the genetically determined B-cell defect ultimately leads to the generation of a suppressor cell population (Blaise et al., 1975).

Clinical Features

The usual history in X-linked infantile agammaglobulinemia is one of recurrent bacterial infections becoming apparent after the protection afforded by maternal antibody subsides. This usually occurs between the ages of 6 and 9 months.

The most common pyogenic infections include chronic otitis media, recurrent otitis externa, acute or chronic sinusitis, bronchiectasis, pyoderma, and osteomyelitis. These infections are usually caused by pneumococci. *Hemophilus influenzae*, streptococci, and *Pseudomonas aeruginosa*. Additionally, these patients may show varying degrees of growth failure, nonrheumatoid arthritis, and conjunctivitis. Despite these infections they do not demonstrate lymphadenopathy, splenomegaly, or prominent tonsil or adenoid tissue.

The otologic manifestations may be particularly resistant to topical therapy, may ultimately develop into mastoiditis, and, despite mastoidectomy, continue to exhibit otorrhea and evidence of poor healing (Sasaki et al., 1981)

Diagnostic Findings

The characteristic laboratory finding in this condition is a markedly reduced level of all five immunoglobulin classes, with IgG levels generally less than 200 mg/dL (normal adult mean 1200 mg/dL).

Additional evaluation of these patients should include sensitization with a potent immunogen such as bacteriophage OX174, keyhole-limpet hemocyanin (KLH), pneumococcal polysaccharide vaccine, or typhoid vaccine. Failure to produce specific antibody following antigenic stimulation confirms the diagnosis of X-linked agammaglobulinemia. Supportive evidence may also be obtained from lymph node biopsies that show the absence of germinal centers, lymphoid follicles, and plasma cells. (See Fig 10-1, and chapter 1, Fig 1-11).

Treatment.

After the diagnosis has been made, the mainstay of treatment involves human gamma globulin replacement therapy, with the usual dosage being approximately 100 mg/kg per month. It is essential that these patients avoid live virus and bacterial vaccines, which could, themselves, result in progressive infection. Also of prime importance is the early recognition of infection in these individuals, prompt institution of appropriate antibiotics after cultures have been obtained, and drainage procedures performed as indicated.

Prognosis

Through the judicious use of antibiotics and gamma globulin replacement, patients often do quite well, although most will have persistent low-grade upper respiratory infection. Chronic lung disease, however, may ultimately lead to debilitation later in life, and a shortened life span.

Common Variable Immunodeficiency (Acquired Agammaglobulinemia)

Like X-linked infantile agammaglobulinemia, the acquired form is associated with markedly diminished serum immunoglobulins and recurrent sinopulmonary infections. Usually this disease presents in the second or third decade of life, which distinguishes it from the X-linked form. On occasion, however, this illness may be acquired during infancy, which creates problems in the separation of these two conditions. The etiology of this disease is unknown, although environmental causes, viral illness, or familial factors have been postulated. There have been a number of immune defects identified, including diminished numbers of B lymphocytes, abnormal B-cell maturation, failure to release synthesized immunoglobulin, and serum or T-cell suppressive factors (Geha et al., 1974; Waldmann et al., 1974).

FIG 10-1. Lymph node from patient with X-linked infantile agammaglobulinemia. Note absence of germinal centers, lymphoid follicles, and plasma cells.

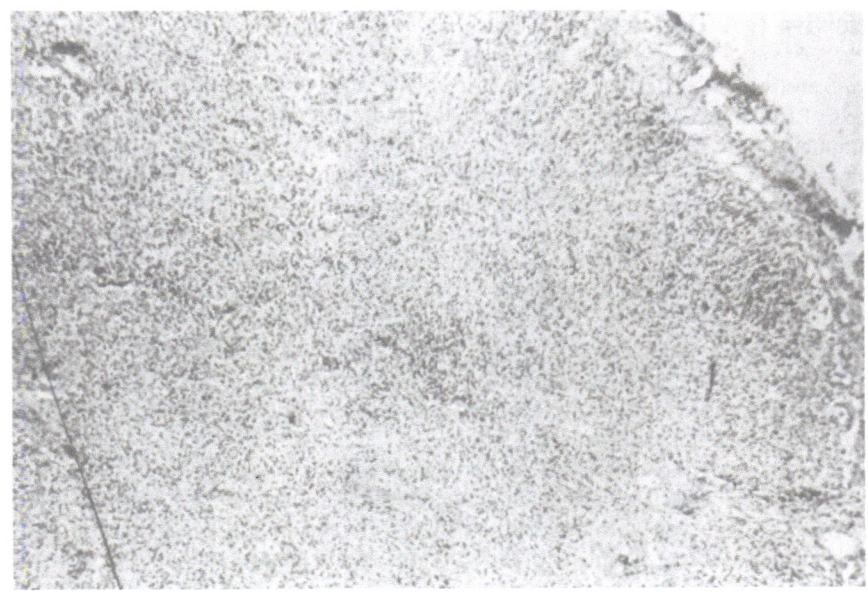

The major head and neck manifestations and their treatment are similar to those occurring in X-linked infantile agammaglobulinemia.

X-Linked Immunodeficiency with Hyper-IgM

This condition is characterized by recurrent pyogenic infections in male children with low or absent levels of IgG, IgA, IgE, and elevated levels of IgM and IgD. Unlike Bruton's agammaglobulinemia, these individuals commonly demonstrate neutropenia, hypertrophied tonsils, and splenomegaly. Oral stomatitis may become prevalent because of the associated neutropenia, in addition to otitis media, tonsillitis, and pneumonia. The etiology of this condition is unknown; however, most consider this to be the result of a defect in the switch mechanism occurring during B-cell development. Normally, there is a switch in the gene expression coding for the constant region of the heavy chains so that a B cell that produces IgM will be the progenitor of cells producing antibody with the same specificity but of a different class (that is, IgG, IgA, IgE). A defect in this switch could, therefore, result in an observed overproduction of IgM, whereas IgG and IgA and

IgE remain deficient. Treatment with adequate levels of gammaglobulin usually is accompanied by a restitution of the IgM to normal levels.

Selective IgA Deficiency

Selective IgA deficiency may be defined as when individuals have abnormally low levels of IgA with normal levels of the other immunoglobulins. IgA is the predominant immunoglobulin contained in the body's secretions and has been shown to protect the mucosal surfaces from invasion by pathogens and from the absorption of antigens or toxins into the general circulation. It is not surprising, therefore, that individuals lacking this immunoglobulin often demonstrate malabsorption and diarrhea. These patients also suffer from a higher incidence of allergies and autoimmune disorders. It has been theorized that because of the lack of the protective effect that this antibody affords, many antigens are absorbed across mucosal surfaces into the general circulation and antibodies are thus formed against them. For example, a high percentage of these individuals demonstrate antibodies to milk as well as autoantibodies (Ammann et al., 1971). Whether these findings are responsible for the development of atopy or cross-reacting antibodies resulting in autoimmunity is not known.

The majority of patients with selective IgA deficiency have relatively mild symptoms unless there are associated cellular immune defects. In fact, one in 500 asymptomatic "normal" patients appear to have this deficiency. The vast majority of patients with this deficiency has absent serum and secretory IgA with normal amounts of secretory component. A very small percentage have absent serum IgA levels, and a few cases have been found with normal IgA, reduced secretory IgA, and absent secretory component. When these patients are symptomatic, they commonly present with diseases of the respiratory and gastrointestinal tracts, of which recurrent pneumonia, chronic bronchitis, obstructive lung disease, various malabsorption syndromes, and chronic diarrhea are most prevalent. The head and neck manifestations may include recurrent rhinitis and sinusitis, serous and chronic otitis media, mastoiditis, adenotonsillitis, and parotitis (Bergal et al., 1976; Kimmelman et al., 1979). As a manifestation of their autoimmune disease, thyroiditis may also be associated.

When treatment is required in this condition, it should be directed toward the specific infectious process or autoimmune condition. Experience with infusing gammaglobulin or fresh-frozen plasma has been both disappointing and potentially dangerous. Gamma globulin contains insufficient quantities of IgA to replace the deficiency yet enough to sensitize the recipient to IgA, thus forming anti-IgA antibodies. Subsequent transfusions, therefore, are fraught with the risk of anaphylaxis. However, topical or oral administration of colostrum, rich in IgA, has been shown to be of benefit in the treatment of malabsorption and some cases of persistent mastoid infections (Sasaki et al., 1981; Krabauer et al., 1975).

IMMUNODEFICIENCY INVOLVING THE T-CELL SYSTEM

Thymic Hypoplasia (DiGeorge Syndrome)

Case History

An infant began to have seizures on the second day of life and was diagnosed as having hypocalcemic neonatal tetany. He responded slowly to calcium therapy. At 6 weeks of age he was admitted with tachypnea, cyanosis, and recurrent seizures. It was noted on physical examination that the baby had a small jaw and mouth, and the ears were low set. Candidal lesions covered the buccal mucosa and extended to a few small areas of the tongue. Muscle tone was increased. Chest x-ray revealed a diffuse interstitial pneumonia. There was a right-sided aortic arch and "narrow waist" configuration of the heart. Thymic shadow could not be delineated on the admission x-ray film because of the pulmonary infiltrate; a review of the neonatal films revealed absence of the thymic shadow on the second day of life. The laboratory studies revealed continued hypocalcemia, normal immunoglobulin levels, lymphopenia, and a lack of blast transformation on PHA stimulation of peripheral blood lymphocytes. The infant failed to improve with antibiotic therapy and was subjected to an open lung biopsy, from which *Pneumocystis carinii* infection was diagnosed. A few cells suggestive of cytomegalovirus infection were also noted. Despite treatment with both trimethoprim sulfa and pentamidine, the pulmonary status continued to deteriorate, and the baby died a month after admission.

Etiology

The thymus gland arises from the third and fourth pharyngeal pouches during the 6th and 8th week of embryonic life. Altered embryogenesis during this time may also result in abnormalities of structures derived from the first, second, and sixth pharyngeal pouches. As a result, there are major variants of this syndrome ranging from an incomplete to a complete form. The thymus gland may range from mildly hypoplastic to totally aplastic. The nature of the immune defect appears to be thymus-dependent and related to a deficiency in the production of a humoral substance that induces and maintains T-cell immunity (Steele et al., 1972). Thymosin has been one such substance isolated from the thymus gland which appears to cause maturation of bone marrow cells or peripheral blood lymphocytes from some individuals with DiGeorge syndrome.

Clinical Manifestations

In both the complete and incomplete forms of DiGeorge syndrome there usually exists a characteristic facial appearance that includes hypertelorism, antimongoloid slanted eyes, low-set ears with notched pinnae and diminished helix development, and micrognathia. (Figs 10-2 and 10-3). In addition, a highly arched palate, bifid uvula, and shortened upper lip philtrum may also be present. The predominant manifestations in areas other than the head and neck include cardiovascular and parathyroid abnormalities.

FIG 10-2. Pinna in patient with DiGeorge syndrome.

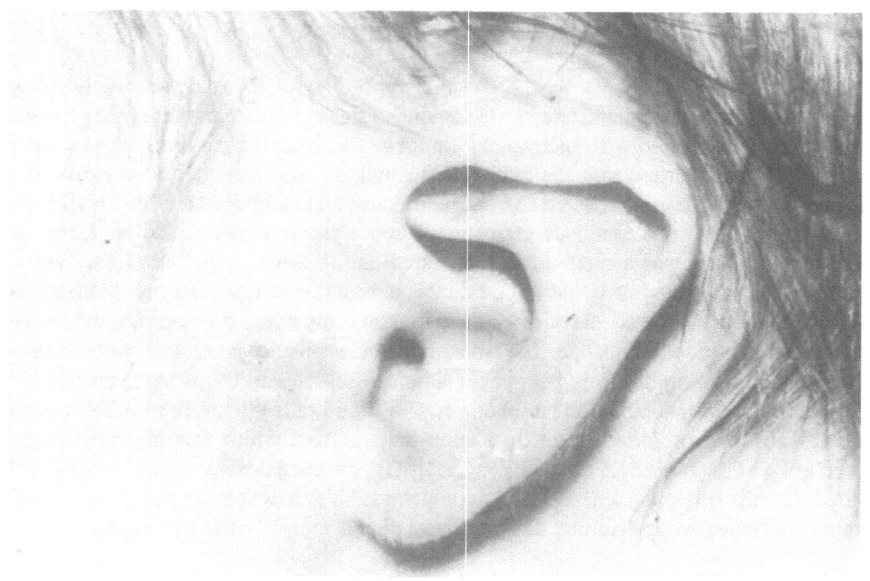

The cardiovascular anomalies may include right-sided aortic arch, ventricular or atrial septal defect, tetralogy of Fallot, right ventricular infundibular stenosis, aberrant left subclavian artery, and pulmonary artery atresia or hypoplasia. The parathyroid deficiency may result in hypocalcemia and tetany in the first few days of life and is associated with an elevated serum phosphorus and absent parathyroid hormone levels.

These infants usually have a stormy neonatal period that becomes complicated by an increased susceptibility to infections. The most prevalent of these are oral candidiasis, chronic rhinitis, recurrent pneumonia (including *Pneumocystis carinii*), and diarrhea. These infants usually fail to thrive.

Diagnostic Findings

The combination of hypocalcemia and congenital heart disease should make one strongly suspicious of the presence of this syndrome and warrant further investigation. One of the most useful preliminary studies is a chest x-ray to demonstrate an absent thymic shadow or malformation of the great vessels. Studies of T-cell immunity should then be considered and include the following assays: total peripheral blood lymphocyte count, T-cell rosettes, lymphocyte blastogenesis to mitogens, mixed leukocyte culture response, and delayed hypersensitivity skin tests. The response of these assays, however, must be analyzed in the context of the entire clinical picture. Lymph node biopsy reveals the absence of lymphocytes in the perifollicular and cortical areas (Fig 10-4).

FIG 10-3. Characteristic facial appearance in patient with DiGeorge syndrome. Note low-set ears, micrognathia, and upturned nose.

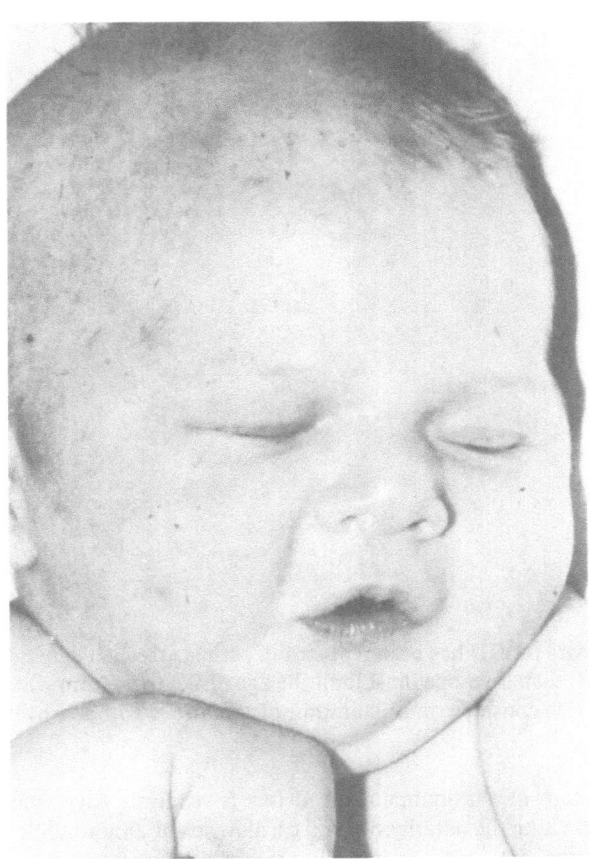

Treatment

Management of hypoparathyroidism is of paramount importance in supporting life. Intravenous calcium gluconate may be given to control tetany, followed by long-term oral vitamin D, a low phosphorus diet, and calcium supplementation. Correction of the T-cell defect may be achieved by fetal thymus transplantation. Thymus tissue fragments are obtained from an aborted 10 to 14-week-old human fetus and transplanted intraperitoneally through a catheter or intramuscularly. Evidence of immunologic reconstitution may be seen as early as six hours post-transplantation (Cleveland, 1975). Fatal

FIG 10-4. Lymph node from patient with DiGeorge syndrome. Note absence of lymphocytes in perifollicular and deep cortical areas.

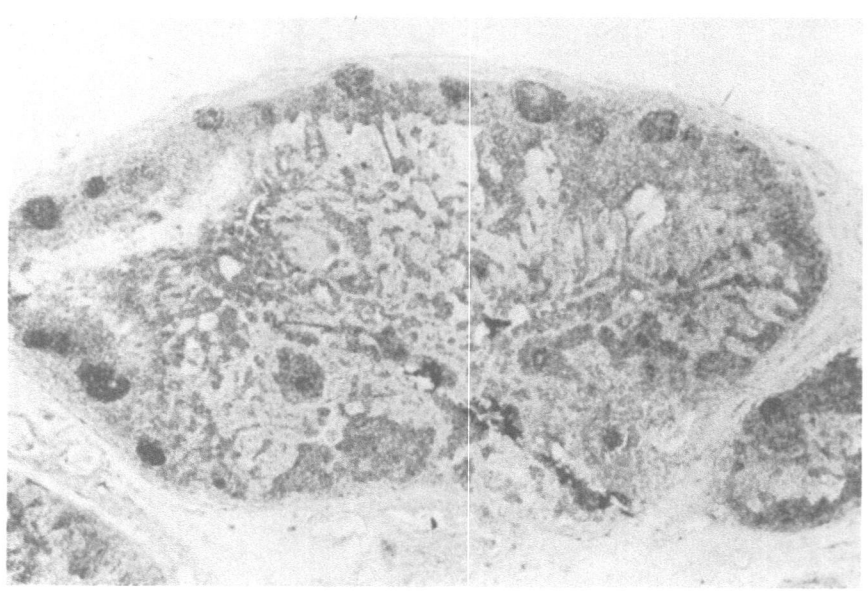

graft *v* host disease (GVH) has been reported in patients receiving greater than 14-week-old fetal thymus; therefore, one must limit the age of the fetus from which thymic tissue is harvested or else consider transplantation of this tissue within a Millipore chamber.

Prognosis

The correction of the immunologic defect is relatively easy compared with the difficulty in correcting the parathyroid and cardiovascular abnormalities. If they can be managed, however, long-term survival is occasionally seen. Spontaneous correction of both the hypoparathyroid state and the T-cell immune defect have been reported if longevity is achieved.

Chronic Mucocutaneous Candidiasis (CMC)

Etiology

The major immunologic defect in this condition is an abnormal T-cell response to *Candida* antigen. This is manifested by anergy to *Candida* skin testing and absent or abnormal lymphocyte blastogenesis to *Candida* antigen in vitro. Additionally, attempts to sensitize patients within 2, 4-dinitrofluorobenzene (DNFB) intradermally have been unsuccessful, further suggesting a basic T-cell defect. Despite these findings there does not appear to be susceptibility to other nonfungal infectious agents. Numerous defects and serum factors have been discovered in these patients that disappear after treatment, causing one to speculate that they were merely epiphenomena rather than that which caused the underlying immune defect. CMC may also be associated with endocrinopathies and in such cases autoimmunity appears to be more prevalent.

Clinical manifestations

This condition may affect individuals during their infancy or may be delayed until they are somewhat older. Candidiasis most commonly presents in the head and neck with involvement of the oral mucous membranes (Fig 10-5). These may appear as superficial whitish plaques easily scraped away with a tongue blade or may be the more invasive granulomatous form, which is ulcerative and vegetative. The latter is more commonly associated with endocrinopathies. Perleche (involvement of the labial commissures with fissuring and crusting) may also occur, resulting in marked discomfort, with the patient having a tendency to avoid eating or talking (Fig 10-6). Dysphagia may be a prevalent symptom solely from the oral lesions but may also represent involvement of the hypopharynx, larynx, and esophagus and should be excluded by examination.

Manifestations in areas other than the head and neck often include *Candida* infection of the skin and nailbeds of the fingers and toes, which are particularly recalcitrant to treatment.

The endocrinopathies associated with CMC include hypoparathyroidism (70%), Addison's disease (37%), and, less commonly, hypothyroidism and diabetes (Blizzard et al., 1968). These patients often exhibit susceptibility to other types of fungal infections as well as *Candida*.

Laboratory Findings

Culture of the lesions readily reveals *Candida*; however, biopsy provides evidence for its depth of tissue invasion and degree of host responsiveness.

Autoantibodies against all of the endocrine organs may be present and may precede the onset of endocrine dysfunction (Blizzard et al., 1968).

Antibodies to *Candida* as well as other antigens are usually found to be normal; however, delayed hypersensitivity skin test reactions are negative to *Candida* and rarely vigorously positive to other antigens. T-cell numbers and phytohemagglutinin (PHA) responses are usually normal, yet lymphocyte transformation and migration inhibition factor production (MIF) is deficient when exposed to *Candida*.

Treatment

Antifungal agents usually must be given continually. Topical agents such as nystatin (Mycostatin) usually will contain the lesions; however, intravenous amphotericin B is required for eradication or improvement. Relapses eventually occur and the toxicity of amphotericin precludes its continuous use. Ketoconazole, a recently approved antifungal agent for oral administration, has been shown to be beneficial.

FIG 10-5. Mucocutaneous candidiasis involving the oral mucous membranes.

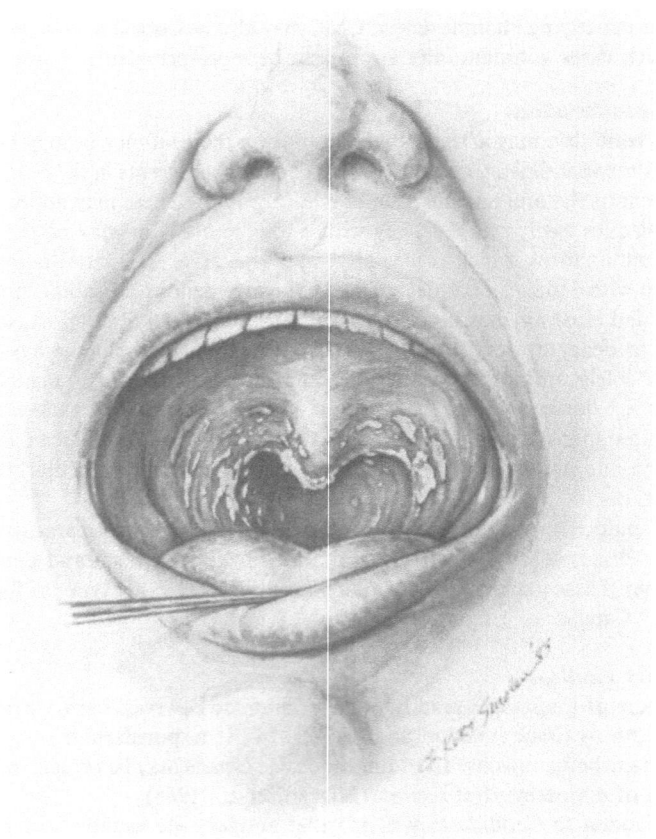

Transfer factor, made from lymphocyte preparations of *Candida*-sensitive donors, has been shown to be of some value in prolonging remission after treatment with amphotericin. Other forms of therapy with limited trials include thymosin, levamisole, matched lymphocyte transfusions, and transplanted fetal thymus.

Treatment of the endocrinopathies is along standard lines and is unaffected by therapy directed toward the immune deficit.

FIG 10-6. Fissuring and crusting of labial commissures (perleche) in patient with mucocutaneous candidiasis.

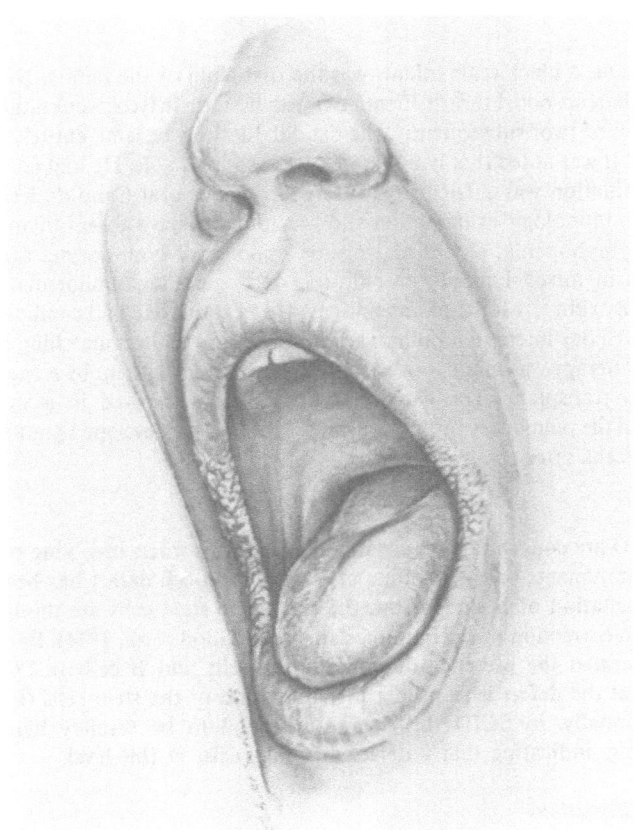

Prognosis
This is a chronic debilitating disease that disfigures patients and is associated, in its severest form, with a shortened life span. Endocrine disorders frequently complicate their care and may lead to death. The mild forms are not associated with a shortened life span but may have a significant psychological effect on their victims.

IMMUNODEFICIENCY INVOLVING BOTH T-CELL AND B-CELL SYSTEMS

Severe Combined Immunodeficiency Diseases (SCID)

Case History

The patient, a black male infant, was the first child of the family. He was 5 weeks old when his parents noted thrush. Treatment with nystatin (Mycostatin) produced clearing for only a day or two; subsequently, the candidal lesions became entirely refractory to local therapy. It was noted that lymph nodes were not palpable. He had no visible tonsils but the examination was difficult because of extensive oral *Candida* lesions. He was referred for immunologic examination and was found to have absent thymic shadow on x-ray films, lymphopenia, absent blastogenic response of lymphocytes after mitogenic stimulus and in mixed lymphocyte cultures, and agammaglobulinemia. His delayed hypersensitivity skin test for *Candida* antigen was negative. He had candidal esophagitis and a mild perihilar interstitial pulmonary infiltrate. He had no matching bone marrow donor so an attempt was made to reconstitute his immune system by a specially treated bone marrow transplant. The Candidiasis completely resolved in a week after the procedure, and the pulmonary infiltrate cleared. However, he developed graft-*v*-host disease and died 3 weeks after the transplant.

Etiology

The SCID are congenital and usually hereditary disorders involving both the T-cell and B-cell components of the immune system. A stem-cell defect has been postulated since transplantation of bone marrow, the site where stem cells are thought to reside, has resulted in correction of the immunodeficiency (Good et al., 1974). Surface markers have demonstrated the presence of immature T cells and B cells in SCID patients, suggesting that the defect is in proper differentiation of the stem cells (Buckley et al., 1976). Additionally, in SCID the thymus is found to be severely hypoplastic and nonfunctioning, indicating that a defect also may exist at this level.

Clinical Manifestations

This illness is associated with the most widespread and devastating infections that occur with the immunodeficiency diseases. Bacterial, viral, and fungal illnesses are prevalent and resist common forms of therapy. Common manifestations of these infections include chronic oral candidiasis, overwhelming pneumonia secondary to *Pneumocystis carinii*, cytomegalovirus or measles virus, ulcerations of the tongue, palate, and buccal mucosa from which herpes virus or pseudomonas can be cultured, chronic diarrhea with malabsorption, chronic active hepatitis, and chronic encephalitis.

FIG 10-7. Lymph node from patient with SCID. Note absence of germinal centers, deep cortical areas, and lymphocytes.

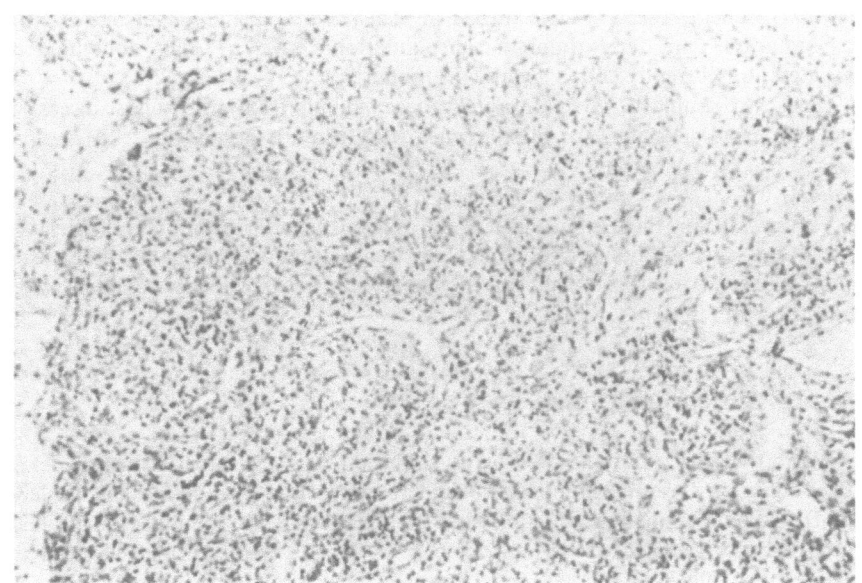

Laboratory Findings

The tests of T-cell function discussed previously also demonstrate various abnormalities in SCID. While lymphocyte counts, E rosettes, and PHA responses are all usually low this is not absolute (Buckely et al., 1976). However, in vitro lymphocyte unresponsiveness to antigens appears to be a universal finding.

The immunoglobulin levels are usually low, with IgA and IgM undetectable by routine analysis and IgG < 200 mg/dL. Occasionally, immunoglobulin levels may only be slightly depressed and the patient's sensitization to antigens is helpful, since this has been associated with a weak or absent antibody response in all cases of SCID. Thymic biopsy demonstrates a small hypoplastic gland with absent lymphocytes and Hassall's corpuscles. Lymph node biopsy reveals absence of lymphocyte and discernible germinal (B-cell) centers and deep cortical (T-cell) areas. (Fig 10-7)

Treatment

Bone marrow transplantation appears to offer the greatest chance of correcting the immune defect in SCID. When bone marrow is obtained from a histocompatible sibling donor (especially matched at the HLA-D focus), the 6-month survival rate is 62.5% (Bortin et al., 1977). Other less successful treatments are fetal liver transplantation, thymic epithelial transplantation, and fetal thumus transplantation; however, only bone marrow transplantation currently shows significant promise.

Great care should be given to protect these patients from graft-v-host disease by giving only irradiated blood or plasma when transfusion is necessary.

Prognosis

Without therapy these infants usually die of overwhelming infection in the first year of life. Prompt recognition and bone marrow transplantation appears to offer greater longevity; however, insufficient numbers of patients have been treated to accurately predict overall survival rates.

Wiskott-Aldrich Syndrome

Wiskott-Aldrich syndrome (WAS) is an X-linked recessive disorder displaying defects in T-cell function, abnormal immunoglobulin levels (increased IgA and IgE and low levels of IgM), and poor antibody production when exposed to antigens. Clinically these patients exhibit petechiae secondary to thrombocytopenia, eczema, and recurrent bacterial and viral infections. The head and neck manifestations include chronic purulent otitis media, mastoiditis, hemotympanum, epistaxis, subconjunctival hemorrhage, mucous membrane petechiae, herpetic lesions, cervical lymphadenopathy, and lymphomas.

Treatment initially is to control the bleeding diatheses and infections with the hope of finding a suitable donor for bone marrow transplantation. If life can be sustained, the later development of lymphoreticular malignancies further threatens survival.

Ataxia-Telangiectasia

This immunodeficiency disorder demonstrates an autosomal recessive inheritance pattern and is characterized by recurrent sinopulmonary infections, telangiectases, progressive cerebellar ataxia, and development of malignancies. The immunologic defect includes IgA deficiency, cutaneous anergy, abnormal response of lymphocytes to mitogens, and autoantibodies. Aside from the upper respiratory infections, the major head and neck manifestation of this disorder involves the development of lymphomas within this region.

The life span of these patients is greatly diminished by the occurrence of malignancy and recurrent infections; in cases where these can be successfully managed, the patient becomes severely disabled by progressive neurologic degeneration.

DISORDERS OF PHAGOCYTOSIS

Neutropenia

Neutropenia is defined as a condition in which there are decreased numbers of circulating polymorphonuclear (PMN) leukocytes. When this level drops below 500/mm^3 these patients are at extreme risk to develop severe infections. This condition may be congenital (autosomal recessive or dominant trait) or acquired (especially as a consequence of drug-induced aplastic anemia). Infections due to *Staphylococcus, Escherichia coli, Pseudomonas, Klebsiella,* and anaerobic organisms are particularly common; however, many of the usual signs and symptoms of infections are absent. For example, abscesses rarely occur since the generation of pus requires PMNs. Treatment consists of appropriate cultures, antibiotics, and prompt attention to seemingly minor infections.

Cyclic neutropenia is a condition in which neutropenia occurs in cycles of 15 to 35 days. During this nadir in granulocyte count, the patient commonly will develop stomatitis, fever, malaise, sore throat, ischiorectal infections, and lymphadenitis (Page et al., 1957). Recognition of this condition is important and treatment is directed toward eradication of the infections.

Chronic Granulomatous Disease of Childhood (CGD)

This disorder follows an X-linked recessive mode of inheritance and is characterized by widespread granulomatous lesions particularly involving the skin, lungs, lymph nodes, liver, and spleen. The immune defect appears to stem from the inability of granulocytes to kill bacteria intracellularly. Studies examining the mechanism by which bacteria survive in granulocytes from CGD patients indicate that there is no activation of NADH or NADPH oxidase during phagocytosis, resulting in no oxygen uptake, no production of superoxide or hydrogen peroxide, and little increase in hexose monophosphate shunt activity; all are considered essential components of microbicidal activity in phagocytes (Quie et al., 1977).

The major manifestations of this illness include persistent rhinitis (56%), ulcerative stomatitis (40%), generalized lymphadenopathy (100%), hepatosplenomegaly (98%), pneumonitis (100%), perianal abscess (36%), and osteomyelitis (28%) (Johnson et al., 1967). The earliest lesions involve eczematoid reactions of the periauricular and nasal skin which progress to purulent dermatitis. Local cervical lymphadenopathy occurs with subsequent necrosis, granuloma formation, and suppuration.

Diagnosis can be made by nitroblue tetrazolium (NBT) reduction test used as a screening procedure, followed by more definitive tests of intracellular killing. Treatment consists of early administration of specific antibiotics, drainage of abscesses, and possible bone marrow transplantation. Recent studies of long-term, low doses of trimethoprim sulfa have shown improvement of the metabolic function of phagocytes and clinical benefit in these patients (Johnston, in press).

DISORDERS OF THE COMPLEMENT SYSTEM

C_1 Inhibitor Deficiency: Hereditary Angioneurotic Edema (HANE)

The HANE is a recurrent, self-limited illness characterized by the sudden swelling and angioedema of the subcutaneous tissues and the upper respiratory and gastrointestinal tracts. It occurs as the result of a genetically determined (autosomal dominant) defect in the biosynthesis of C_1 inhibitor (C_1 IHN).

C_1 is normally activated by tissue trauma or stress, and in individuals in whom C_1 IHN is deficient or nonfunctional, there is an unchecked activation of the complement cascade. This ultimately leads to the liberation of a vasoactive kinin-like peptide believed responsible for angioedema.

The major manifestation of this illness is sudden attacks of abdominal pain due to collections of intestinal wall edema, circumscribed swelling of the hands and feet, and, of greatest potential risk to life, swelling of the mucous membranes of the upper respiratory tract. There is antecedent physical trauma (that is, dental extraction or tonsillectomy) in 54% of cases and evidence of emotional upset in 43% (Frank et al., 1976). The usual clinical course is one to three days with gradual clearing of the edema.

The symptoms in the head and neck generally start out with swelling of the lips, face, palate, and uvula, which may then stabilize or progress to supraglottic, glottic, and hypopharyngeal involvement (Figs 10-8 and 10-9). Complaints of odynophonia, dysphagia, and hoarseness are common with laryngeal involvement and serve as good indicators of impending respiratory distress. These patients must be admitted to a hospital and observed closely for the development of airway obstruction that might necessitate a tracheotomy. Up to a 30% mortality in HANE due to acute respiratory obstruction has been reported. The diagnosis can be made in a suspected individual by a low level of serum C_1 INH with depletion of C_4 and C_2 during symptomatic periods.

The treatment consists of prophylactic methyltestosterone (10 to 25 mg q.d.) which may prevent attacks in up to 50% of treated patients. Danazol has been used quite successfully and has the advantage of not having the masculinizing properties of methyltestosterone (Gelfand et al., 1976). Treatment with epsilon aminocaproic acid has had some success in stopping attacks of angioedema; however, the side effects make its use limited. Tranexamic acid has also been of value in prophylaxis for patients undergoing surgical procedures (Sheffer et al., 1977). Steroids, epinephrine, and antihistamines have not been shown to be helpful in the treatment of these attacks.

A common misconception in the treatment of HANE has been the usefulness of plasma transfusions. The rationale for their use has been that C_1 INH contained in plasma would halt the complement cascade. In practice, however, more complement substrate is provided than inhibitor which, therefore, only serves to heighten the attacks. This form of therapy is therefore contraindicated for this disease.

The C_1 INH deficiency has also been associated with malignant lymphomas. These patients usually have an acquired angioneurotic edema that exhibits all of the clinical symptomatology seen in HANE. Therefore, one must consider an occult lymphoma in the differential diagnosis of these patients.

FIG 10-8. Marked angineurotic edema of face and lips of patient with HANE. (Reprinted with permission of WB Saunders, Philadelphia, 1969. *Atlas of Otorhinolaryngology and Bronchoesophagology***, p 94. Eds: Walter Becker, Richard Buckingham, Paul Holinger, Gunter Korting, Francis Lederer).**

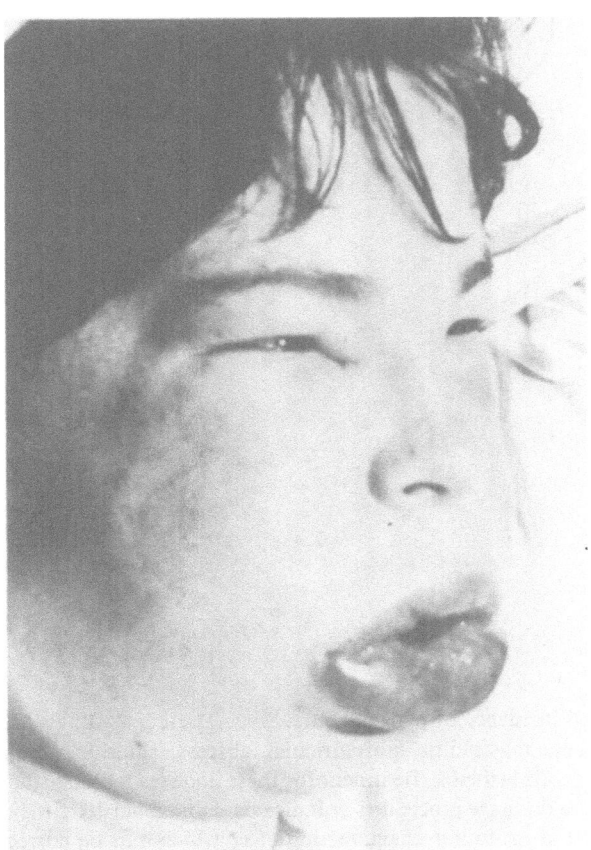

Other Complement Disorders

A number of complement deficiencies (C_{1q}, C_{1r}, C_2 to C_8) have been described with varying degrees of resultant immunodeficiency. For the most part these appear to be inherited disorders with family members also demonstrating similar deficiencies. Defects in complement-mediated functions such as reduced hemolytic and bactericidal activity or failure of chemotaxis and opsonization of endotoxin may be demonstrated in individuals

FIG 10-9. Angioneurotic edema of larynx in patient with HANE. Note normal larynx in upper left for comparison. (Reprinted with permission of WB Saunders, Philadelphia, 1969. *Atlas of Otorhinolaryngology and Bronchoesophagology*, p 94. Eds: Walter Becker, Richard Buckingham, Paul Holinger, Gunter Korting, Francis Lederer.)

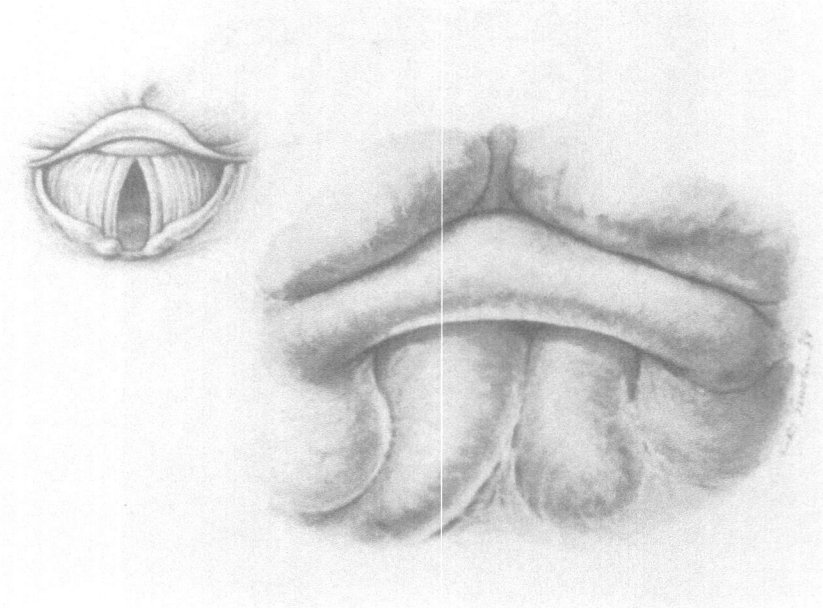

with an increased incidence of pyogenic infections. These individuals may present with otitis media, acute mastoiditis, postauricular abscess, sinusitis, sepsis, pneumonia, meningitis, and septic arthritis. Treatment for these illnesses is along standard lines with specific agents and drainage procedures as indicated. Functional deficiency of C_5 (Leiner's disease) produces a profound chemotactic defect which can be corrected by plasma infusions.

SUMMARY

The otorhinolaryngologist has a great opportunity to see immune-deficient patients early in their course since they often present with serious upper respiratory infections requiring surgical management. The universally available screening tests can point to patients needing referral to an immunologist who must be consulted for the more sophisticated immunologic workup and examination. Management both before and after definitive diagnosis of the immune defect is aimed at scrupulous attention to the surgical and antimicrobial treatment of the infectious processes in these patients.

REFERENCES

Ammann AJ, Hong R: Selective IgA deficiency: Presentation of 30 cases and a review of the literature. *Medicine* 1971; 50:223–236.

Bergal P, Brandzaeg P, Froland SS, et al: Immunodeficiency syndromes with otorhinolaryngological manifestations. *Acta Otolaryngol* 1976; 82:185–192.

Blaise RM, Peng JW, Muchmore A, et al: T-suppressor cells as mediators of infectious agammaglobulinemia. *Fed Proc (abstract)* 1975; 34:1037.

Blizzard RM, Gibbs JH: Candidiasis: Studies pertaining to its association with endocrinopathies and pernicious anemia. *Pediatrics* 1968; 42:231–237.

Bortin MM, Rimm AA: Severe combined immunodeficiency disease: Characterization of the disease and results of transplantation. *JAMA* 1977; 238:591–600.

Buckely RH, Gilbertsen RB, Schiff RI, et al: Heterogeneity of lymphocyte subpopulations in severe combined immunodeficiency. *J Clin Invest* 1976; 58:130–136.

Cleveland WW: Immunological reconstitution in the Di-George syndrome, in Bergsdma D, Good R, Finstad J, Paul N (eds): *Immunodeficiency in Man and Animals. Birth Defects Orig Arb Ser,* vol 11, No 1, Sunderland, Mass, Sinauer Associates, Inc, 1974, pp 352–356.

Cooper MD, Lawton AR: Circulating B-cells in patients with immunodeficiency. *Am J Pathol* 1972; 69:513–528.

Cooper MD, Peterson RDA, South MA, Good RA: The functions of the thymus system and the bursa system in the chicken. *J Exp Med* 1966; 123:75–102.

Frank MM, Gelfand JP, Atkinson JP: Hereditary angioedema: The clinical syndrome and its management. *Ann Intern Med* 1976; 84:580–593.

Geha RS, Schnieberger E, Merler E, et al: Heterogeneity of "acquired" or common variable agammaglobulinemia. *N Engl J Med* 1974; 291:1–6.

Gelfand JA, Sherins RJ, Alling DW, et al: Treatment of hereditary angioedema with danazol. Reversal of clinical and biochemical abnormalities. *N Engl J Med* 1976; 295:1444–1448.

Good RA, Bach FH: Bone marrow and thymus transplants. *Clin Immunobiol* 1974; 2:63–114.

Hobbs JR: Disturbances of the immunoglobulins. *Scientific Basis of Medicine* 1966; 106–127.

Johnston RB: Management of patients with chronic granulomatous disease, in *Advances in Host Defense Mechanism,* in press.

Johnston RB Jr, McMurray JS: Chronic familial granulomatosis: Report of 5 cases and review of the literature. *Am J Dis Child* 1967; 114:370–378.

Kimmelman CP, Postic WP: Immunodeficiency in pediatric otolaryngology. *Am J Otolaryngol* 1979; 1:33–38.

Krabauer R, Zinnemann HH, Hong R: Deficiency of secretory IgA and malabsorption. *Am J Gastroenterol* 1975; 64:319–323.

Medical Research Council Working Party: Hypogammaglobulinemia in the United Kingdom. *Lancet* 1969; 1:163–169.

Owen JJT, Cooper MD, Raff MC: In-vitro generation of B-lymphocytes in mouse fetal liver, mammalian "bursa equivalent." *Nature (London)* 1974; 249:361-363.

Page AR, Good RA: Studies on cyclic neutropenia. *AMA J of Dis Child* 1957; 94:623-660.

Quie PG, Mills EL, Holmes B: Molecular events during phagocytosis by human neutrophils, in Brown EB (ed): *Progress in Hematology*, New York, Grune & Stratton, 1977, vol 10, pp 193-210.

Sasaki CT, Askenase P, Dwyer J, Yanagisawa E: Chronic ear infections in the immunodeficient patient. *Arch Otolaryngol* 1981; 107:82-86.

Sheffer AL, Fearon DT, Austen KF, et al: Tranexamic acid: Preoperative prophylactic therapy for patients with hereditary angioneurotic edema. *J Allergy Clin Immunol* 1977; 60:38-40.

Siegal FP, Siegal M, Good RA: Suppression of B-cell differentiation by leukocytes from hypogamma-globulinemic patients. *J Clin Invest* 1976; 58:109-122.

Squire JR: Hypogammaglobulinemia in the United Kingdom. *Proceedings of Royal Society of Medicine* 1962; 55:393-399.

Steele RW, Limas C, Thurman GB, et al: Familial thymic aplasia. Attempted reconstitution with fetal thymus in a millipore diffusion chamber. *N Engl J Med* 1972; 287:787-791.

Waldmann TA, Durm M, Broder S, et al: Role of suppressor T-cells in pathogenesis of common variable hypogammaglobulinemia. *Lancet* 1974; 2:609-613.

Chapter 11

Cancer

Arnold E. Katz

OUTLINE

INTRODUCTION

Evidence that the immune system is intimately involved in the host-tumor interaction in many animal models as well as in man is impressive. General medical conditions which are associated with decreased effectiveness of the immune system—such as alcoholism, malnutrition, and aging—are associated with an increased risk of developing carcinoma. Moreover, immune deficiencies are more frequent, more severe, and more persistent in patients with carcinoma of the head and neck than in patients with carcinoma involving other regions of the body (Tarpley et al., 1975; Lichtenstein et al., 1980). Many of the approaches now used to treat carcinoma of the head and neck are themselves immuno-suppressive (Wara et al., 1975). It is, therefore, not surprising that the host-tumor interaction in patients with head and neck squamous carcinoma has been a subject of great interest, and design of immunotherapy trials has been attempted (Browder & Chretien, 1977).

Unfortunately, the concept of immunological surveillance (Burnet, 1970) has proved to be somewhat simplistic. It has even been suggested by some that the immune system may be required for the induction of neoplasia (Prehn, 1976), and by others that impaired immunoregulation plays a major role in the development of malignancy (Schwartz, 1975). It now appears that some components of the immune system do indeed prevent the development of malignant disease; whereas, other components seem to impair the host's ability to destroy mutant cells (Katz, 1980). Both humoral and cellular immune responses are involved in this complex interplay, and both are discussed in this chapter.

Since the multifaceted immune system appears to exhibit both potentially beneficial and harmful responses in the face of malignant disease, it is possible that nonspecific immunostimulants, such as BCG, may be reinforcing immunologic responses that are detrimental to the patient. Indeed, it has been suggested that BCG can under certain circumstances accelerate the growth of tumors which has led to the conclusion that this type of immunotherapy not be used except as a "last resort," or in controlled clinical trials (Bast, et al., 1974). Although the present status of immunotherapy is in its infancy, it appears that improvements in prognosis and diagnosis as a result of immunologic methods may be near at hand for patients with head and neck cancer. Tests of cell-mediated immunity appear to be correlated with prognosis in patients with carcinoma of the head and neck (Bosworth et al., 1975; Maisel & Ogura, 1976; Brookes & Clifford, 1981), and detection of Epstein-Barr virus-specific IgA serum antibodies may be extremely helpful in the diagnosis of nasopharyngeal carcinoma (Henle & Henle, 1976; Mathew et al., 1980). These areas are more fully discussed in the text.

CELL-MEDIATED IMMUNITY

It has been shown in a number of experimental model systems that sensitized lymphoid cells are able to destroy neoplastic cells (Hellstrom & Hellstrom, 1972). These cells can be T lymphocytes, macrophages, K or NK cells; however, the T-cell system has been the most studied and appears to be the most important. Sensitized T lymphocytes encounter the neoplastic cell and, in addition to exerting a direct cytotoxic effect, release a host of factors (lymphokines) into the serum. These serve various functions including nonspecific activation of macrophages into cells with cytotoxic capacity. Lymphokines also produce chemotatic effects on macrophages and lymphocytes of various types.

Since cell-mediated immunity to neoplasms is largely a function of the T-cell system, tests designed to measure nonspecific cell-mediated immunity are basically tests of T-cell function. Skin testing to recall or primary antigens (delayed cutaneous hypersensitivity; DCH), enumeration of circulating T-cell levels, and assessment of the in vitro blastogenic reactivity of lymphocytes are the three most common techniques used to assess the status of the T-cell system. Determination of peripheral circulating lymphocyte counts may also be of value because the majority of circulating lymphocytes are T cells.

Skin Testing

It has long been known that the tuberculin skin reaction is frequently negative in patients with neoplastic disease. In a review of over 450 patients, it was shown that negative skin testing was useful in identifying poor risk patients (Israel et al., 1973). Although the patient's immunologic response to his tumor was not being directly assayed, it was felt that if a patient were able to respond to an antigen to which he had previously been sensitized, he was probably also still capable of responding to possible tumor-specific antigens. Conversely, if he could not respond to an antigen to which he had been previously sensitized, he was probably not mounting an effective response against his tumor and his prognosis would be poor.

This idea of determining prognosis in cancer patients on the basis of DCH to non-tumor–specific antigens has followed two major approaches. The earliest approach utilized common antigens to which in all likelihood the patient had been previously exposed (recall antigens). Some of the confounding problems in interpreting skin tests to recall antigens has been whether or not the patient was indeed exposed to the antigens being tested, how long ago, and how intense was the exposure (Browder & Chretien, 1977). Due to the many variables involved, interpretation of DCH results to recall antigens can be misleading.

The second approach utilized the generation of a primary immune response against an antigen to which the patient had never been previously exposed. DNCB (3,4-dinitro-chlorobenzene) is an antigen which can sensitize a patient upon contact. Two weeks after sensitization, patients who are capable of displaying DCH will have a positive skin test upon challenge. Ninety-five percent of normal subjects develop DCH when immunized in this way (Catalona et al., 1972).

Recall Antigens

It has been demonstrated that the tuberculin reaction is frequently negative in patients with malignancies, and an increasing degree of immunological depression has been correlated with spread of tumor and poor prognosis.

Other common recall antigens utilized have included varidase (streptokinase and streptodornase), mumps, trichophytin, histoplasmin, coccidioidin, diphtheria toxoid, blastomycin, mixed tree, dermatophytin, and purified protein derivative. Strepto-kinase-streptodornase (Kopersztych et al., 1976) and *Candida* (Olivari et al., 1976) have been of assistance in predicting survival in various types of carcinoma. Positive skin testing has also been associated with a positive response to chemotherapy (Daly et al., 1979). Anergy to recall antigens has been noted in advanced neoplastic disease (Lamb et al., 1962) and in patients with distant metastasis (Solowey & Rapaport, 1965).

In studies involving patients with carcinoma of the head and neck, a positive reaction to recall antigens was associated with a better short-term prognosis than those who were anergic (Eilber & Morton, 1970). Other investigators, however, have reported that skin testing with recall antigens is of questionable benefit in determining prognosis in patients with carcinoma of the head and neck (Parker et al., 1975; Veltri et al., 1978). On the other hand, response to DCNB testing has been well correlated with stage and clinical course of these patients (Eilber et al., 1975).

DNCB Skin Testing

After demonstrating that impaired immunological reactivity to DNCB was associated with a high incidence of recurrence following cancer surgery (Eilber & Morton, 1970), studies later showed that DNCB reactivity was directly correlated with prognosis and inversely correlated with extent of disease (Wanebo et al., 1975; Maisel & Ogura, 1976; Papenhausen et al., 1979). Inability to respond to DNCB has been documented in patients with multiple primaries, further substantiating that immunosuppression is related to the development of malignancies (Olivari et al., 1976). Although the inability to respond to DNCB has been found in various types of neoplasia, reactivity is most abnormal in squamous cell carcinoma. Furthermore, while DNCB reactivity reverts to normal in patients cured of melanoma and sarcoma, patients with cured squamous cell carcinoma of the head and neck continue to display some impaired ability to respond (Twomey et al, 1974; Browder & Chretien, 1977).

Although the majority of investigators who have examined DNCB reactivity in head and neck cancer patients has found a direct correlation between reactivity and good prognosis, there have been reports to the contrary (Gilbert et al., 1978). Conflicting reports concerning the value of skin testing in determining prognosis can most likely be explained by the lack of standardization in the administration and interpretation of these tests. Although there is some consensus that patients with positive skin testing do better than those who do not respond, this observation has not proved useful in the clinical setting for the following reasons: (1) It is inconvenient; (2) it can delay treatment for at least 2 weeks; and (3) it can be difficult to interpret. For these reasons investigators have been searching for other clinically applicable ways of assessing cellular immune status. Peripheral lymphocyte counts appear to correlate with DNCB skin testing and are more readily available to the clinician (Maisel & Ogura, 1976; Brookes & Clifford, 1981).

Peripheral Lymphocyte Counts

Peripheral T-Cell Counts

In an attempt to more accurately and conveniently monitor defects in the cell-mediated immune system, attempts have been made to correlate the number of circulating T cells with DNCB reactivity and prognosis. T-cell levels have, in fact, been shown to correlate with positive DNCB reactivity in patients with carcinoma (Catalona et al., 1975). Wybran and Fudenberg (1973) documented decreased percentages of circulating T cells which appeared to correlate with clinical status, while others (Olkowski & Wilkins, 1975) have reported that both percentage and absolute number of circulating T cells are helpful determinants of prognosis in patients with carcinoma of the head and neck. The percentage of circulating T cells appears to correlate well with other assays of cell-mediated immunity, although Mason et al. (1977) did not find that the percentage of circulating T cells was of value in predicting survival.

Although the prognostic value of the percentage of circulating T lymphocytes of the total lymphocyte count is controversial, it seems to be widely held that a decreased absolute number of circulating T cells is present in patients who develop carcinoma (Gross et al., 1975), and that this decreased number correlates with increasing stages of the disease (Lundy et al., 1974; Dellon et al., 1975; Kopersztych et al., 1976) and HS clinical course (Veltri et al., 1978). Moreover, absolute T cell levels are more profoundly depressed in patients with carcinoma of the head and neck than in patients with malignancies involving other sites of the body (Lichtenstein et al., 1980). Since T cells comprise the majority of circulating lymphocytes, the total lymphocyte count can be used as a rough measure of the absolute number of T cells and may be of value to the clinician in determining prognosis.

Total Lymphocyte Count

In contrast to skin testing and T-cell blastogenesis assays, the total lymphocyte count (TLC) is an inexpensive, readily available clinical test. It is derived from the complete blood count (CBC), which is available to every practicing physician. The TLC is determined by multiplying the WBC count by the percentage of lymphocytes found in the differential exam; many hospitals now have acquired equipment to determine the TLC automatically.

Riesco (1970) followed 589 cancer patients for 5 years and found a positive correlation between cancer curability and the TLC. Since that time several laboratories have documented that patients with a normal or elevated TLC are likely to have positive skin testing (Brookes & Clifford, 1981), and normal T-lymphocyte counts (Silverman et al., 1975; Papenhausen et al., 1979; Lichtenstein et al., 1980).

Depressed TLCs have been documented in patients with carcinoma of the head and neck (Lichtenstein et al., 1980) and appears to be related to their prognosis (Maisel & Ogura, 1976; Brookes & Clifford, 1981) as well as the prognosis of patients with other solid tumors (Kopersztych et al., 1976; Daly et al., 1979; Bruckner et al., 1982). While some investigators reported that TLC was of no help in determining prognosis, other authors suggested the value of the TLC could be best appreciated when used simultaneously with other immunologic measurements (Maisel & Ogura, 1976; Gilbert et al., 1978). As opposed to the many reports of depressed lymphocyte counts indicating a poor prognosis, data have accumulated to suggest that an elevated total WBC may be associated with a poor prognosis (Snell, 1979). One cannot assume that the TLC is elevated in patients with high total white counts. Lymphocyte elevations per se appear to reflect general immune competence and good nutritional status (Brookes & Clifford, 1981); whereas elevated granulocyte counts may merely reflect the presence of infection and a poor prognosis (Bruckner et al., 1982).

The TLC is the simplest, most reliable, presently available assay of the cell-mediated immune system and appears to have prognostic implications. The TLC by itself, however, may be only of limited value in the clinical situation. It is most useful when combined with other information to appreciate its full prognostic implications (Katz, 1983).

Lymphocyte Reactivity

By far the most complex assays of the cell-mediated immune system are those that monitor lymphocyte reactivity. These tests are in vitro assays of the ability of the patient's lymphocytes to respond to various stimuli. The stimuli may consist of common recall antigens, specific tumor antigens, or nonspecific stimulants (mitogens), such as phytohemagglutinin (PHA), concanavalin A (Con A), or pokeweed mitogen (PWM). It appears that the greater the response of the lymphocytes to the antigen and/or mitogens, the better the prognosis in patients with carcinoma.

It has been shown that lymphocytes in patients with cancer were less likely to respond to common recall antigens than were the lymphocytes from controls. Response to PHA has been shown to be markedly suppressed in patients with cancer of the head and neck (Twomey et al., 1974; Veltri et al., 1978). It is also known that PHA response is more suppressed in patients with inoperable lesions than in operable ones. PHA responses have been shown to remain depressed in treated head and neck cancer patients who have received radiation therapy (Tarpley et al., 1975) and in patients with a poor prognosis (Kopersztych et al., 1976). PHA-induced blastogenesis has been of assistance in determining prognosis specifically in patients with carcinoma of the head and neck (Wanebo et al., 1975; Stefani & Kerman, 1977). Depressed response to PHA has been shown to be more common in elderly patients and patients with multiple primaries. Response to PHA has also been correlated with performance status and survival, as well as with other assays of the delayed hypersensitivity system (Papenhausen et al., 1979).

There are many other types of in vitro assays of T-cell blastogenesis. Some have utilized tumor cells or other lymphocytes as the source of antigenic stimulation. All are highly sophisticated techniques, difficult to perform outside of the research laboratory, and costly. Although the future may see clinical application of these assays, they are presently not widely used in the clinical situation. In view of this, it is extremely fortunate that the

TLC appears to correlate quite well with the more sophisticated assays of cell-mediated immunity (Lichtenstein et al., 1980; Brookes & Clifford, 1981).

HUMORAL IMMUNITY

Humoral factors have been demonstrated in the serum of cancer patients which can inhibit healthy, sensitized lymphocytes from destroying tumor cells (Hellstrom et al., 1971; Currie & Basham, 1972; Giuliano et al., 1979). Immunoglobulins (most frequently in the form of immune complexes) have been shown to be at least partially responsible for this inhibitory effect (Sjogren et al., 1971). Humoral factors may in some cases impair the host response against neoplasia, thereby protecting the tumor.

Other humoral factors are intimately involved with the destruction of tumor. Specific antitumor antibodies have been documented in patients with carcinoma (Gupta & Morton, 1975), and these antibodies have, in some cases, been shown to be essential in augmenting cell-mediated immunity in the destruction of neoplastic cells (Zighelboim et al, 1973).

Two classes of immunoglobulins appear to be involved with the host-tumor interaction in patients with carcinoma of the head and neck. The immunoglobulin A system appears to inhibit the cellular immune system from destroying tumor, while the immunoglobulin E system may be of importance in helping the host (Katz, 1980).

Serum Blocking Factors

It has been well documented in several animal models and in man that specific serum factors can prevent the cytotoxicity of the host's lymphocytes for tumor cells (Hellstrom & Hellstrom, 1974; Mathew et al., 1980). This blocking effect can be abolished by previous absorption of the inhibiting serum with the same type of tumor cells or by removing immunoglobulin (Sjogren et al., 1971). It has been further demonstrated that the most important blocking effect clearly originates in immune complexes in some tumor models (Sjogren et al., 1971; Baldwin et al., 1973).

Baldwin et al. (1972) have shown that the amount of antigen required to produce blocking activity is critical. Blocking activity is lost under conditions of excess antigen, presumably by completely occupying free antibody sites in antigen-antibody complexes. The blocking activity is also lost in serum with very low concentrations of tumor antigen (Baldwin et al., 1973). Fig 11-1 demonstrates how antigen-antibody complexes may prevent lymphocytes from destroying tumor. Under conditions of antigen excess (Fig 11-2), free antibody sites are completely bound and antigen-antibody complexes may not be able to effectively block lymphocytes from reaching the antigens on the surface of the tumor cells. Since the serum no longer exerts a blocking effect, lymphocytes are able to destroy tumor cells. When there is a very low serum concentration of tumor antigen (Figure 11-3),

FIG 11-1. Antigen-antibody complexes producing serum blocking activity.

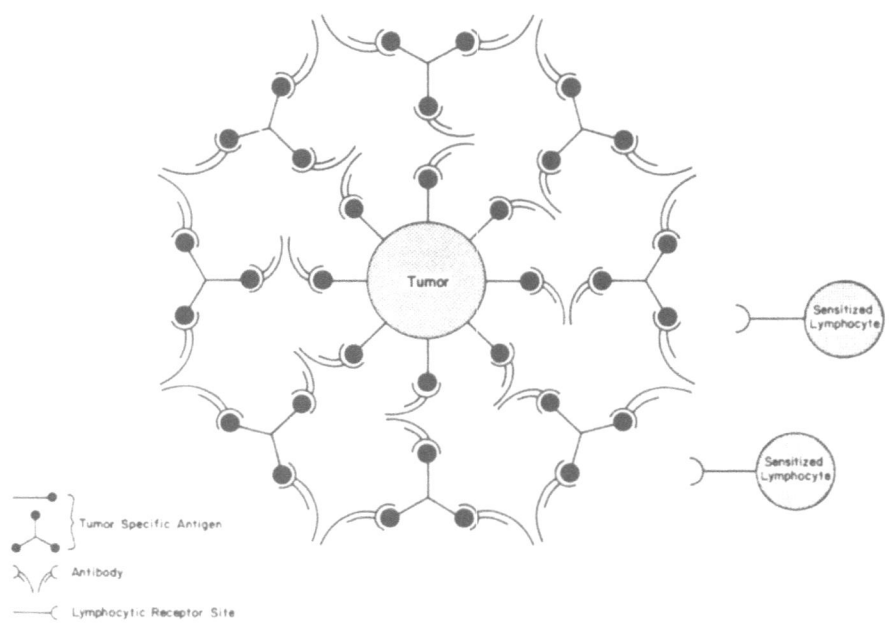

a dynamic equilibrium may exist in which both antibody and lymphocytes are able to reach tumor cells.

While the above summarizes much of what is known about the nature and significance of serum blocking factors, it is not suggested that this is the only, or even most important, mechanism whereby serum components may prevent the host's immune system from destroying tumor. It is possible that immune complexes may directly incapacitate effector lymphocytes, rather than just preventing normal lymphocytes from reaching tumor cells. Serum may also block beneficial host responses against tumor by interfering with antibody-dependent cellular cytotoxicity (ADCC). Indeed, it has been demonstrated that elevated levels of IgA antibodies can block IgG-mediated ADCC in patients with carcinoma of the nasopharynx (Mathew et al., 1980) and these elevated levels of IgA correlate with increasing stage of disease (Wolf et al., 1982).

The Immunoglobulin A (IgA) System

The immunoglobulin A system has several biological roles. There is no doubt that this system is important for its neutralizing activity against viruses. IgA does have other

FIG 11-2. Serum blocking activity lost under conditions of antigen excess.

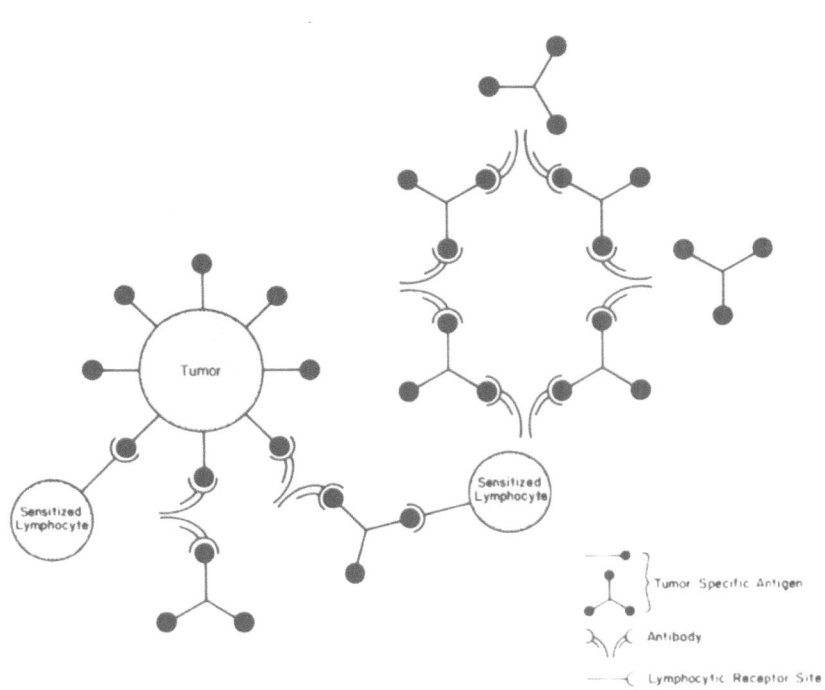

functions, and there is a growing body of data suggesting that IgA may be involved in the prevention of autoimmune disease. IgA may be one of the self-regulatory substances that has evolved to protect the host against its own immune system. However, IgA may, in certain situations, prevent the host from handling foreign antigen "nonself" or neoplastic cells.

Immunoglobulin A and Autoimmunity

Patients who have a selective IgA deficiency have an increased incidence of autoimmune disease, such as systemic lupus erythematosis and rheumatoid arthritis (Ammann & Hong, 1971). There is also an increased incidence of autoantibodies in the IgA deficient population (Hong & Ammann, 1972). The presence of IgA appears to serve as a barrier in preventing the development of an immune response against certain antigens (Cunningham-Rundles et al., 1978).

IgA has been shown to block or interfere with a host of immunologic reactions. Several authors have demonstrated the inhibition of bacteriolysis (Griffiss, 1975) and leukocyte chemotaxis (Ito et al., 1979) by IgA. O'Neill and Romsdahl (1974) demonstrated

266   Katz

FIG 11-3. Serum blocking activity lost when serum tumor specific antigen levels are low.

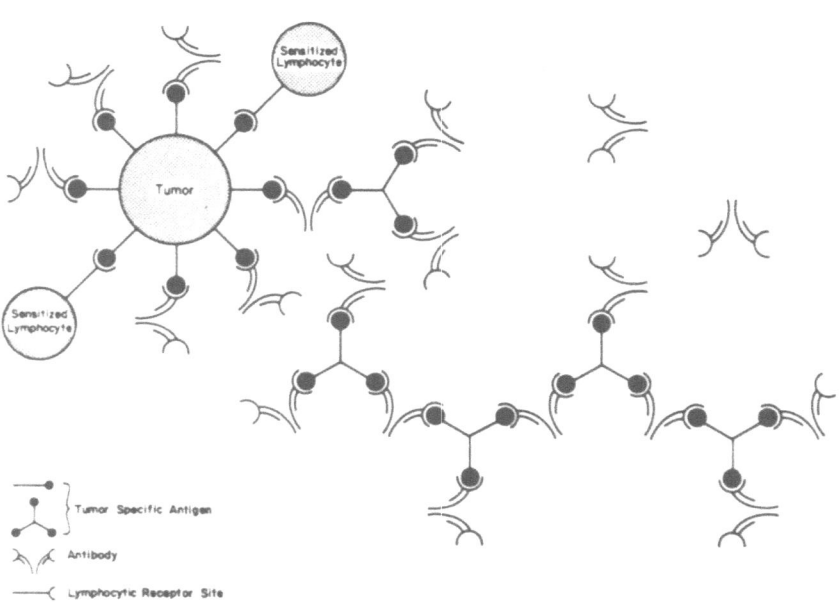

that IgA was capable of abrogating the cytoxic effect of sensitized lymphocytes on human malignant melanoma in vitro and Sipos et al. (1978) reported that the blocking activity seen in the serum of their tumor patients was associated with the IgA subclass. IgA antibodies have also been shown to block IgG-mediated antibody-dependent cellular cytotoxicity of carcinoma of the nasopharynx in humans (Mathew et al., 1980). The IgA system, therefore, appears to play a role in the prevention of the development of autoimmune disease, but this capacity for inhibition of antigen processing can also impair the host's response against all foreign cell-surface antigens, including tumor cells (Mathew et al., 1980; Neel et al., 1982; Wolf et al., 1982).

Immunoglobulin A and Cancer

Elevated levels of total serum IgA have been found in patients with varying types of carcinomas involving mucosal surfaces. Increased serum IgA has also been noted in individuals with precancerous lesions of the larynx (Gierek et al., 1979), as well as in patients with carcinoma of the head and neck (Brown et al., 1975; Tarpley et al., 1975; Katz et al., 1976, 1978, 1980; Khanna et al., 1982).

Elevations of secretory IgA have been reported in the serum or saliva of patients with oropharyngeal and/or bronchopulmonary carcinoma (Brown et al., 1975). Elevated levels of secretory IgA may be helpful in distinguishing benign from malignant lesions in patients with carcinoma of the stomach (Levy et al., 1975b) and/or lung (Mandel et al., 1976). Eluates of various malignant tumors have been shown to contain IgA, and it has been suggested that human carcinomas are capable of producing secretory IgA (deLustig et al., 1980) and SC (Harris & South, 1981).

Elevated levels of total serum IgA have been shown to indicate a poor prognosis in patients with carcinoma of the head and neck. IgA levels rise significantly in the presence of metastatic disease and appear to be directly related to total tumor burden (Khanna et al., 1982). Total serum IgA level has also been correlated with extent of disease in carcinoma of the nasopharynx (Baskies et al., 1979). IgA has been shown to interfere with the destruction of tumor in various types of human malignancies (O'Neill & Romsdahl, 1974; Mathew et al., 1980).

Virus-Specific Immunoglobulin A and Cancer

The association between herpes simplex viruses (HSV) and carcinoma of the head and neck has been documented. A high incidence of antibodies to HSV antigens has been correlated with advanced disease (Silverman et al., 1976). Elevated levels of HSV-specific IgA antibodies have also been documented in patients with a high risk of developing head and neck cancer (Smith et al., 1976a). Furthermore, HSV-specific IgA antibody levels are even higher in patients who have developed carcinoma of the head and neck and appear to be correlated with clinical course (Smith et al., 1976b). HSV-specific IgG or IgM antibody levels do not correlate with clinical course.

Similarly, antibodies to the Epstein-Barr virus (EBV) have been well documented in nasopharyngeal carcinoma as well as other malignancies (Neel, 1982). Once again, it is the IgA class of EBV antibodies that is associated with the presence of carcinoma (Desgranges & de-The, 1979) and is correlated with tumor burden and clinical outcome (Henle & Henle, 1976). EBV-specific IgA antibodies have been shown to block IgG-mediated tumor destruction (Mathew et al., 1980).

Although some authors have described normal or low levels of IgA associated with malignancy, the weight of evidence supports the hypothesis that IgA levels are elevated in some patients with carcinoma of the head and neck and the elevated levels indicated a poor prognosis (Katz, 1983)

The Immunoglobulin E (IgE) System

IgE is the immunoglobulin responsible for mediating type I hypersensitivity, associated with such diseases as atopy, anaphylaxis, urticaria, and angioedema. Because of the dearth of IgE in the blood (0.004% of the total serum immunoglobulin) it escaped detection until the late 1960s (Ishizaka et al., 1966). Even before its discovery, however, the relationship between atopy and the development of malignancy had been a subject of great interest. Several authors had questioned whether the mechanisms which mediate allergic disease in the human may have had some positive evolutionary effect and may assist in the prevention of the development and/or spread of malignant disease.

Atopy and Cancer

Fisherman (1960) reported that the incidence of allergy in cancer patients was significantly below the incidence of atopic disease in a control group. This observation contradicted an earlier report by Logan and Saker (1953) that allergy was more common in patients with malignancies. Other authors, however, have confirmed Fisherman's observations of a decrease in the incidence of allergic disease in patients with malignancy (Allegra et al., 1976; Cockcroft et al., 1979). Ford (1978) reported that cancer develops less frequently in patients suffering from allergic diseases, and Alderson (1974) reported that mortality from malignant diseases is much less in the allergic population. The controversy continues, however, since several authors have not confirmed a negative correlation between the development of malignant disease and the development of allergy (Shapiro et al., 1972). Moreover, others have questioned the significance of the correlation even if it did exist (Madsen, 1975). Some authors, however, believe that the IgE biologic system may be one of the immunologic defense mechanisms in the prevention of the development of malignant disease (Rosenbaum & Dwyer, 1977; Katz, 1980, 1983).

Immunoblobulin E and Cancer

It was hoped that the enigma which surrounded the relationship between the development of allergy and the development of malignancy would be resolved with the discovery of IgE as a reagenic antibody. It was felt that if IgE did, indeed, suppress the development of malignancy, IgE levels would probably be low or absent in patients who develop malignant disease. Early reports did demonstrate low levels of IgE in patients with malignant disease (Rosenbaum & Dwyer, 1977), and a debate soon arose as to the mechanisms by which the IgE system might suppress the development of neoplastic cells (Jacobs et al., 1973). Other laboratories, however, were unable to confirm thse reports (Waldman et al., 1974; Winters & Heiner, 1976). Mander et al. (1975) reported that the site of the development of the tumor may influence the serum IgE levels. Serrou et al. (1975) and Katz et al. (1980) documented elevated levels of IgE in a surprisingly large proportion of patients with carcinoma of the head and neck. Horak and Hussarek (1979) further demonstrated that IgE levels appear to rise as an early response to the presence of malignancy.

It has been suggested that the IgE system has evolved to provide an anaphylactic-type reaction to suppress the development of solid tumors (Lynch et al., 1978). In cancer patients, elevated IgE levels do not appear to correlate well with a history of clinical atopy (Hallgren et al., 1981). It is possible that the elevated levels of IgE in some cancer patients may be directed against tumor-specific antigens, and several mechanisms whereby IgE could enhance tumor immunity have been described (Rosenbaum & Dwyer, 1977; Lynch et al., 1978).

IMMUNOSUPPRESSION IN HEAD AND NECK CANCER PATIENTS

Immunosuppression is more frequent, more profound, and more persistent in head and neck cancer patients than in patients with carcinoma involving other sites of the body (Tarpley et al., 1975; Browder & Chretien, 1977; Lichtenstein et al., 1980; Johnson et al., 1982). Patients who develop carcinoma of the head and neck are also frequently suffering from other general medical conditions such as alcoholism, malnutrition, and aging. These conditions are associated with immunosuppression even in the absence of carcinoma (Katz, 1982).

Alcoholism

The head and neck cancer incidence rate for alcoholics is over five times the rate for the general population, and alcohol has been implicated as a cofactor in the etiology of cancer (Schottenfeld, 1979). Impaired response to DNCB skin testing (Straus et al., 1971) and decreased numbers of circulating T cells (Van Epps et al., 1975) have been documented in the alcoholic patient, even in the absence of cancer.

Serum IgA levels have been shown to be elevated in patients with alcoholic liver disease (Tomasi & Tisdale, 1964). Iturriaga et al. (1977) demonstrated that the elevated levels of serum IgA are directly related to the amount of liver failure present, even in the absence of head and neck cancer. The immunosuppression seen in alcoholic liver disease appears to improve in the recovered alcoholic (Lundy et al., 1975). One might speculate that the poor prognosis seen in patients with immunosuppression, alcoholic liver disease, and carcinoma of the head and neck might be improved by treating the underlying liver disease and thereby improving the general status of the patient.

Malnutrition

Malnutrition is another very common accompanying condition of patients with head and neck cancer (Sobol et al., 1979). Malnutrition may be a complication of alcoholism (Levy et al., 1975) or may be the result of insufficient nutritional intake secondary to the presence of the tumor (Lawrence, 1979). Suskind (1977) has described the effect of malnutrition on the immune response and has demonstrated that almost all parameters are depressed (Suskind et al., 1976). Nutritional status does appear to be closely correlated with immunocompetence in head and neck cancer patients (Brookes & Clifford 1981). Serum IgA levels have been noted to be elevated in malnourished children and have been shown to return to normal with treatment (Suskind et al., 1976). Nutritional repletion appears to restore immune competence (Law et al., 1974) and may reduce mortality and morbidity in cancer patients (Smale et al., 1981). Again, one can only speculate on the potential immunotherapeutic role of nutritional repletion and its effect on prognosis in patients with cancer of the head and neck.

Aging

Cellular immunity is impaired in the elderly. Johnston et al. (1963) demonstrated that skin reactivity to recall antigens decreased with advanced age, while Gross (1965) and Waldorf et al., (1968) demonstrated impaired responses to DNCB in this population. T-cell depletion and impaired lymphocyte reactivity have also been documented in the elderly (Kay & Makinodan, 1976).

Immunoglobulin levels do not decrease in the elderly. In fact, IgA levels rise with advancing age (Cassidy & Nordby, 1975) as do immune complexes (Rossen et al., 1979). As has been previously discussed, elevated levels of IgA and/or immune complexes have been associated with impaired tumor immunity. Age-related changes in both the cellular and humoral immune systems suggest that prognosis in patients with cancer may be impaired with advancing age.

The most prominent factor determining susceptibility to cancer is age. Age is related to an increased duration of exposure to a wide variety of carcinogenic stimuli, and death rates due to cancer increase proportionately with age. Teller et al., in 1964 demonstrated a correlation between old age, depressed immune function, and spontaneous tumor incidence. Willis (1967) showed that elderly people accounted for 85% of the fatal carcinomas found at autopsy, although they comprised only 38% of the population studied. In contrast to a recent report of decreased recurrence rate in patients with cancer of the larynx over age 60 (Harwood et al., 1981), increased age has been correlated with an increasingly poor prognosis in patients with carcinoma of the head and neck (Katz, 1983).

DISCUSSION

Although one can be optimistic about the increasing value of immunological techniques in the diagnosis and prognosis of patients with head and neck cancer, the role of immunotherapy does not appear to be close at hand. It has been suggested that nonspecific immunostimulants, such as BCG, *C parvum*, and MER, may be helpful when only minimum residual disease is present in the treatment of smaller lesions (Browder & Chretien, 1977). This has not yet been proven effective. These types of therapies must still be evaluated in carefully controlled clinical trials because of the very real possibility of stimulating immune responses which may not be in the best interest of the host (Bast et al., 1974), such as the suppressor cell network.

It has also been suggested that immunorestorative agents such as levamisole, thymosin, and transfer factor may be helpful in the treatment of larger lesions (Browder & Chretien, 1977). While it is true that these patients are usually the most immunosuppressed and that surgery and radiation therapy further suppress the immune system, it has not been established that nonspecific restoration of the immune system is beneficial to these patients. It seems reasonable to propose that modulation of specific parts of the immune system may indeed improve survival rates, since malignant neoplasms appear to be more frequent in the immunosuppressed patient (Penn, 1976; Harris & Penn, 1981) and multiple primaries have been well documented in patients with carcinoma of the head and neck (McGuirt, 1982). It is likely, however, that effective modulation of the immune system will be possible only after more is understood about the immunoactive glycoproteins, immunoregulatory antibodies, and the role of the immunoglobulin subclasses. The role of serum blocking factors has been discussed and remains an intriguing avenue for research (Baldwin, 1982; Bansal & Bansal, 1982), as does the possible role of plasma exchange in these patients (Israel et al., 1982). Finally, one can only at present speculate about the beneficial effects of treating alcoholic liver and/or malnutrition in patients with carcinoma of the head and neck.

REFERENCES

Alderson M: Mortality from malignant disease in patients with asthma. *Lancet* 1974; 2:1475.

Allegra J, Lipton A, Harvey H, et al: Decreased prevalence of immediate hypersensitivity (atopy) in a cancer population. *Cancer Res* 1976; 36:3225.

Ammann AJ, Hong R: Selective IgA deficiency. Presentation of 30 cases and a review of the literature. *Medicine* 1971; 50:223.

Baldwin RW: Immune mechanisms in cancer, in Beyer J-H, Borberg H, Fuchs C, Nagel GA (eds): *Plasmapheresis in Immunology and Oncology* New York, S. Karger, 1982, pp 80–90.

Baldwin RW, Embleton MJ, Robins RA: Humoral factors influencing cell-mediated immune responses to tumor-associated antigens. *Proc R Soc Med* 1973; 66:466.

Baldwin RW, Price MR, Robins RA: Blocking of lymphocyte-mediated cytotoxicity for rat hepatoma cells by tumor-specific antigen-antibody complexes. *Nature (London)* 1972; 238:185.

Bansal SC, Bansal BR: Serum-blocking factors in tumor host, in Beyer J-H, Borberg H, Fuchs C, Nagel GA (eds): *Plasmapheresis in Immunology and Oncology*. New York, S. Karger, 1982, pp 91–101.

Baskies AM, Chretien PB, Yang C-S, et al: Serum glycoproteins and immunoglobulins in nasopharyngeal carcinoma: Correlations with Epstein-Barr virus-associated antibodies and clinical tumor stage. *Am J Surg* 1979; 138:478.

Bast RC Jr, Zbar B, Borsos T, et al: BCG and cancer *N Engl J Med* 1974; 290:1413–1458.

Bosworth JL, Ghossein NA, Brooks TL: Delayed hypersensitivity in patients treated by curative radiotherapy. *Cancer* 1975; 36:353.

Brookes GB, Clifford P: Nutritional status and general immune competence in patients with head and neck cancer. *J Royal Soc Med* 1981; 74:132.

Browder JP, Chretien PB: Immune reactivity in head and neck squamous carcinoma and relevance to the design of immunotherapy trials. *Seminars in Oncol* 1977; 4:431.

Brown AM, Lally ET, Frankel A, et al: The association of the IgA levels of serum and whole saliva with the progression of oral cancer. *Cancer* 1975; 35:1154.

Bruckner HW, Lavin PT, Plaxe SC, et al: Absolute granulocyte, lymphocyte, and monocyte counts. Useful determinants of prognosis for patients with metastatic cancer of the stomach. *JAMA* 1982; 247:1004.

Burnet FM: The concept of immunological surveillance. *Progr Exp Tumor Res* 1970; 13:1.

Cassidy JT, Nordby GL: Human serum immunoglobulin concentrations: Prevalence of immuno-globulin deficiencies. *J Allergy Clin Immunol* 1975; 55:35.

Catalona WJ, Tarpley JL, Potvin C, et al: Correlations among cutaneous reactivity to DNCB, PHA-induced lymphocyte blastogenesis and peripheral blood E rosettes. *Clin Exp Immunol* 1975; 19:327.

Catalona WJ, Taylor PT, Chretien PB: Quantitative dinitrochlorobenzene contact sensitization in a normal population. *Clin Exp Immunol* 1972; 12:325.

Cockcroft DW, Klein GL, Donevan RE, et al: Is there a negative correlation between malignancy and respiratory atopy? *Ann Allergy* 1979; 43:345.

Cunningham-Rundles C, Brandeis WE, Good RA, et al: Milk precipitins, circulating immune complexes, and IgA deficiency. *Proc Natl Acad Sci USA* 1978; 75:3387.

Currie GA, Basham C: Serum mediated inhibiting of the immunological reactions of the patient to his own tumor: A possible role for circulating antigen. *Br J Cancer* 1972; 26:427.

Daly JM, Dudrick SJ, Copeland EM III: Evaluation of nutritional indices as prognostic indicators in the cancer patient. *Cancer* 1979; 43:925.

Dellon AL, Potvin C, Chretien PB: Thymus-dependent lymphocyte levels in bronchogenic carcinoma: Correlations with histology, clinical stage, and clinical course after surgical treatment. *Cancer* 1975; 35:687.

DeLustig ES, Matos E, Spector C, et al: Secretory IgA content in human normal and tumoral bronchial mucosa "in vitro." *Oncology* 1980; 37:16.

Desgranges C, de-The G: Epstein-Barr virus specific IgA serum antibodies in nasopharyngeal and other respiratory carcinomas. *Int J Cancer* 1979; 24:555.

Eilber FR, Morton DL: Impaired immunologic reactivity and recurrence following cancer surgery. *Cancer* 1970; 25:362.

Eilber FR, Nizze JA, Morton DL: Sequential evaluation of general immune competence in cancer patients: Correlation with clinical course. *Cancer* 1975; 35:660.

Fisherman EW: Does the allergic diathesis influence malignancy? *J Allergy* 1960; 31:74.

Ford RM: Primary lung cancer and asthma. *Ann Allergy* 1978; 40:240.

Gierek T, Lisiewicz J, Astaldi G, et al: Lymphocytes, neutrophils and serum immunoglobulins in patients with precancerous states of the larynx. *Laryngoscope* 1979; 89:1145.

Gilbert HA, Kagan R, Miles J, et al: The usefulness of pretreatment DNCB in 85 patients with squamous cell carcinoma of the upper aerodigestive tract. *J Surg Oncol* 1978; 10:73.

Giuliano AE, Rangel D, Golub SH, et al: Serum-mediated immunosuppression in lung cancer. *Cancer* 1979; 43:917.

Griffiss JM: Bactericidal activity of meningococcal antisera: Blocking by IgA of lytic antibody in human convalescent sera. *J Immunol* 1975; 114:1779.

Gross L: Immunological defect in aged population and its relationship to cancer. *Cancer* 1965; 18:201.

Gross RL, Latty A, Williams EA, et al: Abnormal spontaneous rosette formation and rosette inhibition in lung carcinoma. *N Engl J Med* 1975; 292:439.

Gupta RK, Morton DL: Suggestive evidence for "in vitro" binding of specific antitumor antibodies of human melanomas. *Cancer Res* 1975; 35:58.

Hallgren R, Arrendal H, Hiesche K, et al: Elevated serum immunoglobulin E in bronchial carcinoma: Its relation to the histology and prognosis of the cancer. *J Allergy Clin Immunol* 1981; 67:398.

Han T, Takita H: Impaired lymphocyte response to allogeneic cultured lymphoid cells in patients with lung cancer. *N Engl J Med* 1972; 286:605.

Harris JP, Penn I: Immunosuppression and development of malignancies of the upper airway and related structures. *Laryngoscope* 1981; 91:520.

Harris JP, South MA: Secretory component: A glandular epthelial cell marker. *Am J Path* 1981; 105:47.

Harwood AR, Deboer G, Kazim F: Prognostic factors in T_3 glottic cancer. *Cancer* 1981; 47:367.

Hellstrom I, Hellstrom KE: Cell-mediated immune reactions to tumor antigens with particular emphasis on immunity to human neoplasms. *Cancer* 1974; 34:1461.

Hellstrom KE, Hellstrom I: Immunologic defenses against cancer, in Good RA, Fisher DW (eds): *Immunobiology,* Stamford, Conn, Sinauer Associates, Inc, 1972, pp 209–218.

Henle G, Henle W: Epstein-Barr virus-specific IgA serum antibodies as an outstanding feature of nasopharyngeal carcinoma. *Int J Cancer* 1976; 17:1.

Hong R, Ammann AJ: Selective absence of IgA. Autoimmune phenomena and autoimmune disease. *Am J Path* 1972; 69:491.

Horak F, Hussarek M: Serum-immunoglobulin-E bei leukoplakiepatienten. *HNO* 1979; 27:185.

Ishizaka K, Ishizaka T, Hornbrook MM: Physiochemical properties of reaginic antibody: V. Correlation of reaginic activity with gamma-E-globulin antibody. *J Immunol* 1966; 97:840.

Israel L, Edelstein R, Samok R: Repeated plasma exchanges in patients with metastatic cancer, in Beyer J-H, Borberg H, Fuchs CH, et al (eds): *Plasmapheresis in Immunology and Oconology,* New York, S Karger, 1982, pp 196–203.

Israel L, Mugica J, Chahinian P: Prognosis of early bronchogenic carcinoma survival curves of 451 patients after resection of lung cancer in relation to the results of pre-operative tuberculin skin test. *Biomedicine* 1973; 19:68.

Ito S, Mikawa H, Shinomiya K, et al: Suppressive effect of IgA soluble immune complexes on neutrophil chemotaxis. *Clin Exp Immunol* 1979; 37:436.

Iturriaga H, Pereda J, Estevez A, et al: Serum immunoglobulin A changes in alcoholic patients. *Ann Clin Res* 1977; 9:39.

Jacobs D, Houri M, Landon J, et al: Circulating levels of IgE in patients with cancer. *Lancet* 1973; 1:102.

Johnson JT, Rabin BS, Hirsch BE, et al: Quantification of T-cell subpopulations in patients with head and neck cancer. *Otolaryngol* 1982; Head Neck Surg. 90(5, Sect 2):219.

Johnston RN, Ritchie RT, Murrary IHF: Declining tuberculin sensitivity with advancing age. *Brit Med J* 1963; 2:720.

Katz AE: Advances in the immunology of head and neck cancer. *Otol Clin N Amer* 1980; 13:431.

Katz AE: Immunity and aging. *Otol Clin N Amer* 1982; 15:287.

Katz AE: Immunobiologic staging of patients with carcinoma of the head and neck. *Laryngoscope,* 1983; 93:445.

Katz AE, Nysather JO, Harker LA: Major immunoglobulin ratios in carcinoma of the head and neck. *Ann Otol Rhinol Laryngol* 1978; 87:412.

Katz AE, Yoo T-J, Harker LA: Serum immunoglobulin A (IgA) levels in carcinoma of the head and neck. *Tr Am Acad Ophth Otol* 1976; 82:131.

Katz AE, Yoo T-J, Nysather JO, et al: Serum immunoglobulin concentrations in carcinoma of the head and neck, in Neiburgs HE (ed): *Prevention and Detection of Cancer, Part II, Detection,* vol 2, *Cancer Detection in Specific Sites.* New York, Marcel Dekker, Inc, 1980, pp 1335–1349.

Kay MMB, Makinodan T: Immunobiology of aging: Evaluation of current status. *Clin Immunol Immunopathol* 1976; 6:319.

Khanna NN, Dao SN, Khanna S: Serum immunoglobulins in squamous cell carcinoma of the oral cavity. *J Surg Oncol* 1982; 20:46.

Kopersztych S, Rezkallah MT, Miki SS, et al: Cell-mediated immunity in patients with carcinoma. *Cancer* 1976; 38:1149.

Lamb D, Pilney F, Kelly WD, et al: A comparative study of the incidence of anergy in patients with carcinoma, leukemia, Hodgkin's disease and other lymphomas. *J Immunol* 1962; 89:555.

Law DK, Dudrick SJ, Abdou NI: The effects of protein-calorie malnutrition on immune competence of the surgical patient. *Surg Gynecol Obstet* 1974; 139:257.

Lawrence W Jr: Effects of cancer on nutrition. Impaired organ system effects. *Cancer* 1979; 43:2020.

Levy CM, Tamburro CH, Zetterman R: Liver disease of the alcoholic. *Med Clin N Amer* 1975a; 59:909.

Levy M, Petreshock EP, Mandell C, et al: The response of the local immunoglobulin system to malignant lesions of the stomach: A new diagnostic test. *Cancer* 1975b; 36:1991.

Lichtenstein A, Zighelboim J, Dorey F, et al: Comparison of immune derangements in patients with different malignancies. *Cancer* 1980; 45:2090.

Logan J, Saker D: The incidence of allergic disorders in cancer. *N Z Med J* 1953; 52:210.

Lundy J, Raff JH, Deakins S, et al: The acute and chronic effects of alcohol on the human immune system. *Surg Gynecol Obstet* 1975; 141:212.

Lundy J, Wenebo H, Pinsky C, et al: Delayed hypersensitivity reactions in patients with squamous cell cancer of the head and neck. *Am J Surg* 1974; 128:530.

Lynch NR, Salomon J-C, Turner KJ: Evolutionary development of IgE and the role of anaphylactic-type reactions in resistance to solid tumours. *Cancer Immunol Immunother* 1978; 4:223.

McGuirt WF: Panendoscopy as a screening examination for simultaneous primary tumors in head and neck cancer: A prospective sequential study and review of the literature. *Laryngoscope* 1982; 92:569.

Madsen SN: Asthma and cancer. *Lancet* 1975; 1:166.

Maisel RH, Ogura JH: Dinitrochlorobenzene skin sensitization and peripheral lymphocyte count: Predictors of survival in head and neck cancer. *Ann Otol Rhinol Laryngol* 1976; 85:517.

Mandel MA, Dvorak KJ, Worman LW, et al: Immunoglobulin content in the bronchial washings of patients with benign and malignant pulmonary disease. *N Engl J Med* 1976; 295:694.

Mander AM, Bolton PM, Davidson JM, et al: IgE serum levels in cancer patients. *Lancet* 1975; 1:396.

Mason JM, Kitchens GG, Eastham RJ III, et al: T-lymphocytes and survival of head and neck squamous cell carcinoma. *Arch Otolaryngol* 1977; 103:223.

Mathew GD, Qualtiere LF, Neel HB III, et al: Immunoglobulin A antibody to Epstein-Barr viral antigens and prognosis in nasopharyngeal carcinoma. *Otolaryngol Head Neck Surg* 1980; 88:52.

Neel HB III, Pearson GR, Taylor W, et al: Application of Epstein-Barr virus serology to the diagnosis and staging of North American patients with nasopharyngeal carcinoma. *Otolaryngol Head Neck Surg* 1982; 90 (No 5, Sect 2):176.

Olivari A, Pradier R, Feierstein J, Guardo A, Glait H, Rojas A: Cell-mediated immune response in head and neck cancer patients. *J Surg Onc* 1976; 8:287.

Olkowski ZL, Wilkins SA: T-lymphocyte levels in the peripheral blood of patients with cancer of the head and neck. *Am J Surg* 1975; 130:440.

O'Neill PA, Romsdahl MM: IgA as a blocking factor in human malignant melonoma. *Immunol Comm* 1974; 3:427.

Papenhausen PR, Kukwa A, Croft CB, Borowiecki B, Silver C, Emerson EE: Cellular immunity in patients with epidermoid cancer of the head and neck. *Laryngoscope* 1979; 89:538.

Parker R, Alexander S, Shaheen OH, Parkes P: On the immunology of head and neck cancer—a prognostic index. *J Laryngol Otol* 1975; 89:687.

Penn I: Second malignant neoplasms associated with immunosuppressive medications. *Cancer* 1976; 37:1024.

Prehn RT: Do tumors grow because of the immune response of the host? *Transplant Rev* 1976; 28:34.

Riesco A: Five year cancer cure: Relation to total amount of peripheral lymphocytes and neutrophils. *Cancer* 1970; 25:135.

Rosenbaum JT, Dwyer JM: The role of IgE in the immune response to neoplasia: A review. *Cancer* 1977; 39:11.

Rossen RD, Reisberg MA, Singer D, Suki WN, Duffy J, Hersh EM, Schloeder FX, Hill LL, Eknoyan G: The effect of age on the character of immune complex disease: A comparison of the incidence and relative size of materials reactive with C18 in sera of patients with glomerulonephritis and cancer. *Medicine* 1979; 58:65.

Schottenfeld D: Alcohol as a co-factor in the etiology of cancer. *Cancer* 1979; 43:1962.

Schwartz RS: Another look at immunological surveillance. *N Engl J Med* 1975; 293:181.

Serrou B, Dubois JB, Robinet-Levy M: IgE serum-levels in cancer patients. *Lancet* 1975; 1:396.

Shapiro S, Heinonen OP, Siskind V: Cancer and allergy. *Cancer* 1971; 28:396.

Silverman NA, Alexander JC, Hollinshead AC, Chretien PB: Correlation of tumor burden with "in vitro" lymphocyte reactivity and antibodies to herpes viral tumor-associated antigens in head and neck squamous carcinoma. *Cancer* 1976; 37:135.

Silverman NA, Potvin C, Alexander JC, Chretien PB: In vitro lymphocyte reactivity and T-cell levels in chronic cigarette smokers. *Clin Exp Immunol* 1975; 22:285.

Sipos J, Gabor V, Toth Z: Inhibition of leukocyte migration by tumour-associated antigen and its modification by serum; IgA as a blocking factor. *Neoplasia* 1978; 25:181.

Sjogren HO, Hellstrom I, Bansal SC, Hellstrom KE: Suggestive evidence that the "blocking antibodies" of tumor bearing individuals may be antigen-antibody complexes. *Proc Nat Acad Sci USA* 1971; 68:1372.

Smale BF, Mullen JL, Buzby GP, Rosato EF: The efficacy of nutritional assessment and support in cancer surgery. *Cancer* 1981; 47:2375.

Smith HG, Horowitz N, Silverman NA, Henson DE, Chretien PB: Humoral immunity to herpes simplex viral-induced antigens in smokers. *Cancer* 1976a; 38:1155.

Smith HG, Chretien PB, Henson DE, Silverman NA, Alexander JC: Viral-specific humoral immunity to herpes simplex-induced antigens in patients with squamous cell carcinoma of the head and neck. *Am J Surg* 1976b; 132:541.

Snell NJC: Leukocyte-counts and survival in unresectable lung cancer. *Lancet* 1979; 1:383.

Sobol SM, Conoyer JM, Zill R, Thawley SE, Ogura JH: Nutritional concepts in the management of the head and neck cancer patient. I. Basic concepts. *Laryngoscope* 1979; 89:794.

Solowey AC, Rapaport FT: Immunologic responses in cancer patients. *Surg Gynecol Obstet* 1965; 121:756.

Stefani SS, Kerman RH: Lymphocyte response to phytohaemagglutinin before and after radiation therapy in patients with carcinomas of the head and neck. *J Laryngol Otol* 1977; 91:605.

Straus R, Berenyi MR, Huang J-M, Straus E: Delayed hypersensitivity in alcoholic cirrhosis. *Am J Dig Dis* 1971; 16:509.

Suskind RM, Sirishinha S, Vithayasai V, Edelman R, Damrongsak D, Charupatana C, Olson RE: Immunoglobulins and antibody response in children with protein-calorie malnutrition. *Am J Clin Nutr* 1976; 29:836.

Suskind RM: *Malnutrition and the Immune Response.* New York, Raven Press, 1977.

Tarpley JL, Potvin C, Chretien PB: Prolonged depression of cellular immunity in cured laryngopharyngeal cancer patients treated with radiation therapy. *Cancer* 1975; 35:638.

Teller MN, Stohr G, Curlett W, Kubisek ML, Curtis D: Aging and cancerigenesis. I. Immunity to tumor and skin grafts. *JNCI* 1964; 33:649.

Tomasi TB Jr: Secretory immunoglobulins. *N Engl J Med* 1972; 287:500.

Tomasi TB Jr, Tisdale WA: Serum gamma-globulins in acute and chronic liver diseases. *Nature (London)* 1964; 201:834.

Twomey PL, Catalona WJ, Chretien PB: Cellular immunity in cured cancer patients. *Cancer* 1974; 33:435.

Van Epps DE, Strickland RG, Williams RC, Jr: Elevated IgE levels in liver disease. *Clin Res.* 1975; 23:106A.

Veltri RW, Sprinkle PM, Maxim PE, Theofilopoulos AN, Rodman SM, Kinney CL: Immune monitoring protocol for patients with carcinoma of the head and neck. *Ann Otol* 1978; 87:692.

Waldmann TA, Bull JM, Bruce RM, Broder S, Jost MC, Balestra ST, Suer ME: Serum immuno-globulin E levels in patients with neoplastic disease. *J Immunol* 1974; 113:379.

Waldorf DS, Willkens RF, Decker JL: Impaired delayed hypersensitivity in an aging population. Association with antinuclear reactivity and rheumatoid factor. *JAMA* 1968; 203:111.

Wanebo HJ, Jun MY, Strong EW, Oettgen H: T-cell deficiency in patients with squamous cell cancer of the head and neck. *Am J Surg* 1975; 130:445.

Wara WM, Phillips TL, Wara DW, Ammann AJ, Smith V: Immunosuppression following radiation therapy for carcinoma of the nasopharynx. *Am J Roetgen Rad Ther Nuclear Med* 1975; 123:482.

Willis RA: *Pathology of Tumors.* 4th Ed, pp. 67–91, 1967. Butterworth, London.

Winters WD, Heiner DC: IgE levels in sera of cancer patients. *J Allergy Clin Immunol* 1976; 57:181.

Wolf GT, Wolfe RA, Chretien PB: Circulating immune complexes in patients with nasopharyngeal carcinoma. *Otolaryngol Head Neck Surg* 1982; 90 (No. 5, Sect. 2):226.

Wybran J, Fudenberg HH: Thymus-derived rossette-forming cells in various human disease states: cancer, lymphoma, bacterial and viral infections, and other diseases. *J Clin Inv* 1973; 52:1026.

Zighelboim J, Bonavida P, Fahey JL: Evidence for several cell populations active in antibody dependent cellular cytoxicity. *J Immunol* 1973; 111:1737.

Chapter 12

Transplantation in Otolaryngology

Wim Kuijpers
Jan E. Veldman

OUTLINE

INTRODUCTION

**HISTOPHYSIOLOGY AND CELL BIOLOGY OF
TYMPANOPLASTY**
  Myringoplasty
  Ossiculoplasty
**IMMUNOHISTOPHYSIOLOGY AND
ALLOGRAFT-TYMPANOPLASTY**
  Origin and Fate of Immunologically Competent Cells
    Lymphocytes and lymphoid cell traffic
    The immune response in the lymph node
    X-irradiation and the allograft reaction
  Otologic Tissue Grafting—Its Place in the Immunohistophysiology
    of Lymphoid Tissue
    Privileged site or privileged tissue
    Analyses of the antigenicity of tympanoossicular grafts
     in animal models
  Clinical Immunopathology of Human Middle Ear Implants
    Serology and immunofluorescence studies in human
     allograph/tympanoplasty

DISCUSSION
  Cell Biological Considerations

Immunological Considerations
The middle ear: A privileged site for tolerogenesis in allograft tympanoplasty?

REFERENCES

INTRODUCTION

Since the first attempt of Marcus Banzer in 1640 to erase the deleterious effect of a persisting perforation in the tympanic membrane with a piece of pig bladder mounted on an ivory tube, a variety of techniques have been used to close a perforated tympanic membrane. Especially during the last 100 years numerous methods have been introduced for reconstructing the sound-conducting system. However, many of them were abandoned because of unsatisfactory results.

A revolutionary development in reconstructive ear surgery was the introduction of tympanoplasty by Von Moritz (1952), Wullstein (1952) and Zollner (1952). Their concept resulted in the use of a large variety of biological tissues—even alloplastic materials—for the reconstruction of a tympanic membrane and/or ossicular chain. A comparable development can be observed in the search for new methods and materials in rhinoplasty. Since the first report on restoring the contour of the nose by Rousset in 1828, an endless series of metals, plastics, autologous, allogenous, and xenogenous grafts have been applied for this purpose. New techniques with new grafts have been introduced, but within a few years were followed by reports of disappointing results. Comprehensive reviews on this matter have been given by McDowell (1952) and Bloom (1960). At present satisfactory results are obtained with biological grafts like bone and cartilage, autologous and allogenous. Cartilage seems to be superior to any other auto- or allograft (Huizing, 1974).

In contrast to reconstructive ear and rhinosurgery, only very recently have attempts been made to transplant a larynx in laryngectomized patients. This is understandable because of the technical problems involved in reanastomosing nerves and blood vessels on the one hand, and the immunological rejection problem on the other. In the era of successful kidney and cornea transplantations—even early promising reports on long-standing heart transplants appeared in the literature—human larynx transplantation does not seem to have a future at present. An occasional attempt has been disastrous. Failure was said to be mainly due to unsolved immunological problems (Kluyskens and Ringoir, 1970). Also in experimental larynx transplantations rejection of the allograft remains a source of surgical frustration (Ogura et al., 1966, 1970).

A survey of the literature on reconstructive surgery in otolaryngology reveals a scarcity of fundamental data on the immunobiological behavior of the materials used, particularly the rhino- and laryngology. This leaves us with the field of otology. During the past two decades various experimental studies, accompanying or following the introduction of new techniques in tympanoplasty, have been performed to study the sequelae of grafts used in reconstructive middle ear surgery. A review of our own work and that of others is presented, and special emphasis is given to transplantation-immunology in relation to allograft-tympanoplasty (part B).

HISTOPHYSIOLOGY AND CELL BIOLOGY OF TYMPANOPLASTY

Myringoplasty

The introduction of tympanoplasty in the early 1950s changed the treatment of chronic middle ear disease from eradication of the diseased tissue to an improvement of hearing by a subsequent reconstruction of the sound-conducting system. Initially only the tympanic membrane was reconstructed. For that purpose autologous external body skin was used. However, a few years after its introduction the usefulness of such a graft was already very doubtful. The long-term results appeared to be quite unsatisfactory (Beickert, 1958; Thorburn, 1960; House & Sheehy, 1961; Wright, 1963; Örtegren, 1964). Inflammation and excessive desquamation often occurred and in many cases cholesteatoma developed from the graft. Persistence of the original character of the graft for a long period of time, as well as climatological conditions in the deeper parts of the meatal skin, are together presumably responsible for these phenomena. The humidity and temperature are much higher in the meatus than at the retroauricular region from which the grafts usually originated. This assumption may explain the more successful use of skin grafts in myringoplasty from the deeper parts of the external meatus (Frenckner, 1955, Mulcahy & McAffe, 1964; Sheehy, 1964; Sooy, 1964).

The disappointing results with external body skin gave rise to the search for other biological grafts. Many autologous tissues have been used and are still in use. From the excellent results reported with autologous tissues of mesodermal-origin, like fascia (Heermann, 1962; Ortegren, 1964; Patterson et al., 1967; Smyth, 1976), vein (Austin, 1965), perichondrium (Goodhill et al., 1964), and fat (Ringenberg, 1962) it can reasonably be concluded that they are very useful in myringoplasty.

Simultaneously with the autologous grafts, allogenous tissues have been introduced to close a tympanic membrane perforation, like perichondrium (Jansen, 1963), pericardium (Nickel, 1963), tympanic membrane (Chalat, 1964; Marquet, 1966, 1968), dura (Albrite & Leigh, 1966; Smyth, 1976), fascia (Smyth, 1976), and even xenogenous grafts, like cardiac valves (Cornish & Scott, 1968), calf's tympanic membrane, and calf's serosa (Jansen, 1973). With many of these grafts satisfactory results were obtained.

However, it must be noted that apart from Chalat (1964) no real allografts have been used. In fact only nonvital allogenous tissues, physicochemically preserved in various manners, are transplanted. The successful use of a large variety of tissues from different origin in myringoplasty is an intriguing problem and needs further explanation. To understand these observations one has to consider the condition of the tympanic membrane with a persisting perforation as a consequence of a healed chronic ear disease, as well as the course of events after covering the perforation with a graft. In contrast to a traumatically induced perforation, a perforation resulting from past chronic middle ear disease usually fails to heal spontaneously. In these cases the tympanic membrane is generally partly atrophic, poorly vascularised, and contains scar tissue. It has been known for years that etching of the rim of a perforation or removal of the scar tissue at the edge can stimulate the membrane to proliferate and narrow or even close small perforations (Dunlap & Schuknecht, 1974). However, large perforations fail to heal with these techniques. Covering the perforation with a tissue graft has been shown to be necessary for closing these perforations. From experimental studies and clinical observations more insight is gained about the role played by the graft itself (Salen, 1968; Reijnen & Kuijpers, 1971; Marquet et al., 1973). The general feeling is that the graft's function is as a scaffold for guiding the epithelium that migrates from the perforation edges that have been stimulated to proliferate by removing the scar tissue. Evidence for this assumption is derived from the observation that healing of a subtotal perforation with the use of an allogenous tympanic membrane graft results in a new membrane with a conical shape, while a spontaneously healed, subtotal, traumatically-produced perforation often results in a completely flat membrane.

However, a second and even more important role of the graft is that it gives mesenchymal cells and capillaries the opportunity to grow into and along the graft. In this way the epithelium, which migrates along the graft, may proliferate as has been shown in an animal model using (^{3}H)-thymidine (Reijnen & Kuijpers, 1971). Bridging of the perforation by the epithelium is no longer exclusively dependent on a cell supply from distant proliferative centers as occurs with perforations which are not closed with a graft (Fig 12-1a, 1b). After closure of the gap the mitotic activity decreases rapidly and a reorganization occurs. The lamina propria arises from fibroblasts migrating into and along the graft; it gradually becomes thinner by resorption of the graft. Grafts composed mainly of collagenous fibers, like fascia and tympanic membrane, have been shown to be highly resistant to resorption. Remnants of these tissues may persist for years (Fig 12-2a, 2b). No apparent differences have been found between the healing of a perforation with the use of autologous or preserved allogenous grafts. The conclusion seems to be justified that vitality of the graft is of no importance to the healing process. Although preservation has an effect on the antigenic properties of an allogenous graft (van den Broek & Kuijpers, 1974; Veldman et al., 1979; Veldman & Kuijpers, 1981), the way in which immunological interference occurs—not reported in most clinical cases—remains an unsolved problem in allograft-myringoplasty. Furthermore, the use of preserved grafts can be assumed to have an additional advantage in preventing early graft perforation as compared to fresh autologous tissues. While in fresh autografts the autolytic enzymes are an important factor in early graft destruction, such enzymes are inhibited or even destroyed by some of the currently used preservation methods.

Ossiculoplasty

With the introduction of tympanoplasty initially only the tympanic membrane was reconstructed. The graft was directly positioned on the remnants of the ossicular chain

FIG 12-1. Micrographs of cat tympanic membrane after traumatically produced perforation:

a. Edge of perforation consisting of migrating epithelial cells, after 4 days (haemotoxyline-eosin staining (HE, × 200).

b. Perforation closed with fat graft, after 4 weeks. Note ingrowth of fibrous tissue (HE, × 70).

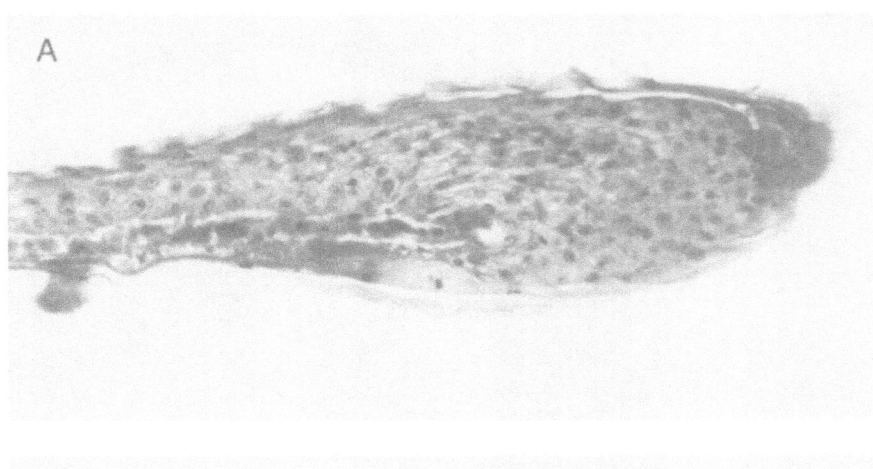

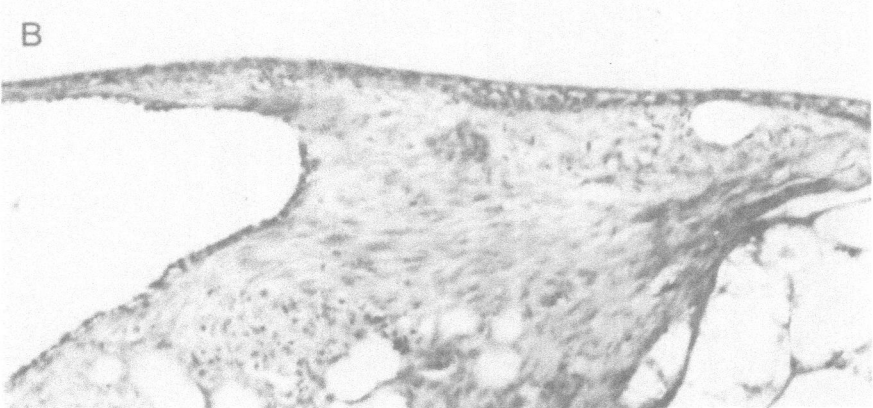

and no attempts were made to reconstruct the ossicular chain. However, during the following years a wide variety of techniques were introduced to restore the ossicular chain to obtain better hearing results. This development was forced by the progressive tendency to avoid the cavity problem and to maintain a normal middle ear space. During the first period various artificial prostheses were used for reconstruction, encouraged by the

FIG 12-2.   Micrographs of tympanic membrane sections after myringoplasty:
a. Human specimen, 3 years after closing a perforation with an autogenous fascia graft. F: remnant of fascia graft, S: sclerotic patch (HE, × 150).
b. Rat specimen, one year after closing traumatic perforation with Cialit® preserved allogenous tympanic membrane graft. G: graft (Azran, × 200).

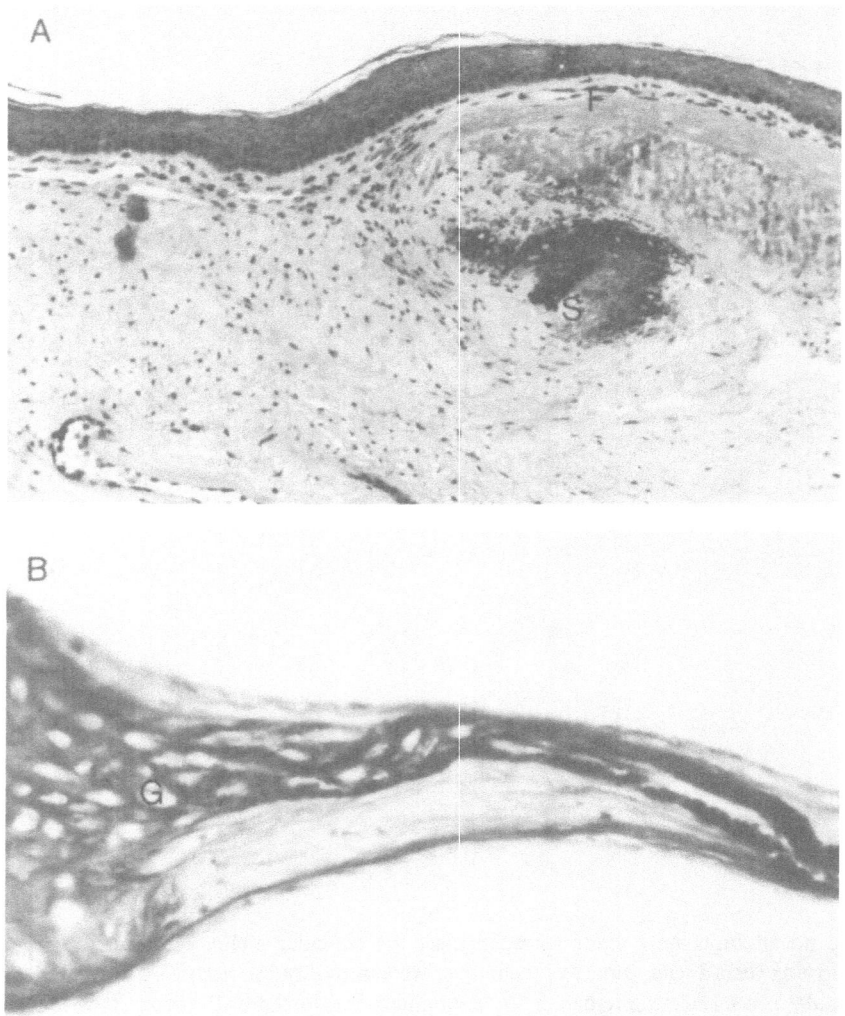

excellent results obtained with these prostheses in stapes surgery. Although the initial results were promising, most of these prostheses were discarded because of instability and extrusion. Apart from cytotoxic effects, the main cause of failure must be ascribed to the local pressure exerted by the prostheses of the malleus handle and tympanic membrane, causing necrosis and perforations, together with the lack of a firm biomechanical union between prosthesis and the middle ear structures. The recent development of porous implants, allowing ingrowth of connective tissue and bone, seems to answer these problems (Homsey et al., 1973). Encouraging results have been reported both from experimental and clinical studies (Kuijpers & Grote, 1977; Shea & Emmett, 1978). However, after a few years clinical use, the question arises again whether these materials are really the most appropriate ones as an alloplastic strut in tympanoplasty. There is an increasing number of reports recommending the use of cartilage between the porous implant and the tympanic membrane to avoid extrusion (Brackman & Sheehy, 1979; Strauss, 1979).

In the first efforts for ossiculoplasty with biological tissues cortical bone chips from the mastoid or from the cortex of the skull, shaped into a columella or incus, were used (Zollner, 1960; Plester & Steinbach, 1977). However, this technique has never become very popular. Final results were often quite unsatisfactory, presumably due to bone resorption. Far better success was obtained with autologous cartilage (Jansen, 1962) and preserved allogenous septal cartilage (Smyth, 1976; Altenau & Sheehy, 1978). Up to the present cartilage has proven its validity for ossicular chain reconstruction. Histological studies of cartilage—obtained during revision surgery—that had been in the middle ear for more than 2 years revealed that a major part of the prosthesis remains unchanged (Fig 12-3a-d). In a minor number of cases resorption and replacement by fibrous tissue has been reported (Kerr et al., 1973; Strauss & Schreiter, 1979).

Simultaneously with the introduction of cartilage the use of repositioning the patients' own incus has enjoyed increasing popularity in tympanoplasty since the first report of it by Hall and Rytner (1957). It resulted in the development of many new techniques in which the intact or remodeled ossicles were used for ossicular reconstruction. Many authors have reported their results and consider it as one of the most valuable methods.

From experimental studies as well as from histological examination after revision surgery, it appears that the gross structure of the ossicle is retained even after years. However, there is no unanimity in opinion on the vitality of the graft (Stengl & Hohmann, 1964; van den Broek & Kuijpers, 1967; Smith & Overton, 1968; Kerr & Smyth, 1971; Fig 12-4). A controlled experimental study on rats revealed that the vitality of the transposed incus was strongly related to the time lag between removal and repositioning. Moreover, it appeared that storage of the dislocated ossicle in the wound fluid during the surgical procedure preserved the osteocytes to a great extent (van den Broek & Kuijpers, 1967). Generally it can be stated that in transposing ossicles a varying initial cell decay occurs, which is highly dependent on the surgical procedure. This is followed within a few weeks by an extensive formation of new bone if the periostal cells survive (Fig 12-5). Whether complete revitalization ever occurs, remains very doubtful.

FIG 12-3.   Allogenous alcohol preserved cartilage grafts, removed at revision surgery because of dysfunction (a,b,d) and infection (c) (HE, × 150).
a. Underlay of tympanic membrane, after 1 year.
b. Columella, after 3 years.

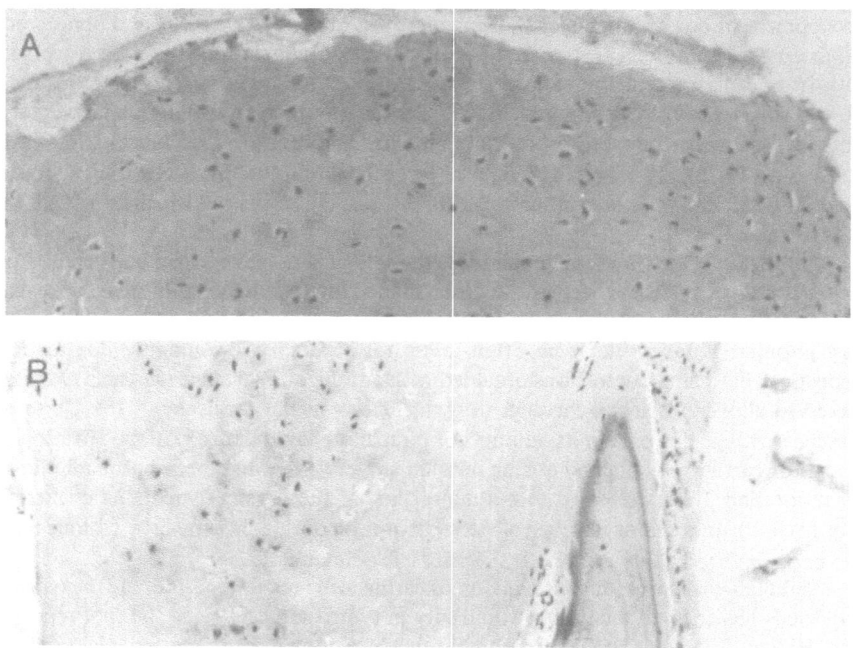

Shortly after the introduction of the ossicular repositioning technique, the use of preserved allogenous ossicles was advocated by House et al (1966) and Glasscock and House (1968). This was performed in patients in whom, eg, the incus was absent or in cases where an ossicle had to be replaced to avoid the risk of reintroducing the preexistent disease (Bellucci & Wolff, 1966). In the next years the use of preserved allogenous ossicles became widespread, and comparable results have been reported as with the use of autologous ossicles. This development finally resulted in the introduction of the tympano-ossicular monobloc implant, which is considered the ideal physiological reconstruction of the sound transmission system (Glasscock et al., 1972; Marquet et al., 1973). As in the case of allogenous grafts from myringoplasty different methods are applied for the preservation of allogenous ossicles. Since various authors attribute their results to the use of a certain method of preservation it seems useful to give a short analysis of its modalities. The preservatives that have received most attention are: Cialit® (Marquet, 1966), alcohol (Kerr & Smyth, 1971; Wehrs, 1976), formaldehyde (Perkins, 1975ab;

FIG 12-3.   continued
c. Columella with local infective erosion, after 2 years.
d. Columella showing distortion and fibrosis, after 5 years.

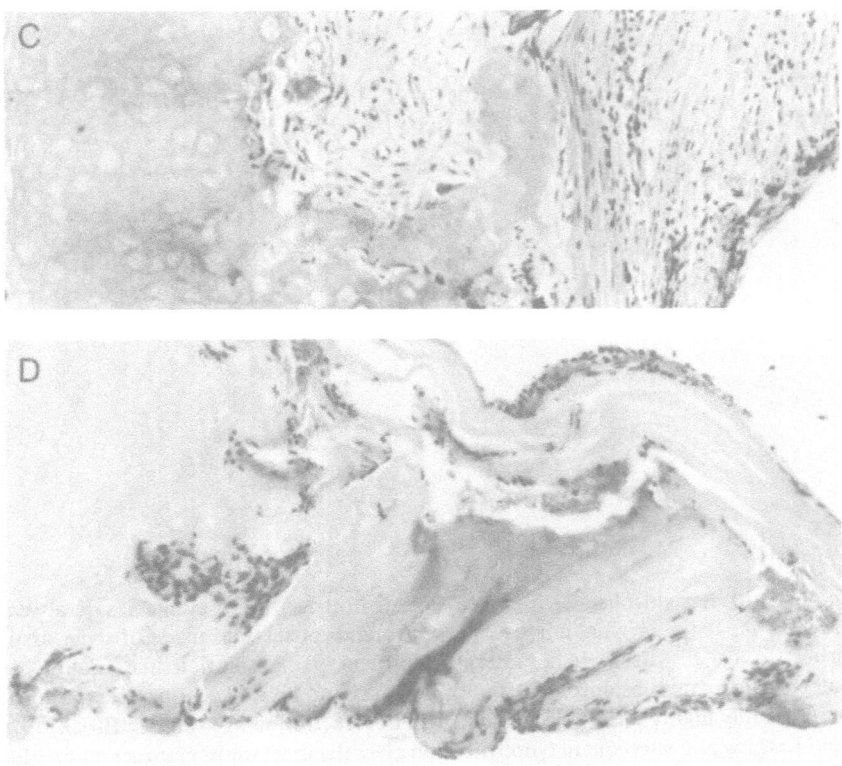

Marquet, 1976) and thiomersalate (McKinnon, 1972). In addition, freeze-drying and subsequent sterilization of the otologic allograft is also advocated as a reliable preservation method (Lacher, 1971; Smith, 1977, 1980). These procedures have in common that microorganisms are killed and no graft cells will survive. They differ, respectively, in their effect on the morphological and biochemical properties of the tissues. Alcohol and formaldehyde affect the molecular structure of the proteins. Alcohol changes the protein structure profoundly with resultant coagulation, while formaldehyde is a noncoagulant fixative that does not separate water from the tissue proteins. Due to these properties, preservation in alcohol results in shrinkage and hardening of the tissues, while formaldehyde hardens,

FIG 12-4. Remodeled autogenous incus, placed between stapes and malleus, removed because of dysfunction after 1 year. The major part of the bone is avital (HE, × 70).

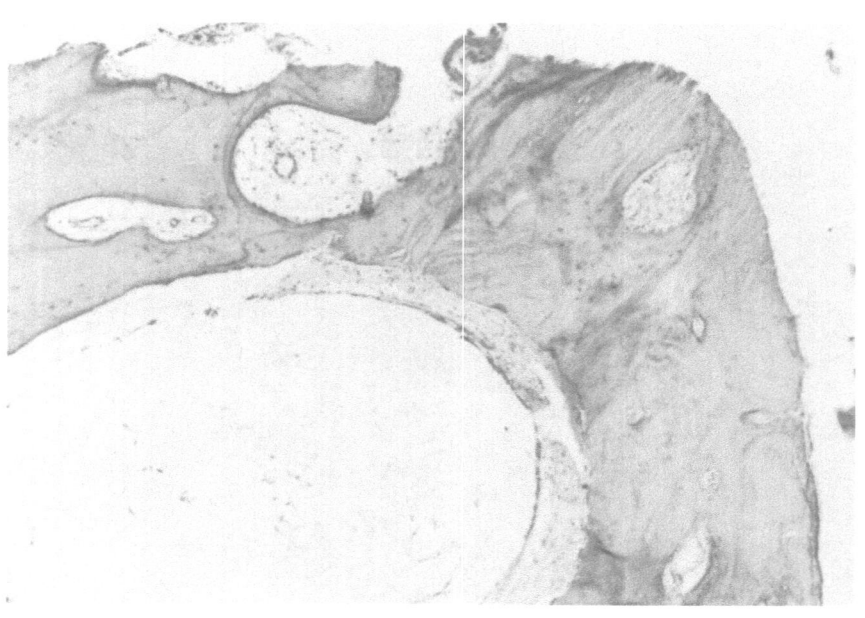

although with less shrinkage. Prolonged storage in these fluids, even for several years, does not change the original microscopic appearance of sections made of these tissues. During storage of tissues in a watery nonprotein fixing solution like Cialit® and thiomersalate many substances leak out of the grafts, and it is likely that after prolonged storage mainly highly unsoluble elements will be left (Kuijpers & van den Broek, 1975). Rapid freezing and subsequent lyophylization gives the most optimal preservation of the tissue components and the biochemical properties of the graft. The effects of some preservatives on the microscopical structure of ossicles and tympanic membrane are shown in Fig 12-6a, 6b, and Fig 12-21a.

An evaluation of experimental studies on the behavior of preserved allogenous ossicles transplanted into the middle ear reveals that the first reaction of the middle ear is apparently not different from that to the transposed autologous ossicles (van den Broek, 1968). Within a few weeks the grafts become covered with an epithelial lining. Blood vessels grow into the haversian canals. Longer survival periods of several months show a limited amount of new bone formed around the haversian canals and scattered along the periphery. From serial sections it appeared that the major part of the bone remained avital without clear signs of resorption through an observation period of 2 years. Except for the incidence of new bone formation no differences were seen in the behavior of the

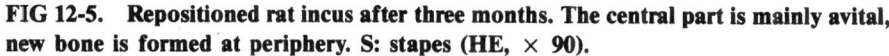

FIG 12-5.   Repositioned rat incus after three months. The central part is mainly avital, new bone is formed at periphery. S: stapes (HE, × 90).

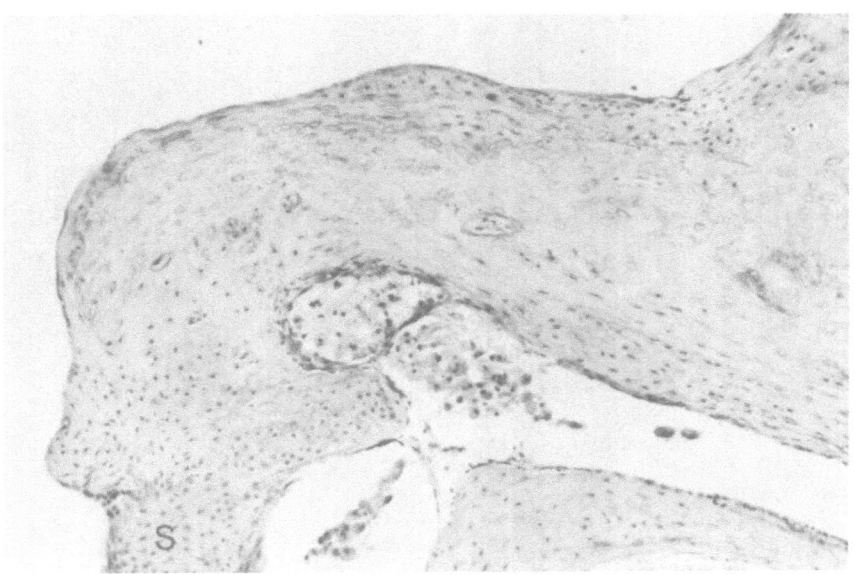

ossicles preserved in various manners (Fig 12-7; Wilson et al, 1966; Smith & Overton, 1968; Touma & Maguda, 1973; van den Broek & Kuijpers, 1974; Christiansen & Hohmann, 1975). Comparable observations, also with a variable degree of osteoneogenesis, have been reported from microscopic studies of ossicles obtained at revision operations (Fig 12-8a, 8b) (Kerr & Smyth, 1971; Strauss & Ickler, 1980). Generally it can be assumed that osteoneogenesis in preserved avital allogenous ossicles can occur in two manners. The first source is the periosteum of the middle ear, which will proliferate as a consequence of the surgical procedure and extend to the ossicular implant. A second possibility is the preservation of a bone-inducing property of the graft. The so-called bone morpho-genetic protein (BMP) stimulates undifferentiated cells into bone-forming cells. The preservation of this BMP has been shown to be highly dependent on the way grafts have been treated (Urist et al., 1967). This might explain the difference in the amount of new bone formed in ossicular grafts that have been preserved in various manners.

Apart from the difference in amount of new bone formed, some specimens from unsuccessful clinical cases show resorption, sometimes only microscopially visible. However, in other cases large parts of the graft can be eroded, often without signs of inflammation. One can only speculate on the cause (Fig 12-8) (Kuijpers & van den Broek, 1975; van den Broek & Kuijpers, 1976; Strauss & Ickler, 1980). The recovered specimen

FIG 12-6.   Micrographs of rat malleus with adhering pars tensa, stored in Cialit® for 1 year (a) and a pars flaccida stored in alcohol for 3 years (b). Note absence of nuclei, except for a few cartilaginous cells, in the Cialit® preserved specimen (HE, × 200).

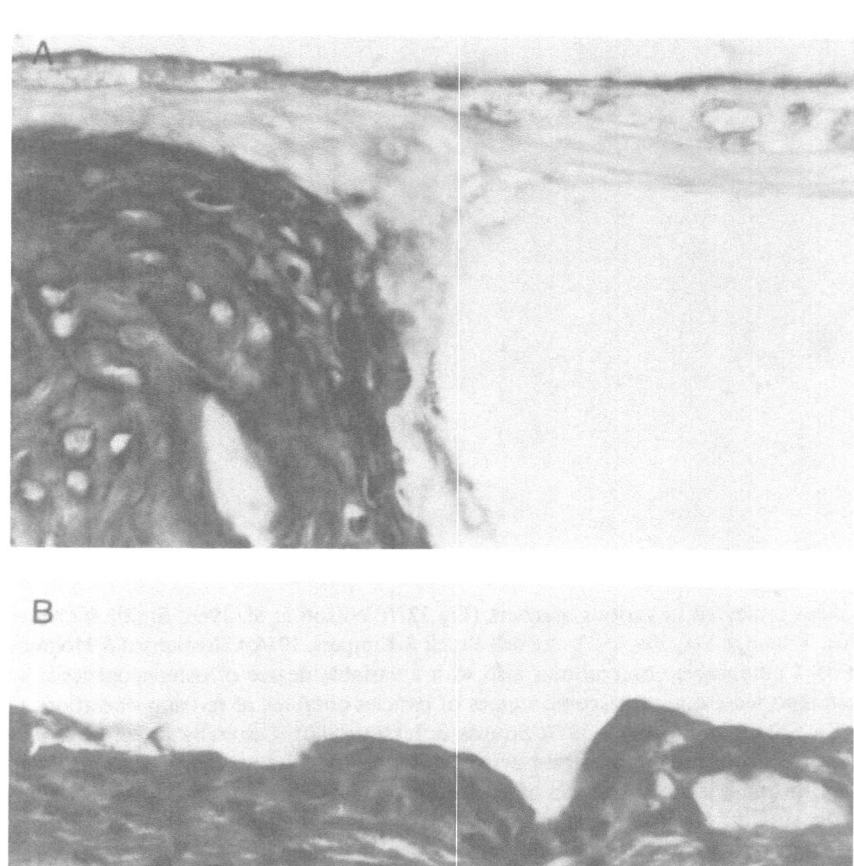

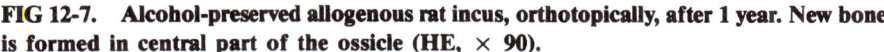
FIG 12-7. Alcohol-preserved allogenous rat incus, orthotopically, after 1 year. New bone is formed in central part of the ossicle (HE, × 90).

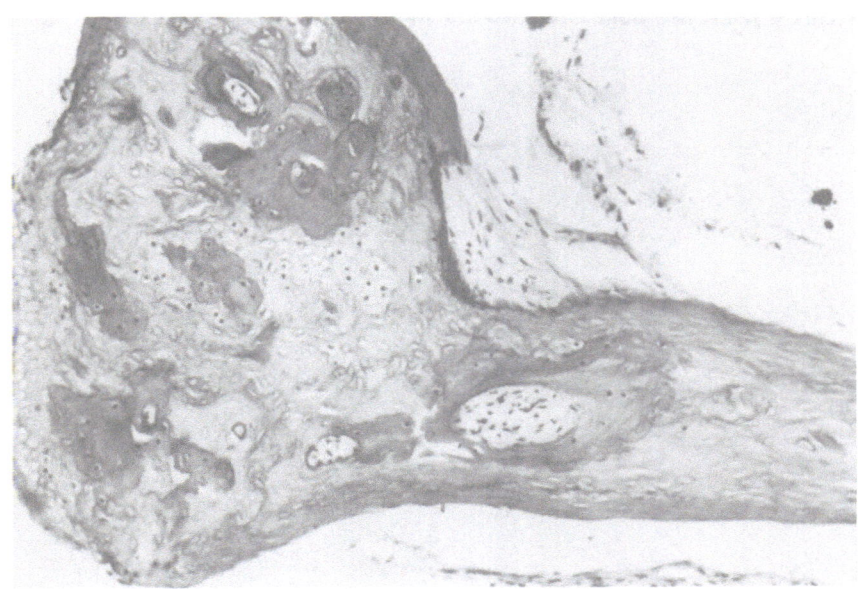

from revision operations cannot be assumed to be always representative for allograft-ossiculoplasty. Such specimens constitute a minor percentage of the total number of transplanted ossicles, the rest of which function very well. However, the crucial question remains what the ultimate fate of the only partially revitalized ossicle will be. In other sites of the body avital bone grafts have been shown to be resorbed within a certain amount of time. The same process has been observed with preserved ossicles in animal experiments (Fig 12-9) (van den Broek & Kuijpers, 1974). Therefore, is this process in the middle ear only retarded? Time will presumably give us a final answer.

A second intriguing observation in allograft-tympanoplasty is the apparent absence of a serious interference of the immunological reflex, although there is substantial evidence that preservation does not abolish the antigenic properties of the grafts (van den Broek & Kuijpers, 1974; Veldman et al., 1979; Veldman & Kuijpers, 1981). This phenomenon is discussed in the next section. Because of the complexity of transplantation immuno-biology a general survey is given; it is the backbone of our experimental studies on allograft-tympanoplasty as far as immunology is applied to it.

FIG 12-8. Alcohol-preserved allogenous incudes, removed at revision surgery, because of dysfunction.
a. After 1 year; bone is avital and lenticular process resorbed (HE, × 70).
b. After 4 years; new bone is formed around lacunae (HE, × 150).

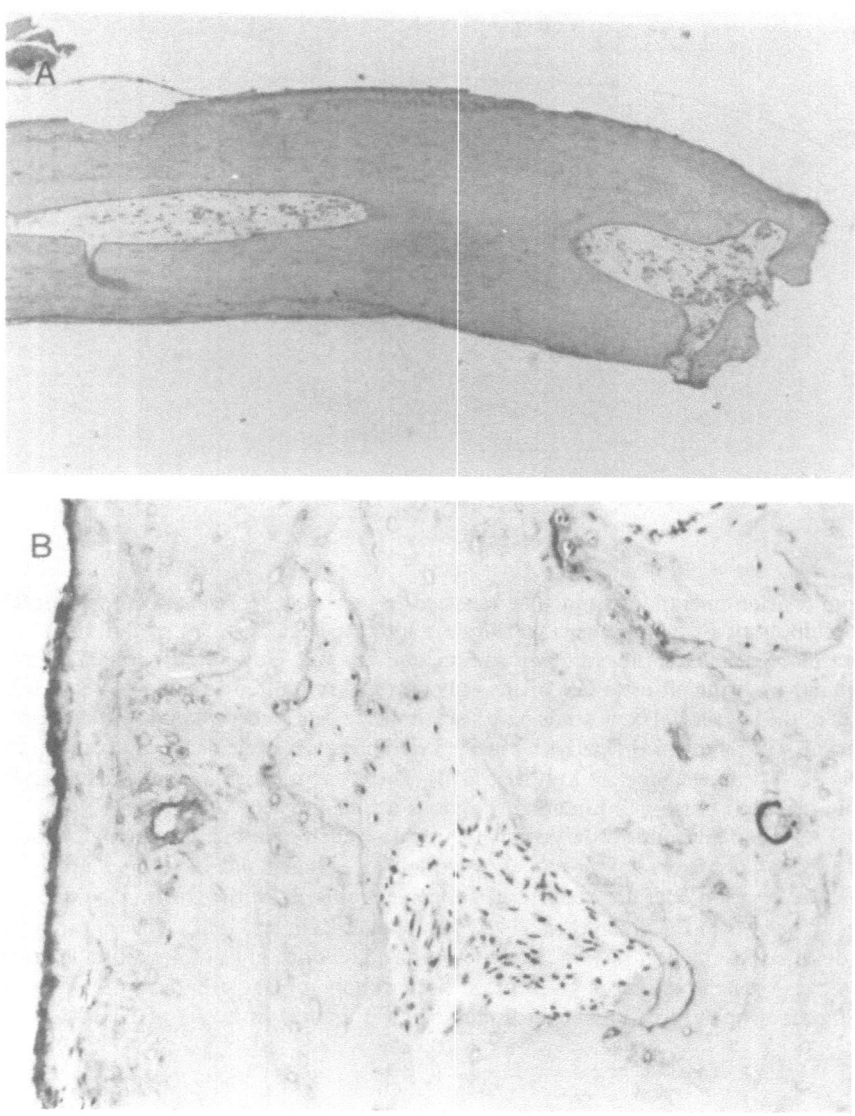

FIG 12-9. **Formaldehyde-preserved allogenous rat incus, transplanted ectopically, showing extensive resorption after 1 year (HE, × 70).**

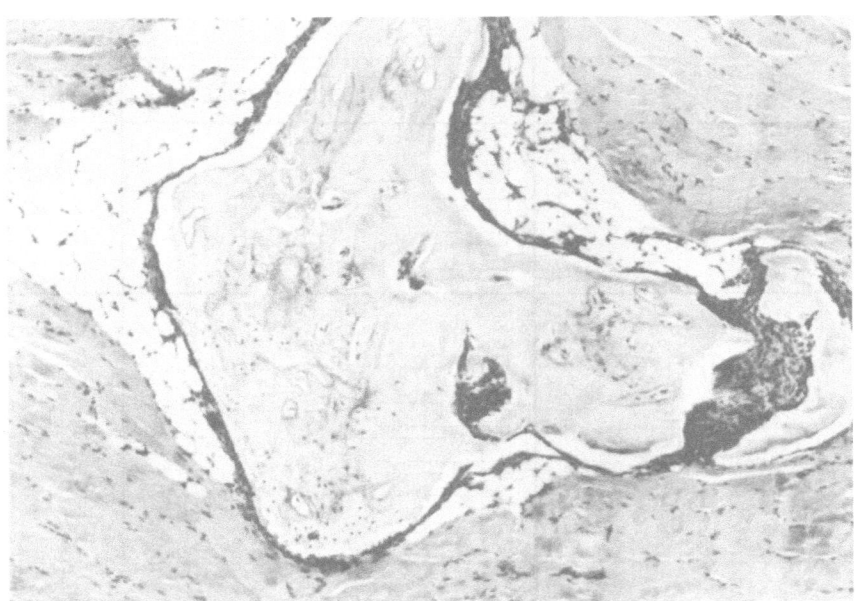

IMMUNOHISTOPHYSIOLOGY AND ALLOGRAFT-TYMPANOPLASTY

An extremely efficient and developed protective immune system recognizes the allograft and mobilizes its cellular defenses to destroy the invader. The diversity of antigenicity within a species is remarkable. To most surgeons involved in transplantation these histocompatibility antigens are a source of great frustration.

Cells rather than humoral antibodies are necessary for an allograft reaction under normal conditions (Table 12-1). Allografts enclosed within millipore chambers will not be rejected as long as the pores are not large enough to allow host cells to reach the graft (Algire et al., 1957). Mitchison (1953) provided evidence at an early date that transplantation immunity could be transferred by cells rather than serum. Billingham et al., (1954) demonstrated that the best adoptive transfer could be obtained with lymph nodes draining the graft directly. Histological analyses of these nodes revealed strong immunoblast reactions of—as has been demonstrated—T- and B-lymphocytic origin. Further experimental analysis by means of sublethal total body x-irradiation in rabbits showed that the characteristic thymus-dependent area (TDA-bound; Parrot et al., 1966) immunoblast reaction was primarily responsible for cellular immunity (allograft rejection

TABLE 12-1. Skin allograft rejection in normal (B and T cells present) and B-cell deprived rabbits (only T cells present) rejection period : _____.
(From Veldman & Keuning, 1978).

EXPERIMENTAL SYSTEM		"TRANSPLANTATION RESPONSE"	SURVIVAL TIME
controls	1	7 days	11 days
	2		11 „
	3		12 „
	4		15 „
B-cell deprived rabbit	1		16 „
	2		12 „
	3		15 „
	4		16 „
	5		12 „
	6		13 „

and delayed sensitivity; Fig 12-10) (Micklem & Brown, 1961; van der Slikke & Keuning, 1964; Veldman, 1970; Veldman & Keuning, 1978). In B-cell deprived rabbits, reconstituted with recently thymus-derived lymphocytes, skin allografts were rejected within 12 to 16 days (Table 12-1). Through autoradiography it could be demonstrated—in an analogous experimental model—that these TDA-bound immunoblast reactions have a progeny of committed T lymphocytes responsible for skin graft rejection or delayed sensitivity (Veldman, 1970; Veldman & Keuning, 1978; Veldman et al, 1980).

Origin and Fate of Immunologically Competent Cells

During the past two decades the morphology of lymphoid tissue has been clarified in terms of population dynamics and migration streams. It has been generally recognized that the lymphocyte population of peripheral lymphoid tissue is not static, but one that is continuously exchanged. Mature cells within the lymphoid system have in addition the capacity to arrange themselves in clear-cut microenvironments of peripheral lymphoid organs (Parrot et al., 1966; Veldman, 1970; Veldman et al., 1978a; Veldman & Keuning, 1978; deSousa, 1978).

FIG 12-10.   T-immunoblast reaction on skin allograft in axillary lymph node of B-cell deprived rabbit.
(methyl-green pyronin staining (MGP) × 140; insert × 700)
(From Veldman & Keuning, 1978).

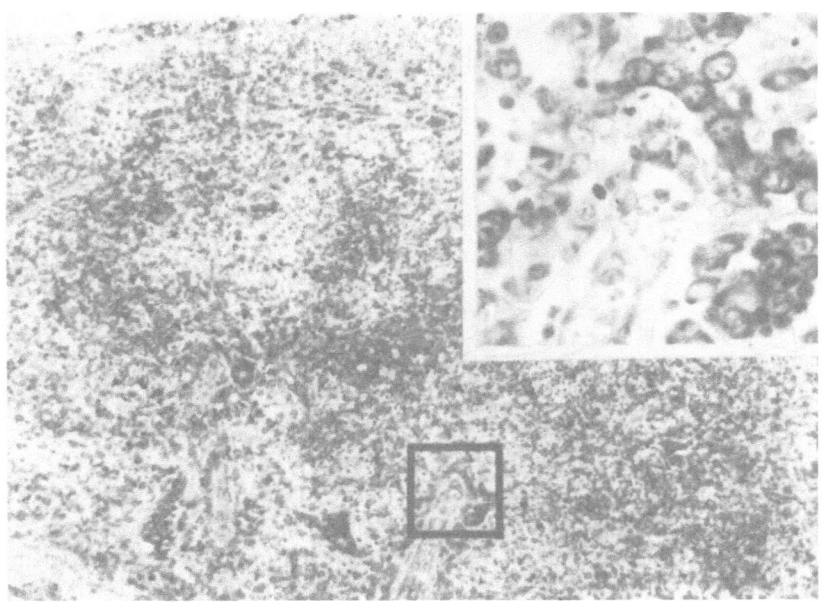

Lymphocytes and lymphoid cell traffic (Fig 12-11)

The existence of a pool of recirculating lymphocytes which alternate between circulating as blood lymphocytes and residing in lymphoid tissue, are consequently continuously redistributed among the various lymphoid organs, has been definitely demonstrated by Gowans (1959). The basic observation was an enormous decrease of lymphocyte output by the cannulated thoracic duct in rats after a few days of lymph drainage and when the collected lymph was returned without cells, and its restoration to normal values when the cells were reinjected intravenously. Lymphoid cell traffic could be further analyzed in detail by means of ^{3}H-labeling experiments—both in vivo and in vitro—in different animal species (Gowans & Knight, 1964; Weissman, 1967; Ford, 1969; Nieuwenhuis, 1971; Nieuwenhuis & Ford, 1976). Upon chronic drainage of thoracic duct lymph, particular areas—designated as thymus-dependent areas—are specifically depleted, whereas after in vitro labeling with ^{3}H-adenosine of these thoracic duct cells the major portion of immigrant lymphocytes are found histologically again in these same areas (Gowans & McGregor, 1965). Thymus dependency applies to these areas since the

FIG 12-11.   Diagram of (re)circulation pathway of T and B lymphocytes.

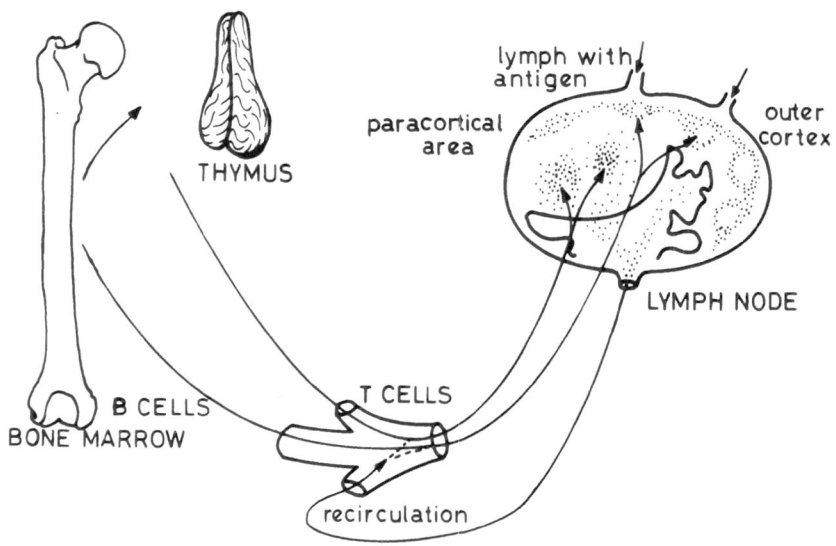

same pattern of depletion is observed in different animal species after neonatal thymectomy (Waksman et al., 1962; Parrot et al., 1966) or thymectomy at a later stage in life combined with total body x-irradiation (Veldman, 1970; Veldman et al., 1978a; Veldman & Keuning, 1978). Peripheral lymphoid organs (e.g., spleen, lymph nodes, tonsils, adenoids, etc.) can be divided into thymus-dependent (T) and thymus-independent (B) areas, which contain predominantly thymus-derived (T) and bone marrow-derived (B) cells, respectively (Parrot et al., 1966; Veldman, 1970; Veldman & Keuning, 1978; Veldman et al., 1978a, b). Their spatial distribution and microarchitecture in peripheral lymphoid organs is clearly defined topographically (Fig 12-11). Immunologically, elimination of the thymus-derived (T) cell population has been found to result in a long-lasting immunological unresponsiveness regarding transplantation immunity (Miller, 1961, 1962; Veldman, 1970; Veldman et al., 1978a, b). On the other hand, humoral immunity reactions against various antigens— although often impaired—remains present in these T-cell depleted animals. Sophisticated chromosome-marker techniques have demonstrated that an ultimately bone marrow- derived, thymus-independent lymphoid (B) cell is the antibody forming cell precursor (Miller & Mitchell, 1969). These cells are considered to be antigen-specific and clonally determined via cell-surface antigen-specific receptors (Burnet, 1959; Byrt & Ada, 1969; Cooper et al., 1972), whereas thymocytes bear a ø-positive, specific thymus alloantigen in their cell membrane (Raff & Cantor, 1971). Through modern immunohistochemical techniques both cell types can be demonstrated histologically in a variety of tissues.

The immune response in the lymph node.

The lymph node is representative of peripheral lymphoid tissue as to structure, functions, and cell-interactions. When dealing with transplantation immunity these are features of importance for the subsequent fate of any allograft reaction. The lymph node can be considered as a continuously operating mechanism, permanently kept ready for an immune response. Its structural organization at any given moment depends on a more-or-less basic pattern of specialized reticular cells, blood cells, and other nonlymphoid elements (Veldman et al., 1978a, b; deSousa, 1978; Veldman & Kaiserling, 1980). In this basic structure two main types of lymphoid cell traffic precipitate distinct morphological, though essentially dynamic, entities (Fig 12-11). These structural dynamics form the basis of immune responses induced by immunogens, which have been carried along with the lymph in afferent lymph vessels. Within certain limits the route of administration of an antigen determines which of the lymphoid organs will be the site of the ensuing immune response.

Immune reactions in lymphoid tissue comprise three antigen-induced processes: the plasma cell reactions representing antibody formation, cellular immunity reactions leading to cell-mediated immunity (e.g., the allograft reaction), and the germinal center reaction. This latter process has been shown to be a source of "memory cells," the plasma cell precursors of secondary response antibody formation (Wakefield & Thorbecke, 1968), as well as a site of generation and amplification of antibody forming cell precursors in general (Nieuwenhuis & Keuning, 1974; Opstelten et al., 1980). Their ultimate bone marrow origin is established beyond doubt (Balner & Dersjant, 1964; Mitchell & Miller, 1968; Miller & Mitchell, 1969).

These immune reactions occur simultaneously following the majority of antigenic stimuli. The bias of the response may be toward the cellular or humoral side, depending on the type of antigenic stimulus. Foreign proteins may elicit heavy cellular as well as humoral immunity reactions. The same holds for vital tissue graft, although the rejection of an allograft is particularly a consequence of the cellular immunity component (Scothorne & McGregor, 1955; Burwell, 1962; Veldman, 1970; Veldman & Keuning, 1978). If memory cells recirculate after a first challenge, these reactions accelerate even more after a second challenge with the same antigen (secondary response or second-set transplantation reaction). Extensive structural analyses of plasma cell and cellular immunity reactions as well as immunohistophysiological research on the population dynamics of T and B cells have demonstrated that the site of initiation of these complex immunoblast reactions is topographically restricted in the microarchitective of peripheral lymphoid tissue (Veldman, 1970; Nieuwenhuis, 1971; Veldman & Keuning, 1978; Veldman et al., 1978a, b; Veldman & Kaiserling, 1980).

Histological analyses of lymph nodes draining the site of tissue grafting, reveal strong immunoblast reactions in two distinct areas of the regional lymph node: a cellular immune response with production of small lymphoid cells in the paracortical area, as well as a humoral immune response initiated in the outer cortex. This is followed at ± four days after antigen administration by a germinal center reaction. The lymphoid end-cells of the cellular immunity reactions are responsible for specificity when dealing with a transplantation response.

Neonatal thymectomy has been found to result in a long-lasting immunological unresponsiveness regarding transplantation immunity. Adult thymectomy on the other hand has only negligible immediate effects in this respect. However, severe impairment of immunological function could also be caused in adult mammals if thymectomy was combined with potentially lethal x-irradiation (Veldman, 1970; Veldman et al., 1978a). Adult thymectomy in rabbits was without direct immunological effects, but in combination with repeated sublethal x-irradiation it completely abolished the ability to reject skin allografts for periods up to 150 days. A tentative conclusion from the available evidence has been that the immunological incompetence induced by neonatal thymectomy was due to a complete absence of thymus-derived lymphocytes in lymph nodes and other peripheral lymphoid organs. In adult animals thymectomy, although it cuts off any new supply of these cells, does not affect those already present in the periphery, unless total body x-irradiation has been added.

X-Irradiation and the allograft reaction.

Inhibition and disturbance of cell mitosis is the main effect of ionizing radiation on living cells. Radiosensitivity of any tissue is therefore primarily determined by the mitotic rate of its cells. Lymphoid tissue is affected in still another, rather specific way, viz by interphase death of small lymphocytes. There appears to be a certain differentiation in radiosensitivity between the different T- and B-cell populations.

An x-irradiation dose of $\pm$ 800 rads, which as a total body irradiation is lethal within 10 days in most mammals, destroys nearly all lymphocytes in blood and lymphoid tissues within 12 hours. Already committed and dividing offspring of these lymphocytes are only subject to a dose-dependent mitotic inhibition and are radioresistent as far as interphase death is concerned.

If local x-irradiation of a lymph node is performed ($\pm$ 750 rads) the same general rules apply. However, the complete destruction of lymphocytes, brought about in that node within eight to 12 hours, is overcome by an influx of blood-born lymphocytes at the same time. This influx appears to encompass two distinct territories: a T-cell repopulation in the paracortex and a B-cell influx in the outer cortex of that node (Fig 12-11, Fig 12-12a, b). Immunologically this influx into the locally irradiated lymph node has been found to have restored the immune capacity of that node. If challenged 24 hours after local x-irradiation with an antigen, immune reactivity is related to this antigen, particularly when this influx has been restricted to 24 hours by means of further total body x-irradiation and lymph node shielding at the time of antigenic stimulation. This tool has been applied to our animal experiments in rabbits, both in primary and secondary response transplantation reactions, in order to analyze the antigenicity of tympano-ossicular allografts of the middle ear (cf Fig 12-14).

FIG 12-12.
a. Normal lymph node with outer cortex, paracortical areas and medulla (cf FIG 12-11) (HE × 20) (From Veldman et al., 1978a).
b. Lymph node, 24 h after local x-irradiation (750 rads). F: follicle; PCA: paracortical area (MGP × 80) (From Veldman et al., 1978a).

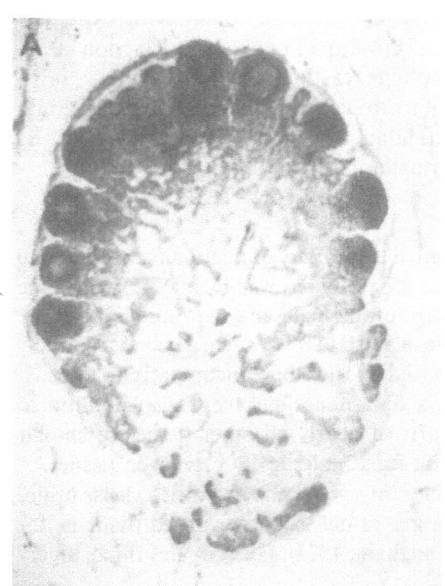
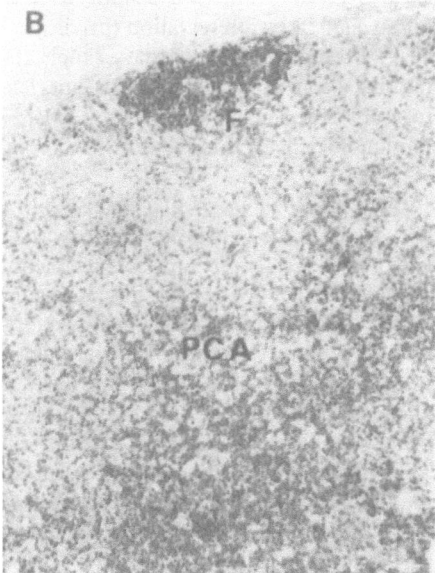

Otologic Tissue Grafting—Its Place in the Immunohistophysiology of Lymphoid Tissue

The clinical importance of allograft-tympanoplasty lies in the fact that successful transplantations can restore an excellent sound transmission mechanism to persons suffering from serious conductive hearing loss. The reported success rate in tympanoplasty with preserved allogenous tympanic membranes and tympano-ossicular bloc grafts (Marquet et al., 1973; Perkins, 1975a, b; Smith & Ballantyne, 1975; Plester & Steinbach, 1977; Smith, 1977, 1980; Marquet, 1976, 1980; Pulec & Reams, 1977) makes it, with the good results with viable corneal transplants in keratoplasty, almost unique in the field of clinical tissue and organ transplantation. However, by analogy to keratoplasty in ophthalmology, graft failures do occur. If failure occurs in allograft-tympanoplasty, it has been attributed to defects in operative techniques, secondary infection, or recurrence of the middle ear disease. Important immunobiological factors leading to graft failure have usually not been taken into account. To explain the apparent inability of a recipient to recognize the presence of an allogenous preserved tympanic or tympano-ossicular bloc graft, the idea has originated that the middle ear is a privileged site (discussed below) and that allograft reactions do not occur in it. Furthermore, it has been suggested by various authors that tissue antigens are no longer expressed, or at least extremely diminished, after preservation (privileged tissue?) (Marquet et al., 1973; Gagnon et al., 1979). Presumably it is not that a simple all-or-nothing reaction occurs, as with skin grafts, but that a concurrence of several factors leads either to success or failure. Although certain interdependencies undoubtedly exist, particular emphasis is placed upon the immunological factors relevant to allograft-tympanoplasty.

Privileged site or privileged tissue?

Tissue grafts have been repeatedly transplanted to a variety of anatomically unnatural sites of genetically incompatible recipients. The longevity enjoyed by allografts in some of these sites has given rise to the concept that some of these sites may be "immunologically privileged," or favored in the sense that grafts transplanted to them are in some way partially or fully exempted from the normal rigors imposed by their histoincompatible status. It has also been found, often empirically, that a few tissues survive transplantation to allogenic hosts under conditions in which grafts of nearly all other tissues of similar genetic makeup would suffer prompt rejection: immunologically privileged tissues.

Known natural privileged sites are the anterior eye chamber, cornea, lens, brain, hamster's cheek pouch, and decidual tissue in gravid uterus. A privileged tissue is, for instance, assumed to be cartilage (Barker & Billingham, 1973). For oto- and rhinosurgery this latter fact is important.

There is little or no clinical or experimental evidence to assume that the middle ear, mastoid cavity, and/or external ear canal belong to this first category. The privileged status of cartilage is ascribed to quarantining properties of its matrix, which is thought to have a capacity comparable to that of a cell-impermeable millipore membrane (Heyner, 1969). Chondrocytes isolated from cartilage are immunogenic and display normal susceptibility to transplantation immunity. The statement that tympanic membrane, external ear skin—even deepithelialized—or ossicles, after various preservation procedures, would belong to this category of privileged tissue being the explanation for successful allograft-tympanoplasty cannot stand. Recent experimental analyses of the immunogenicity of these grafts clearly demonstrates that at least part of the original histoincompatibility remains after using the currently applied preservatives (Veldman, 1971; Veldman & Kuijpers, 1977, 1978, 1981; Veldman et al., 1979). Reconsidering the existence of an afferent and efferent loop of the immune response in the middle ear complex, the following experimental data are strong arguments against the middle ear being a privileged site. In rats, vital xenogenous incudes, transplanted into the middle ear are rejected during a primary response (Kuijpers & van den Broek, 1975). Although

FIG 12-13.   Immunobiological consequences of experimental orthotopic incus transplantation: I vital or preserved allograft (primary response); II vital xenograft (primary response); III vital allograft (secondary response).

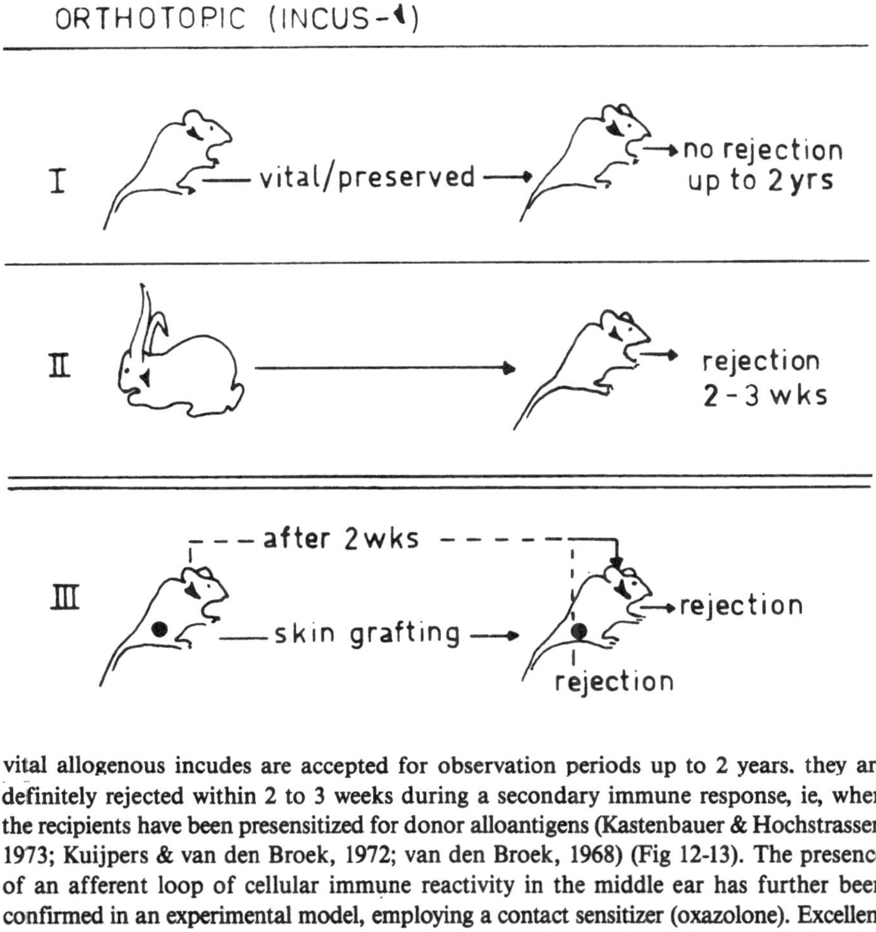

ORTHOTOPIC (INCUS-◀)

vital allogenous incudes are accepted for observation periods up to 2 years. they are definitely rejected within 2 to 3 weeks during a secondary immune response, ie, when the recipients have been presensitized for donor alloantigens (Kastenbauer & Hochstrasser, 1973; Kuijpers & van den Broek, 1972; van den Broek, 1968) (Fig 12-13). The presence of an afferent loop of cellular immune reactivity in the middle ear has further been confirmed in an experimental model, employing a contact sensitizer (oxazolone). Excellent delayed reactions could be elicited in the abdominal skin of guinea pigs and rabbits after prior application of this chemical sensitizer to the middle ear mucosal lining (Veldman et al., 1978c, 1979). The presence of a normal immunological reflex in the middle ear has further recently been confirmed by Frootko and Fabre (1980). Both histologically and immunologically there is no doubt any more that an intact immune mechanism exists in the middle ear complex.

FIG 12-14. Experimental analyses of antigenicity of tympanic membrane. First (I,) and second (II,) set transplantation experiments (ectopically).

AG: antigen (vital or preserved tympanic membrane).

$\not$: local x-irradiation (750 rads) of axillary (ax) lymph (ly) node.

$\square$: time of allograft implantation.

$\nearrow$: time of lymphadenectomy.

● : identity in genetic makeup.

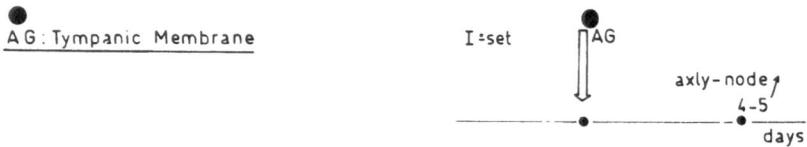

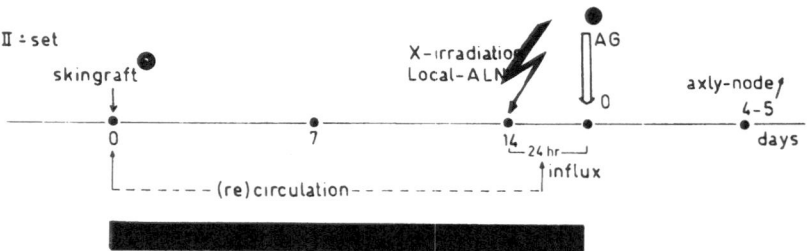

Analyses of the antigenicity of tympano-ossicular grafts in animal models.

In rats (Wistar and Osborne-Mendel) ortho- and ectopic transplantations were performed. In rabbits only ectopic transplantation experiments were done. To eliminate in rabbits the background activity present in a regional lymph node, the earlier developed technique of local lymph node x-irradiation was applied (Veldman, 1970; Veldman et al, 1978a; Veldman & Kaiserling, 1980) (cf Fig 12-12a, b). The group of animals transplanted orthotopically with a middle ear allograft were killed 6 weeks later.

After ectopic implantation of viable or preserved allografts (tympanic membrane, external ear skin and/or incudes), axillary lymph nodes were removed four to five days after allograft implantation, five to six days after local x-irradiation of the axillary lymph node. In controlled studies the immune response on viable and preserved middle ear autografts was analyzed. Axillary lymph nodes were also removed four to five days after transplantation. Second set reactions were performed through prior full-thickness skin grafting (Fig 12-14).

In rats and rabbits an immunoblast reaction is seen in the T-dependent paracortical areas of the regional axillary lymph node after ectopic implantation of viable or preserved

FIG 12-15.   Immune response in first (I, II) and second (III, IV) set transplantation experiments—ectopic implantation of tympanic membrane (vital or preserved):
PCR: plasma cell reaction (B cells).
CMI: cell-mediated immunity (T cells).
GCR: germinal center reaction (B cells).

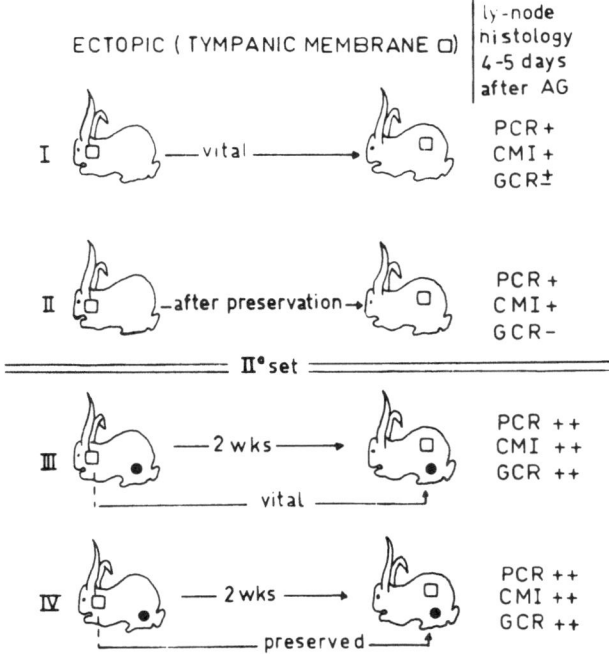

allografts (Figs 12-14, 12-15). At the same time, a plasma cell response is seen in the outer cortex. Germinal center reactions are present. The strongest immune response is observed after ectopic implantation of either a tympanic membrane or an external ear skin manchet. Less outspoken, though still present, are the reactions on ossicles. Comparing the various preservation methods used, the immune response in the regional lymph node is more pronounced after tissue preservation in formaldehyde than in alcohol or Cialit® (Fig 12-16a, b). Reactivity after formaldehyde preservation seems to be even greater than after ectopic implantation of viable specimens. The immune response on Cialit® -preserved tympanic membrane or external ear skin is quite evident (Fig 12-17). Outer cortical B-cell reactivity (plasma cell reaction and germinal center reaction) as well as paracortical T-cell reactivity is intense.

Whereas orthotopic ossicular transplantation of viable or preserved allografts showed no signs of graft rejection during a primary response up to observation periods of 6 to

FIG 12-16.
a. Antigen: formaldehyde preserved tympanic membrane (rabbit). First set. Outer cortical
   B-cell reactivity (⟶) (MGP × 1500).
   (from Veldman and Kuijpers, 1981).

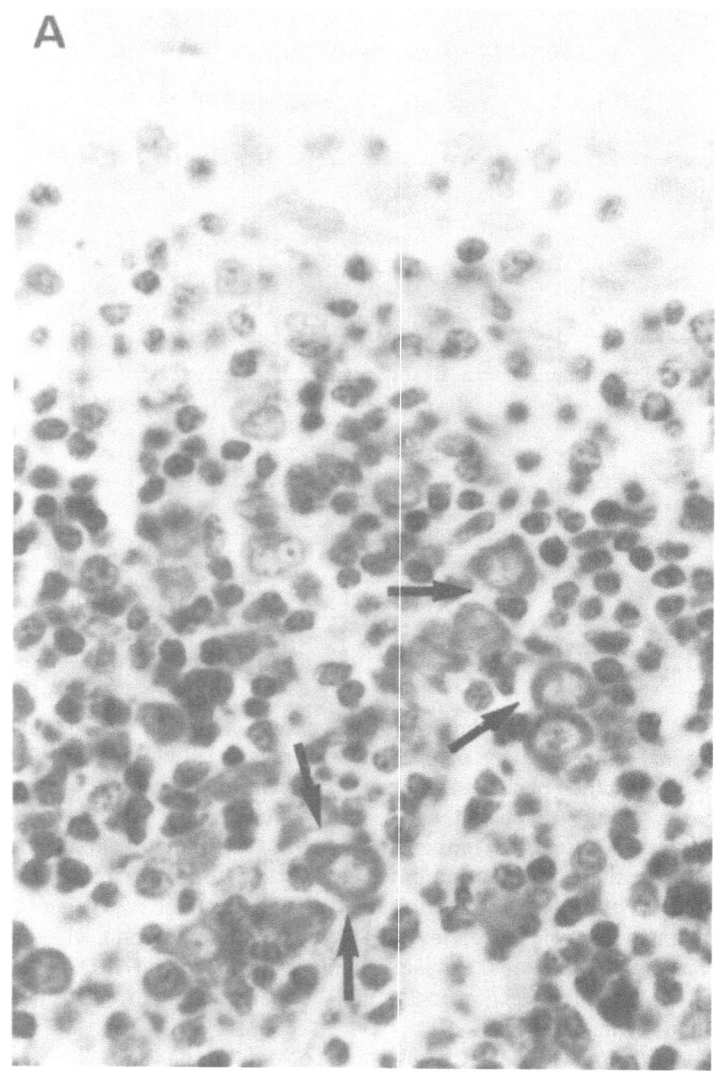

FIG 12-16.
b. Antigen: formaldehyde preserved tympanic membrane (rabbit). Paracortical T-cell reactivity (→)
(MGP × 1500)
(from Veldman & Kuijpers, 1981).

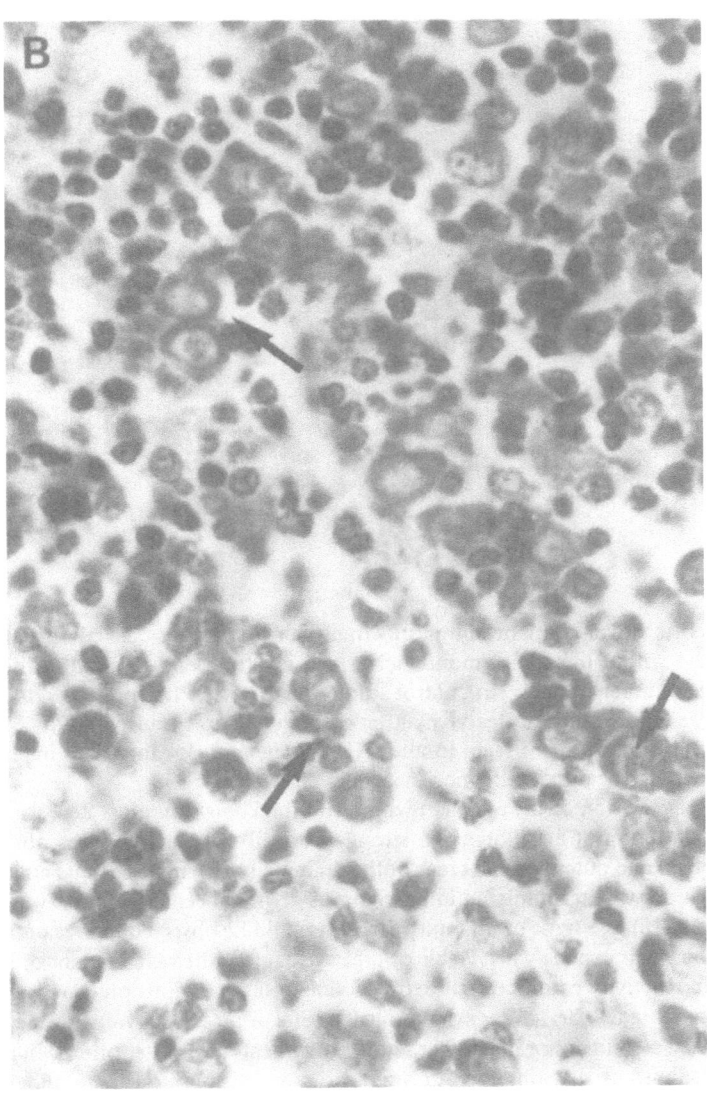

FIG 12-17.   Antigen: Cialit® preserved external ear manchet (rabbit). First set. Outer cortex: germinal center reaction (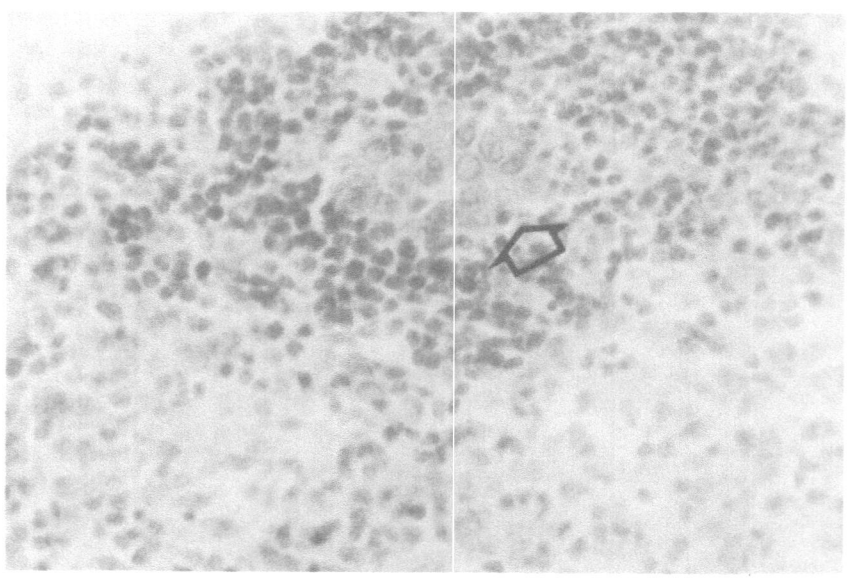) (MGP × 900).

8 weeks after transplantation, orthotopically transplanted tympano-meatal–flap allografts demonstrated within 6 weeks a mononuclear cell infiltrate and tissue resorption in a considerable number of cases. In control studies neither vital nor preserved autografts revealed any sign of recipient's reactivity after ortho- or ectopic transplantation. In other words, preservation does not seem to alter HLA-tissue antigens in such a manner that immune reactivity against "self" now occurs.

After sensitization of the recipient with a full-thickness skin graft 2 weeks prior to ectopic implantation of an allograft, a strong T- and B-cell reactivity was observed in the paracortical and outer cortical areas of the draining lymph nodes of rats and rabbits. At four to five days after implantation a vigorous germinal center reaction was usually present (Fig 12-18). No signs of immune reactivity could be observed in the contralateral control axillary lymph node when viable or preserved autografts were implanted. No clear difference in reactivity could be seen between vital and the various preserved allografts (tympanic membrane, external ear skin, or incus). Vital or preserved tympanic membranes of an unrelated second donor in another set of experiments gave, after prior skin grafting, a similar response as that observed during a primary response on these allografts.

FIG 12-18. Antigen: Cialit® preserved tympanic membrane (rabbit), second set (cf FIG 12-14). Outer cortex: germinal center reaction (▷) (MGP × 900).

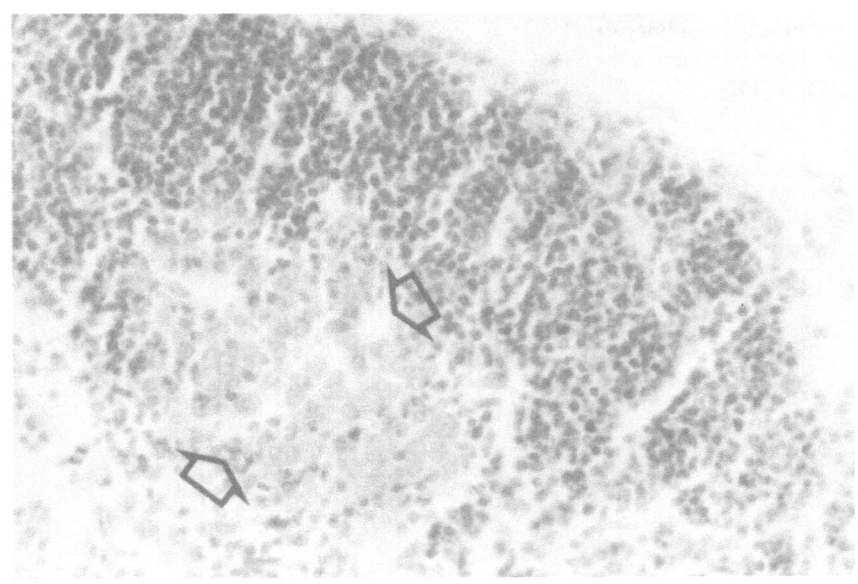

As in Kastenbauer and Hochstrasser's (1973) experiments graft rejection was observed in all orthotopically transplanted cases. Around the preserved grafts—particularly the tympano-meatal allografts—a heavy (perivascular) accumulation of mononuclear cells was seen. The reactions of formaldehyde-preserved tissues were significantly more outspoken than on alcohol 70% or Cialit® 1:5.000 preserved allografts (Fig 12-19a, b).

Clinical Immunopathology of Human Middle Ear Implants

The high success rate in middle ear transplantation, claimed by some otologists, might imply that little or no immunological interference occurs at all. On the basis of recent experimental immunological data (Veldman, 1977; Veldman & Kuijpers, 1977, 1978, 1981; Poliquin et al., 1979; Frootko & Fabre, 1980), however, this is very unlikely. The histopathology of different specimens of middle ear allografts, obtained after unsuccessful surgery, show signs of immunological interference. Microscopy revealed the presence of a large accumulation of small lymphoid cells and mononuclear phagocytes, perivascularly and close to the lamina propria of the tympanic membrane allograft (Fig 12-20). Even

FIG 12-19.
a. **Antigen: formaldehyde preserved incus. Second set reaction in SPF rat after orthotopic implantation:**
I: Incus allografts; ME: middle ear cavity.
Ex: external auditory canal.
Ty: tympanic membrane
(HE × 175).

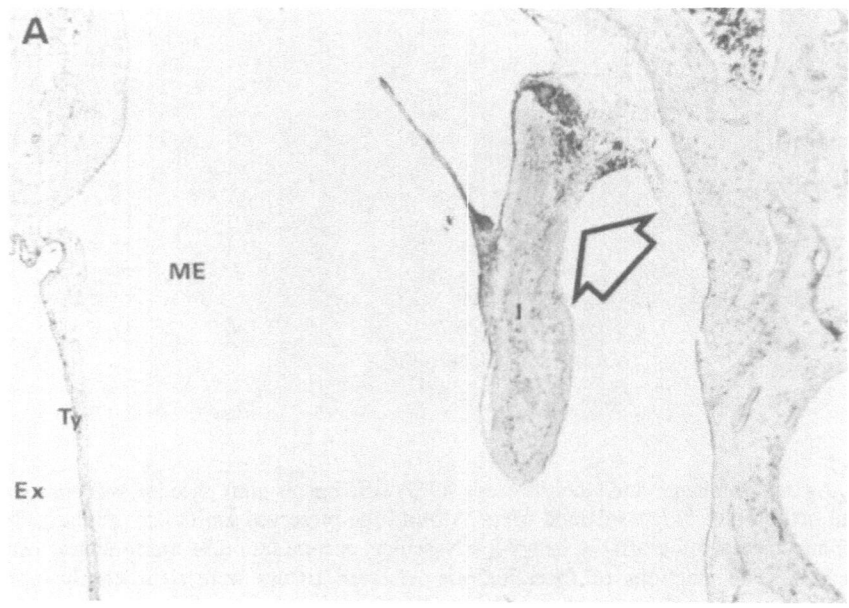

when minimal contact exists in the middle ear cavity between recipient and ossicle, this phenomenon of graft rejection can occur. Theoretically one may expect that this immunological event would rarely occur if prior tissue typing had been performed. Figure 12-21a shows the microanatomy of an allograft that has been preserved in formaldehyde-Cialit® for 2 weeks, whereas Fig 12-21b illustrates the incorporated allograft-core in the new tympanic membrane (allograft not rejected). In this latter case part of the newly formed tympanic membrane was removed ±9 months after transplantation during a second stage of surgery. The donor-allograft seems to act as a scaffold for mucosa at one side and fibroblasts and epithelium at the other side. Vascular infiltration occurs, whereas the Cialit-preserved allograft continues to exist. In this case no active mononuclear cell infiltration has been seen.

FIG 12-19. continued
b. Detail of indicated area (◇) in Fig 12-19a. Mononuclear infiltrate (◢) (HE × 450)
(From Veldman & Kuijpers, 1980).

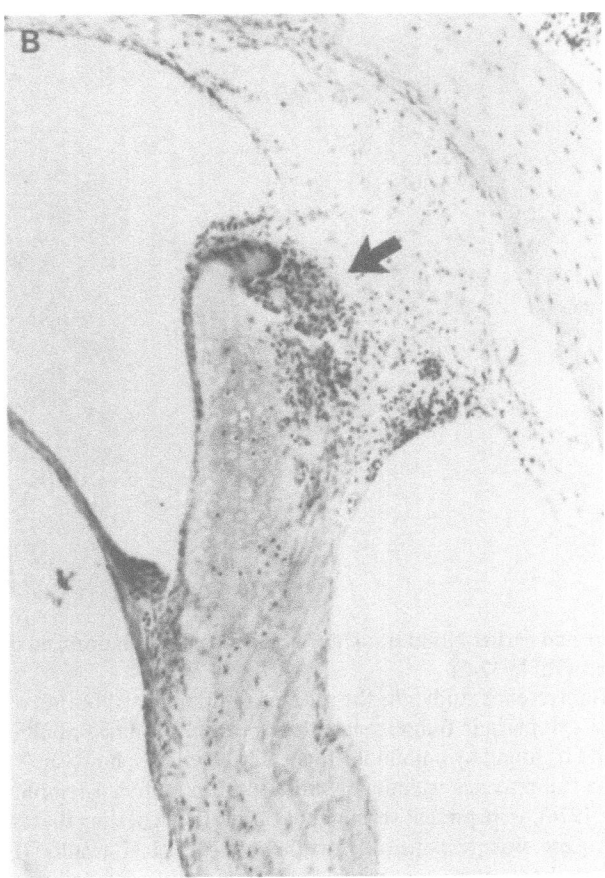

Serology and immunofluorescence studies in human allograft/tympanoplasty.
Since our experimental data reveal that both B- and T-cell reactivity can occur after ectopic allograft implantation, antileukocyte antibodies were determined in eight clinical allograft-tympanoplasty cases, prior to implantation and 3 - 6 months after surgery (none

FIG 12-20.   Human tympanic membrane-allograft
One year after implantation. Rejected. Note perivascular mononuclear infiltrate (→)
(HE × 20) (From Veldman et al., 1978c).

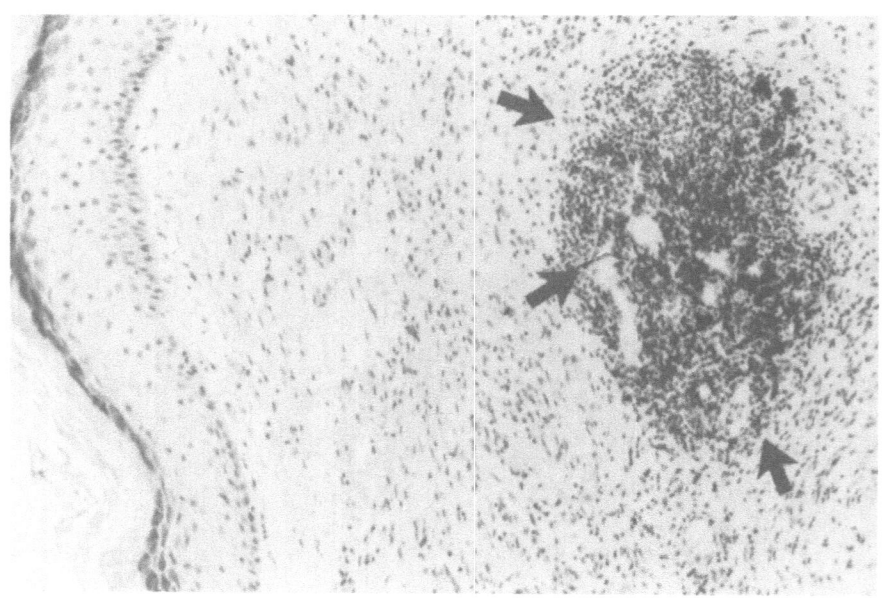

of the recipients had earlier blood transfusions). Both agglutination and cytotoxicity tests
were performed (Table 12-2).

Immunofluorescence studies of the rejected tympanic membranes of patients 1 and
8 failed to show cytoplasmic fluorescence for any of the immunoglobulin classes. Hardly
any B cells could be found by immunohistochemical methods; however, T cells, identified
by a membrane fluorescence technique with a specific human T-lymphocyte antiserum
(Schoorl et al., 1976), were present throughout the graft, suggesting that immunologically
a rejection process was responsible for the poor clinical results (Fig 12-22a, b).
Antileukocyte antibody titers were negative at the time of graft failure. Surveillance of
these antibodies in the rejected tissue grafts has not been performed before. However,
it does not mean that anti-HLA antibodies were not produced against the graft shortly
after transplantation. This may have occurred, although T-cell reactivity remains primarily
responsible for allograft rejection.

FIG 12-21.
a. Human tympanic membrane after several weeks of formaldehyde–Cialet® preservation (basic fuchsin-methylene blue × 350)
  1. mucosal lining
  2. lamina propria
  3. epithelial remnant

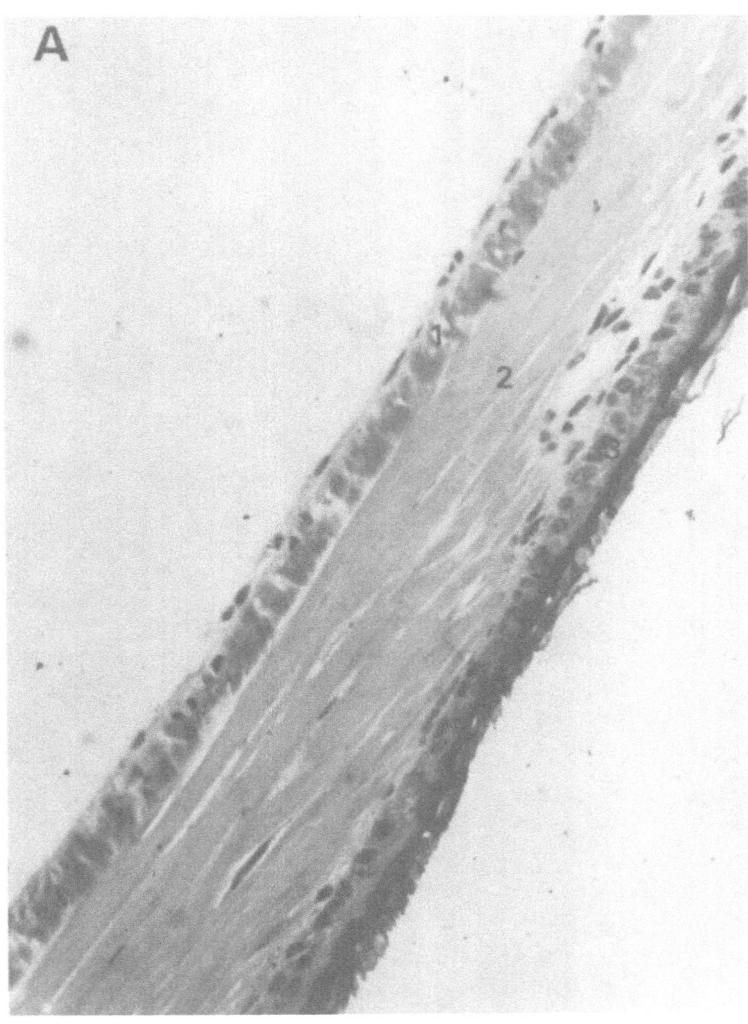

FIG 12-21. continued
b. Core (▷) of human tympanic membrane allograft - as in Fig 21a - ±9 months
after successful transplantation capillaries : (◢)
(basic fuchsin-methylene blue × 350).

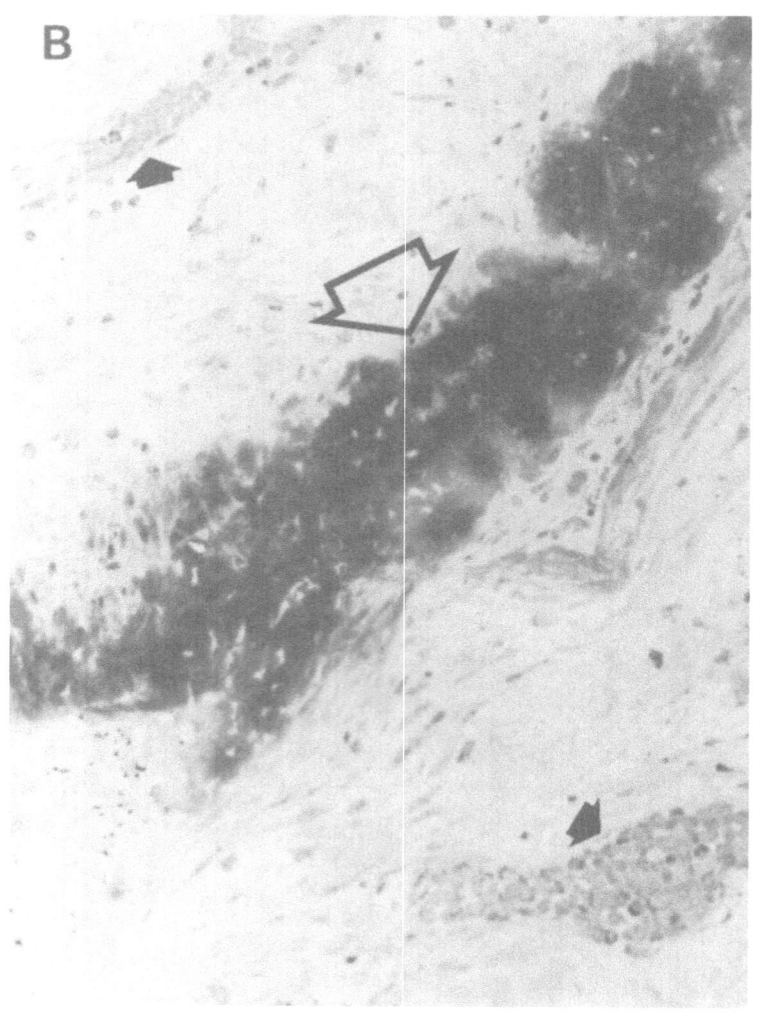

TABLE 12-2.

Patient	♂ / ♀	Age (Years)	Tympanoplasty	Results‡	AB a b
1	♂	32	TMO	rejected[1]	— / —
2	♀	56	TM (2×)	intact	— / —
3	♂	56	TMO	intact	— / —
4	♀	34	TMO	intact	— / —
5	♂	21	TMO	intact	— / —
6	♀	44	TMO	perforation	— / —
7	♂	51	TMO	intact	— / —
8	♀	23	TMO	rejected[2]	— / —

NOTE:

‡	: short-term results (after 6 to 12 months);
AB a,b	: antileukocyte antibody titer prior (a) and 3 to 6 months after (b) transplantation;
TMO	: tympano-ossicular bloc;
TM	: tympanic membrane;
[1] and [2]	: histopathology and tissue immunofluorescence of TM performed.

DISCUSSION

Cell Biological Considerations

Successful reconstruction of the sound transmission system of the ear can be obtained with the use of fresh and preserved tissues from different origin. In myringoplasty the grafted tissues contribute in various ways to the healing of a persisting perforation. The graft functions as a guide for the various tissue components proliferating from the residual part of the tympanic membrane. Second, the graft, becoming vascularized and infiltrated by mesenchymal cells, affords the epithelium migrating along the graft the opportunity to proliferate. Furthermore, the mesenchymal cells contribute to a great extent to the formation of a new middle layer. An important requirement of the grafted tissues is to keep the perforation closed until the proliferating tissues have bridged the gap.

In ossicular reconstruction the used ossicular and cartilaginous grafts initially function mainly as an avital sound-conducting system. Subsequently the ossicles become revitalized to a varying extent, although the impression exists that the major part of the ossicle(s) is still avital after 1 or 2 years. Apart from the incidentally observed resorption in a small percentage of the recovered ossicles, it can be assumed that the middle ear reacts in a

FIG 12-22.

a. Human tympanic membrane. Rejected ± 6 months after transplantation (case 1, Table 2); perivascular mononuclear infiltrate (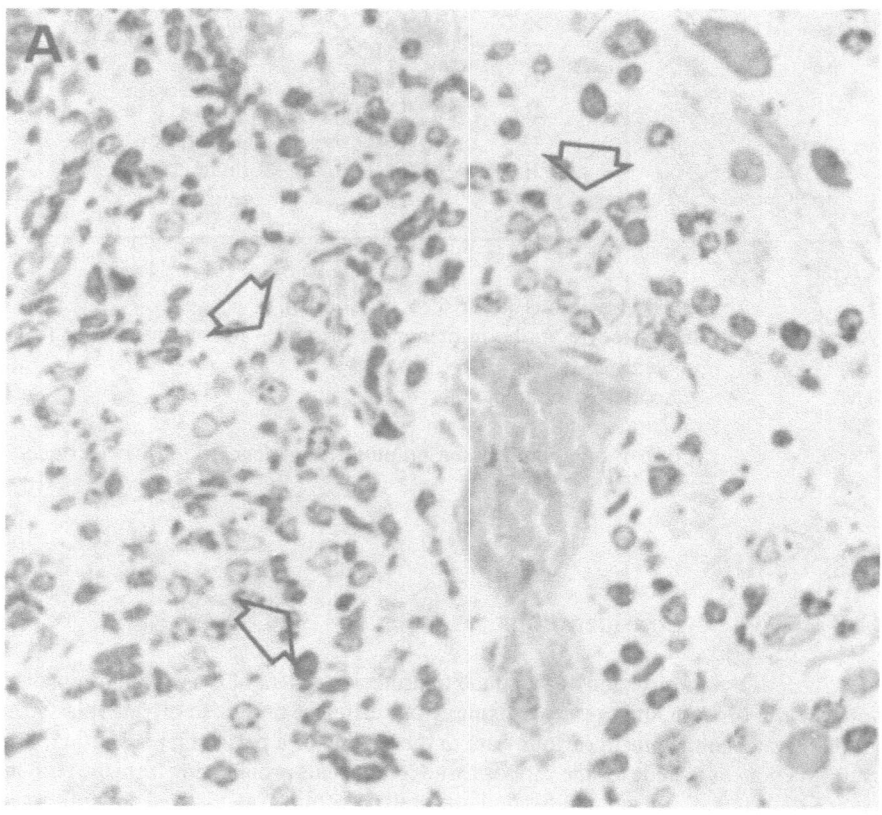) (basic fuchsin-methylene blue × 600) (From Veldman & Kuijpers, 1981).

different way to avital ossicular grafts than do other parts of the body. However, the answer may also be that this process is only retarded. The balance between tissue resorption and possible further revitalization of the grafts will ultimately determine the fate of this borrowed sound-conducting system.

Immunological Considerations

The information on the immunological status of allografts in the middle ear complex has been incomplete and fragmentary. The assumption that lack of antigenicity of the

FIG 12-22. continued
**b. T-cell membrane immunofluorescence with Rhodamine label. Note predominance of
   T cells in rejected tympanic membrane (TM) (case 1, Table 2).
   Same TM as in Fig 12-22a; c: capillary in Tm (× 500).**

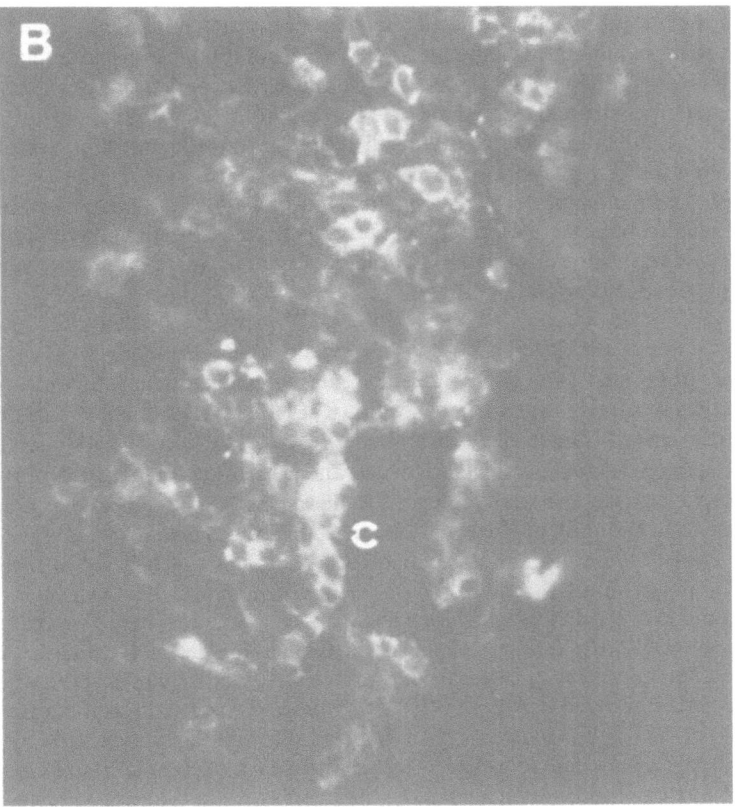

preserved tympanoossicular grafts and all its various components—privileged tissue—is
untenable according to the presented controlled animal experiments and clinical pathology
data of graft failures (Veldman & Kuijpers, 1978; Veldman et al., 1979; Veldman & Kuijpers
1981). Poliquin's recent data (Poliquin et al., 1979) on the antigenicity of guinea pig
tympanic membrane—unpreserved—confirm our experimental immunology achievements
with vital and preserved otologic allografts. The currently used preservatives of allografts
(formaldehyde, alcohol, or Cialet®) do not abolish the tissue histoincompatibility antigens,
although it might affect the concentration and form of the antigen. (Formaldehyde and
Cialit® presumably also act as haptens.) Persistence of the original histoincompatibility

antigens after tissue preservation—also when Cialit was used—could be proven in our second set of transplantation experiments. Sensitization through prior skin grafting resulted in a pool of recirculating B and T lymphocytes with a specific immunological memory for the tissue antigens of that species. Triggering these memory cells out of the circulation through local lymph node x-irradiation has two results: immunological background activity in that node dies out and "virgin" memory cells (B and T) repopulate that node. If, in a vascular bed draining to that regional lymph node, a preserved allograft from the same donor as the skin allograft is implanted and a vigorous immune response (plasma cell, cellular immunity, and germinal center reaction) is elicited—quantitatively exceeding a primary response—the only explanation is that a considerable amount of the original tissue histoincompatibility antigens are still present in the allograft after preservation. This occurs after any of the used preservatives.

Since the immunological reflex functions adequately in the middle ear compartment—in other words, there are no solid arguments for the concept of a privileged site— how does one explain the discrepancy between our experimental findings and the reported successful use of otologic allografts?

The middle ear: A privileged site for tolerogenesis in allograft-tympanoplasty?

Apart from elimination of any foreign agent through an immune response, we know now a variety of mechanisms whereby exposure of lymphocytes to antigen can produce a state of specifically diminished responsiveness. According to Burnet's clonal selection theory (Burnet, 1959), natural tolerance to autoantigens is due to elimination of lymphoid cell clones which recognize "self." Tolerance to these "self" tissue components is generally considered to be the result of clonal deletion of both T and B lymphocytes. When dealing with low antigen concentrations this immunotolerance is usually believed to be the result of T-cell tolerance. B-cell reactivity in terms of production of blocking antibodies might also play an active role in this tolerance phenomenon. To induce a state of immunological unresponsiveness the following mechanisms are thought to operate: (a) clone inactivation or elimination induced by appropriate antigen administration ("classical tolerance"); (b) active suppression by bone marrow- (B-) or thymus- (T-) derived lymphocytes; and (c) blockade by antibody, antigen, or a hapten. One might wonder whether these experimentally known circumstances which facilitate the induction of a state of immuno- tolerance operate in orthotopic allograft-tympanoplasty. No evidence militates against such an extrapolation at present. It would be a solid explanation for successfulness in middle ear transplantation. There are further different situations that have been experimentally applied to induce tolerance: (a) low immunogenicity of antigen— concentrations of antigen too low to immunize, but high enough to induce tolerance ("low zone tolerance"); (b) the form of antigen, the rate and the route of administration— immunization with killed cells—an effect of preservation or freeze-drying of otologic allografts—instead of intact cells favors enhancement over transplantation immunity; and (c) concomitant immunosuppression by irradiation or drugs. This latter condition does not apply to elective surgery such as allograft-tympanoplasty. A combination of altering and diminishing antigenicity through preservation of the graft material as well

FIG 12-23.   Diagram of supposed position of middle ear complex in immune system. Immunological consequences of ortho- and ectopic allograft transplantation (from Veldman et al., 1978c).

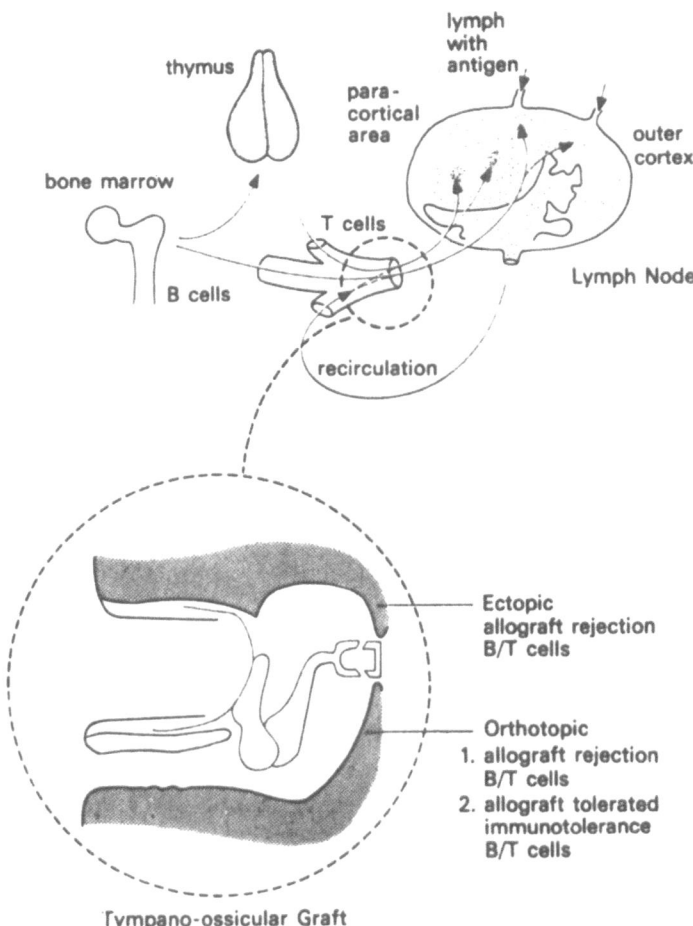

lymph
with
antigen

thymus

para-
cortical
area

outer
cortex

bone marrow

T cells

Lymph Node

B cells

recirculation

Ectopic
allograft rejection
B/T cells

Orthotopic
1. allograft rejection
   B/T cells
2. allograft tolerated
   immunotolerance
   B/T cells

Tympano-ossicular Graft

as the particular site of implantation might together favor a concurrent situation which is responsible for tolerance induction in allograft-tympanoplasty. If, however, these presumably ideal circumstances are not met, graft rejection will follow (Fig 12-23).

The accomplishment of immunotolerance would mean the occurrence of changes in the host, which renders it unable to respond to the donor's histoincompatibility antigens.

FIG 12-24.   Presumable effect of tissue-typing between donor (D) and recipient (R) in otologic allograft-tympanoplasty (from Veldman & Kuijpers, 1981).

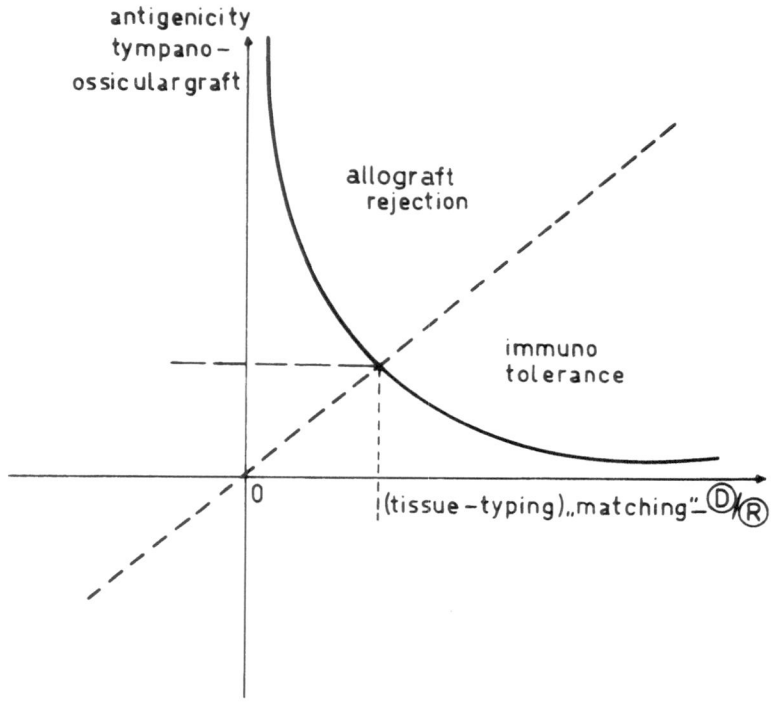

Middle ear transplantations are still performed at random; reports on appropriate matching for tissue antigens—prior to tissue preservation (chemically or by means of freeze-drying)—have not appeared yet in the otology literature. However, according to our experimental data one may predict that, if performed, an augmentation in success rate can be expected in otologic tissue grafting (Fig 12-24) when indications and otomicrosurgical techniques are adequate.

The fact that after several months a primarily successful grafting becomes a graft failure is not in direct conflict with our concept of tolerogenesis in otologic tissue grafting. A delayed rejection phenomenon is a well-known fact in clinical and experimental transplantations. It is often thought to be the consequence of an assumed breakthrough (of B lymphocytes?) in tolerance. Why this occurs in certain cases is virtually unknown. When it will occur is also unpredictable so long as no better surveillance is available than clinical otologic judgment after surgery. If, indeed, the above-mentioned mechanisms operate in otologic tissue grafting, it may be feasible to perform more successful allograft-tympanoplasties in the near future. The consequences of prior tissue typing seem to be more important than those of chemical tissue preservation, since histoincompatibility remains the main biological issue to deal with in allograft-tympanoplasty.

REFERENCES

Albrite JP, Leigh BC: Dural homograft myringoplasty. *Laryngoscope* 1966; 76:1687.

Algire GH, Weaver JH, Prehn RT: Studies on tissue homotransplantation in mice, using diffusion chamber methods. *Ann NY Acad Sci* 1957; 64:1009.

Altenau MM, Sheehy JL: Tympanoplasty: Cartilage prostheses—A report of 564 cases. *Laryngoscope* 1978; 88:895.

Austin DF: Present status of vein graft tympanoplasty. *Arch Otolaryngol* 1965; 81:20.

Balner H, Dersjant H: Early lymphatic regeneration in thymectomized radiation chimaeras. *Nature (London)* 1964; 204:941.

Banzer M: Cited by Dunlap AM, Schuknecht HF: Closure of perforations of the tympanic membrane. *Laryngoscope* 1947; 57:479.

Barker CF, Billingham RE: Immunologically privileged sites and tissues, in corneal graft failure. Amsterdam/New York, Ciba Foundation Symposium 15, North-Holland, *Excerpta Medica*, pp 79–104.

Beickert P: Das Lappencholesteatom. Eine Spatkomplikation nach Tympanoplastik. *Z Laryngol Rhinol* 1958; 37:567.

Bellucci, RJ, Wolff D: The incus, normal and pathological. *Arch Otolaryngol* 1966; 83:413.

Billingham RE, Brent L, Medawar PB: Quantitative studies on tissue transplantation immunity: II. The origin, strength and duration of activity and adoptively acquired immunity. *Proc Roy Soc B* 1954; 143:58.

Bloom SM: The problems of implants in rhinoplasty. *Arch Otolaryngol* 1960; 71:778.

Brackmann DE, Sheehy JL: Tympanoplasty: TORPs and PORPs. *Laryngoscope* 1979; 89:108.

Broek van den P: The fate of incus grafts. Nijmegen, the Netherlands, PhD thesis, 1968.

Broek van den P, Kuijpers W: Incus autografts and homografts in rats. *Arch Otolaryngol* 1967; 81:287.

Broek van den P, Kuijpers W: The effect of preservation on the behavior of homologous ossicular grafts. *Acta Otolaryngol* (Stockholm) 1974; 77:335.

Broek van den P, Kuijpers W: The preserved tympano-ossicular homograft. *J Laryngol* 1976; 90:907.

Burnet FM: The clonal selection theory of acquired immunity. Cambridge, Mass: Cambridge University Press, 1959.

Burwell RG: Studies of the primary and secondary immune responses of lymph nodes draining homografts of fresh cancellous bone (with particular reference to mechanisms of lymph node reactivity). *Ann NY Acad of Sci* 1962; 99:821.

Byrt P, Ada GL: An in vitro reaction between labelled flagellin or haemocyanin and lymphocyte-like cells from normal animals. *Immunology* 1969; 17:503.

Chalat HI: Tympanic membrane transplant. *Harper Hosp Bull* 1964; 22:27.

Christiansen TA, Hohmann A: The effects of preservation methods on homologous incus transplants in cats. *Trans Am Acad Opthalmol Otolaryngol* 1975; 80:60.

Cooper MD, Lawton AR, Kincade PW: A developmental approach to the biological basis for antibody diversity, in Hanna MG, Jr (ed): *Contemporary Topics in Immunology*, New York, Plenum Press, 1972, pp 33–46.

Cornish CB, Scott PJ: Freeze-dried heart valves as tympanic grafts. *Arch Otolaryngol* 1968; 88:350.

Dunlap AM, Schuknecht HF: Closure of perforation of the tympanic membrane. *Laryngoscope* 1947; 57:479.

Ford WL: The kinetics of lymphocyte recirculation within the rat spleen. *Cell Tissue Kinet* 1969; 2:171.

Frenckner P: Einige Erfahrungen bei Fallen operativer Trommelfellplastik und Tympanoplastik. *Acta Otolaryngol* (Stockholm) 1955; 45:455.

Frootko NJ, Fabre JW: Allograft rejection in the rat middle ear (abstract). *Clinical Otolaryngology* 1980; 5:423.

Gagnon NB, Piche J, Larochelle D, et al: Homografts of the middle ear. Privileged tissue or privileged site. *Arch Otolaryngol* 1979; 105:35.

Glasscock ME, House WF: Homograft reconstruction of the middle ear. A preliminary report. *Laryngoscope* 1968; 78:1219.

Glasscock ME, House WF, Graham M: Homograft transplants to the middle ear. A follow-up report. *Laryngoscope* 1972; 82:868.

Goodhill V, Harris I, Brockmann SJ: Tympanoplasty with perichondrial graft. *Arch Otolaryngol* 1964; 79:131.

Gowans JL: The recirculation of lymphocytes from blood to lymph in the rat. *J Physiol* 1959; 146:54.

Gowans JL, Knight EJ: The route of recirculation of lymphocytes in the rat. *Proc Roy Soc B* 1964; 159:257.

Gowans JL, McGregor DD: The immunological activities of lymphocytes, in Kallos P, Waksman BH (eds): *Progress in Allergy, IX.* Basel/New York, Karger, 1965, p 1.

Hall A, Rytner C: Stapedectomy and autotransplantation of ossicles. *Acta Otolaryngol* (Stockholm) 1957; 46:318.

Heermann J: Experience with free grafts of fascia connective tissues for tympanoplasties and for obliteration of radical cavities: Cartilage bridge from the stapes to the lower margin of the drum. *Z Laryngol Rhinol* 1962; 41:141.

Heyner S: Significance of intercellular matrix in survival of cartilage allografts. *Transplantations* 1969; 8:666.

Homsey CA, Kent JH, Hinds EC: Materials for oral implantation—Biological and functional criteria. *J Am Dental Ass* 1973; 86:817.

House WF, Patterson ME, Linthicum FH: Incus homographs in chronic ear surgery. *Arch Otolaryngol* 1966; 88:148.

House WF, Sheehy JL: Myringoplasty. *Arch Otolaryngol* 1961; 78:291.

Huizing EH: Implantation and transplantation in reconstructive nasal surgery. *Internat Rhinology* 1974; 12: 93.

Jansen C: Stapesersatz durch Knorpel. *Acta Otolaryngol* (Stockholm) 1962; 54:262.

Jansen C: Cartilage-tympanoplasty. *Laryngoscope* 1963; 73:1288.

Jansen C: Heterologous tympanoplasty. *Trans Am Acad Opthalmol Otolaryngol* 1973; 77:111.

Kastenbauer E, Hochstrasser K: Der Einfluss des Konservierungsmittel Cialit auf die Proteinloslichkeit und die Antigenitat von allogenen und xenogenen Gehorknochlchen und Trommelfelltransplantaten. *Arch fur Klin und exp Ohren-Nasen, und Kehlkopfheilkunde* 1973; 203:225.

Kerr AG, Smyth GDL: The fate of transplanted ossicles. *J Laryngol Otol* 1971; 85:337.

Kerr AG, Byrne JET, Smyth GDL: Cartilage homografts in the middle ear: A long-term histological study. *J Laryngol Otol* 1973; 87:1193.

Kluyskens P, Ringoir S: Follow-up of a human larynx transplantation. *Laryngoscope* 1970; 80:1244.

Kuijpers W, van den Broek P: Fundamental aspects of incus transplantation. *Laryngoscope* 1972; 82:2174.

Kuijpers W, van den Broek P: The preserved tympano-ossicular homograft. *J Laryngol* 1975; 90:907.

Kuijpers W, Grote JJ: The use of proplast in experimental middle ear surgery. *Clin Otolaryngol* 1977; 2:5.

Kuijpers W, Veldman JE: Immunology and allograft-tympanoplasty. *J Laryngol and Otol*.

Lacher G: Banque d'osselets pour homogreffe en chirurgie tympanoplastique. *Acta Otorhinolaryngol Belg* 1971; 24:95.

Marquet J: Reconstructive microsurgery of the ear drum by means of tympanic membrane homograft. *Acta Otolaryngol* (Stockholm) 1966; 62:868.

Marquet J: Myringoplasty by ear drum transplantation. *Laryngoscope* 1968; 78:1329.

Marquet J: Ten years of experience in tympanoplasty using homologous implants. *J Laryngol Otol* 1976; 90:897.

Marquet J: *Homografts today.* The 6th Shambaugh Int Workshop on Otomicrosurgery and 3rd Shea Fluctuant Hearing Loss Symposium (abstract). Chicago, March 2-7, p 99, 1980.

Marquet J, Schepens P, Kuijpers W: Experiences with tympanic transplants. *Arch Otolaryngol* 1973; 97:58.

McDowell F, Valone JA, Brown JB: Bibliography and historical note on plastic surgery of the nose. *Plast and Reconstr Surg* 1952; 10:149.

McKinnon DM: Homograft tympanic membrane in myringoplasty. *Ann Otol Rhinol Laryngol* 1972; 81:194.

Micklem HS, Brown JAH: Rejection of skin grafts and production of specific isohaemagglutinins by normal and x-irradiated mice. *Immunology* 1961; 4:318.

Miller JFAP: Immunological function of the thymus. *Lancet* 1961; 11:748.

Miller JFAP: Role of the thymus in transplantation immunity. *Ann NY Acad Sci* 1962; 99:340.

Miller JFAP, Mitchell GF: Cell to cell interaction in the immune response: I. Hemolysin-forming cells in neonatally thymectomized mice reconstituted with thymus or thoracic duct lymphocytes. *J Exp Med* 1968; 128:801.

Miller JFAP, Mitchell GF: Thymus and antigen-reactive cells in Moller G (ed): Antigen sensitive cells, their source and differentiation, *Transplantation Reviews 1:* 1 Munksgaard-Copenhagen, 1969.

Mitchell GF, Miller JFAP: Cell to cell interaction in the immune response: II. The source of hemolysin-forming cells in irradiated mice given bone-marrow and thymus or thoracic duct lymphocytes. *J Exp Med* 1968; 128:821.

Mitchison NA: Passive transfer of transplantation immunity. *Nature (London)* 1953; 171:267.

Moritz von W: Plastische Eingriffe am Mittelohr zur Wiederherstellung der Innenohrschalleitung. *Z Laryngol Rhinol* 1952; 31:338.

Mulcahy HD, McAfee, W: A five year study on the fate of grafts in reconstructive middle ear surgery. *Ann Otol Rhinol and Laryngol* 1964; 73:1020.

Nickel AL: The use of homologous vein grafts in otolaryngology. *Laryngoscope* 1963; 73:919.

Nieuwenhuis P: On the origin and fate of immunologically competent cells. PhD thesis, Groningen. Groningen, The Netherlands, Wolters-Noordhoff Publishing, 1971.

Nieuwenhuis P, Ford WL: Comparative migration of B- and T-lymphocytes in the rat spleen and lymph nodes. *Cell Immunol* 1976; 23:254.

Nieuwenhuis P, Keuning FJ: Germinal centers and the origin of the B-cell system: II. Germinal centers in the rabbit spleen and popliteal lymph nodes. *Immunology* 1974; 26:509.

Ogura JH, Kawasaki M, Takenouchi S, et al: Replantation and transplantation of the canine larynx. *Ann Otol Rhinol and Laryngol* 1966; 75:295.

Ogura JH, Harvey JE, Mogi G, et al: Further experimental observations of transplantation of canine larynx. *Laryngoscope* 1970; 80:1231.

Opstelten D, Stikker R, van der Heijden D, et al: Germinal centres and the B-cell system: IV. Functional characteristics of rabbit appendix germinal centre (-derived) cells. *Virch Arch B Cell Path* 1980; 34:53.

Örtegren U: Myringoplasty. Four year's experience of temporalis fascia grafts. *Acta Otolaryngol* (Stockholm) (Suppl) 1964; 193.

Parrot DMV, De Sousa MAB, East J: Thymus dependent areas in the lymphoid organs of neonatally thymectomized mice. *J Exp Med* 1966; 123:191.

Patterson ME, Lockwood EW, Sheehy JL: Temporalis fascia in tympanic membrane grafting. Tissue culture and animal studies. *Arch Otolaryngol* 1967; 74:985.

Perkins R: Ear bank of project HEAR. *Trans Am Acad Ophthalmol Otolaryngol* 1975a; 80:23.

Perkins R: Otologic homograft indictions, techniques, results. *Trans Am Acad Ophthalmol Otolaryngol* 1975b; 80:41.

Plester D, Steinbach E: Histologic fate of tympanic membrane and ossicle homografts, in Lesinski SG (ed): *Symposium on homograft tympanoplasty. The Otolaryngol Clinics of North America* 1977; 10 (3):487.

Poliquin JF, Catanzaro A, Robb J, et al: Antigenicity of the guinea pig's tympanic membrane. *Otolaryngol Head Neck Surgery* 1979; 87:852.

Pulec JC, Reams CL: Homograft tympanoplasty techniques and results for restoration of hearing, in Lesinski SG (ed): *Symposium on homograft tympanoplasty. The Otolaryngol Clinics of North America* 1977; 10(3):553.

Raff MC, Cantor H: Subpopulations of thymus cells and thymus derived lymphocytes, in Amos B (ed): *Progress in Immunology.* New York, Academic Press, 1971, p 83.

Reijnen CJH, Kuijpers W: The healing pattern of the drum membrane. *Acta Otolaryngol* (Stockholm) (Suppl) 1971; 244.

Ringenberg JC: Fat graft tympanoplasty. *Laryngoscope* 1962; 72:188.

Rousset D; cited by Bloom SM: The problems of implants in rhinoplasty. *Arch Otolaryngol* 1960; 71:778.

Salen B: Tympanic membrane grafts of full thickness skin, fascia and cartilage with its perichondrium (an experimental and clinical investigation). *Acta Otolaryngol* (Stockholm) (Suppl) 1968; 244.

Schoorl R, Brutel de la Riviere A, von den Borne, AEGK, et al: Identification of T- and B-lymphocytes in human breast cancer with immunohistochemical techniques. *Am J of Path* 1976; 84:529.

Scothorne RJ, McGregor IA: Cellular changes in lymph nodes and spleen following skin homografts in the rabbit. *J Anat* (London) 1955; 89:283.

Shea JJ, Emmett JR: Biocompatible ossicular implants. *Arch Otolaryngol* 1978; 104:191.

Sheehy JL: Tympanic grafting: Early and long-term results. *Laryngoscope* 1964; 74:985.

Slikke LB van der, Keuning FJ: Influence of sublethal x-irradiation on the survival time of skin homografts and the reaction of the lymphoid system. *Int J Rad Biol* 1964; 8:279.

Smith MFW: Reconstruction of the open mastoidectomy ear, in Lesinski SG (ed): Symposium on homografts in tympanoplasty. *The Otolaryngol Clinics of North America* 1977; 10(3):549.

Smith MFW: Freeze-dried otologic implants. *J Otolaryngol* (USA) 1980; 3:222.

Smith MFW, Ballantyne JC: The results of an international questionnaire in otologic homografts. *Trans Am Acad Ophthalmol Otolaryngol* 1975; 80:71.

Smith CW, Overton D: The fate of middle ear ossicle grafts. *Laryngoscope* 1968; 78:1002.

Smyth GDL: Tympanic reconstruction. Fifteen-year report on tympanoplasty: Part II. *J Laryngol Otol* 1976; 713.

Smyth GDL, Kerr AG: Homologous graft for ossicular reconstruction in tympanoplasty. *Laryngoscope* 1967; 77:330.

Sooy FA: A clinical and laboratory evaluation of tympanoplasty utilizing canal wall pedicle skin grafts. *Laryngoscope* 1967; 74:979.

Sousa de MAB: Ecotaxis, ecotaxopathy and lymphoid malignancy: Terms, facts and predictions, in Twoney JJ, Good RA (eds): *The Immunopathology of Lymphoreticular Neoplasms*. New York, Plenum Press, 1978, pp 325-359.

Stengl T, Hohmann A: Experimental incus transposition. *Arch Otolaryngol* 1964; 80:72.

Strauss P: Vergelich von Ambossinterposition und Kunststofcolumella bei der Tympanoplastik. *Laryngol Rhinol* 1979; 58:15.

Strauss P, Schreiter K: Konservierte menschliche Knorpelimplantate und korpereigene vitale Transplantate in Nase und Mittelohr. *Laryngol Rhinol* 1979; 53:201.

Strauss P, Ickler P: Knochenneubildung und Knochenabbau konservierter menschlicher Ambosse im Mittelohr. *Laryngol Rhinol* 1980; 59:298.

Thornburn JB: A critical review of tympanoplastic surgery. *J Laryngol Otol* 1960; 74:453.

Touma JB, Maguda TA: Ossicular chain transplantation in cats. *Ann Otol Rhinol Laryngol* 1973; 82:62.

Urist MR, Silverman BF, Buring K, et al: The bone induction principle. *Clin Orthop* 1967; 53:243.

Veldman JE: Histophysiology and electronmicroscopy of the immune response, (part I and II). PhD thesis, Groningen. Drukkerij Dijkstra-Niemeyer, Groningen, The Netherlands, 1970.

Veldman JE: The middle ear: An immunologically privileged site for tolerance induction in otologic tissue grafting? in Mandel TE, Cheers C, Hosking CS, et al (eds): *Proceedings, 3rd Int Congress of Immunology*, workshop: Deletion models of tolerance. Sydney, Australia. *Progress in Immunology III*:805. Amsterdam-New York, North-Holland Publishing, 1977.

Veldman JE, Kuijpers W: Middle ear implantation: An immunologically privileged way of tolerance induction in otologic tissue grafting. *ORL* 1977; 39:346.

Veldman JE, Keuning FJ: Histophysiology of cellular immunity reactions in B-cell deprived rabbits. An x-irradiation model for delineation of an isolated T-cell system. *Virchows Arch B-cell Path* 1978; 28:203.

Veldman JE, Kuijpers W: Experimental and clinical immunopathology of middle ear transplantation. *Clin Otolaryngology* 1978; 3:293.

Veldman JE, Kaiserling E: Interdigitating cells, in Carn I, Deams WT (eds): *The Reticulo-Endothelial System*, vol 1, *Structure in Relation to Function*. New York, Plenum Press, 1980, pp 318–416.

Veldman JE, Kuijpers W: The antigenicity of tympano-ossicular homografts of the middle ear. Analysis of the immune response to viable and preserved grafts in animal models. *Otolaryngol Head Neck Surg* 1981; 89:142.

Veldman JE, Keuning FJ, Molenaar I: Site of initiation of the plasma cell reaction in the rabbit lymph node. Ultrastructural evidence for two distinct antibody forming cell precursors. *Virchows Arch B-cell Path* 1978a; 28:187.

Veldman JE, Molenaar I, Keuning FJ: Electron microscopy of cellular immunity reactions in B-cell deprived rabbits. Thymus derived antigen reactive cells, their micro-environment and progeny in the lymph node. *Virchows Arch B-cell Path* 1978b; 28:217.

Veldman JE, Kuijpers W, Overbosch HC: Middle ear implantation: Its place in the immuno-histophysiology of lymphoid tissue. Review. *Clin Otolaryngol* 1978c; 3:93.

Veldman JE, Boezeman AJ, Overbosch HC, et al: Middle ear transplantation: A new concept in clinical otology, in Muller-Ruchholtz W, Muller-Hermelink HK (eds): *Adv in Exp Biology and Med*, vol 114, *Function and Structure of the Immune System*. New York, Plenum Press, 1979, p 357.

Veldman JE, Nieuwenhuis P, Molenaar I, et al: The graft-versus-host reaction in the rabbit spleen. Ultrastructural evidence for two differentiated T-cell lines. *Virchows Arch B-cell Path* 1980; 33:117.

Wakefield JD, Thorbecke GJ: Relationship of germinal centers in lymphoid tissue to immunological memory: I. Evidence for the formation of small lymphocytes upon transfer of primed splenic white pulp to syngeneic mice. *J Exp Med* 1968; 128:153.

Waksman BH, Arnason BG, Jankovic BD: Role of the thymus in immune reactions in rats: III. Changes in the lymphoid organs of thymectomized rats. *J Exp Med* 1962; 116:187.

Wehrs RE: The homograft tympanic membrane. A five year study. *Trans Am Acad Ophthalmol Otolaryngol* 1976; 82:39.

Weissman IL: Thymus cell migration. *J Exp Med* 1967; 126:191.

Wilson DF, Pulec JL, van Vliet PD: Incus homografts in cats. *Arch Otolaryngol* 1966; 83:554.

Wright WK: Tissues for tympanic grafting. *Arch Otolaryngol* 1963; 78:291.

Wullstein H: Funktionelle Operationen im Mittelohr mit Hilfe des freien Spaltlappen-Transplantates. *Arch fur klin und exp Ohren-Nasen und Kehlkopfheilkunde* 1952; 161:442.

Zollner F: Plastische Eingriffe an den Labyrinthfenstern. *Arch fur klin und exp Ohren-Nasen und Kehlkopfheilkunde* 1952; 161:414.

Zollner F: Technik der Formierung einer Columella aus Knochen. *Z Laryngol Rhinol* 1960; 39:536.

Chapter 13

Clinical and Experimental Immunobiology of the Ear

Jeffrey P. Harris
Allen F. Ryan

OUTLINE

INTRODUCTION

IMMUNOBIOLOGY OF THE EXTERNAL EAR
 Tympanosclerosis
 Myringitis

IMMUNOBIOLOGY OF THE MIDDLE EAR
 Otitis Media
 Type II Collagen Autoimmunity and Middle Ear Disease
 Effect of Middle Ear Immunity on the Inner Ear

IMMUNOBIOLOGY OF THE INNER EAR
 Experimental Inner Ear Immunology
 Autoimmune Inner Ear Disease
 Meniere's Disease
 Type II Collagen Autoimmunity and Inner Ear Disease

CONCLUSION

INTRODUCTION

Recently there has been interest in the possibility that immunological mechanisms play an etiological role in ear disease. Many disorders which have long been considered

Supported by Grants NS 14389 and NS 18643 from the NIH/NINCDS, by the American Otological Society, by the Deafness Research Foundation, and by the Research Service of the Veterans Administration.

idiopathic are now being examined for such an immunologic basis. While it is possible that many of these idiopathic diseases will ultimately prove not to be immunologically mediated, the outcome of these research endeavors will certainly clarify some of the basic mechanisms of host immunity involved in ear disease.

This chapter will examine from both experimental and clinical viewpoints, the immunobiology of diseases which affect the tympanic membrane, middle ear, and inner ear.

IMMUNOBIOLOGY OF THE EXTERNAL EAR

Tympanosclerosis

Tympanosclerosis is a disease state characterized by the slow growth of sclerotic, frequently calcified, plaques in the lamina propria of the tympanic membrane. This condition is often associated with previous chronic otitis media, and it has been recognized that tympanosclerosis is the result of chronic inflammation. Since response to antigen almost invariably involves inflammation to some degree, it is reasonable to speculate that immune responses play a causative role in this disease. Schiff, Catanzaro, Ryan, and Poliquin (1980) hypothesized that tympanosclerosis is an autoimmune phenomenon, mediated by circulating immunoglobulin directed against the connective tissue elements of the tympanic membrane. Injury to the drum resulting in increased vascular permeability would provide access for the antibody to tympanic membrane connective tissue. The resultant antigen-antibody complexes could trigger complement fixation, with subsequent tissue injury and inflammation. This hypothesis was tested experimentally by Poliquin, Cantanzaro, Robb, and Schiff (1980). An antiserum against tympanic membrane connective tissue was first raised by preparing guinea pig tympanic membrane antigen for immunization of rabbits. The resultant antiserum was passively infused into normal guinea pigs and, after a brief interval, their tympanic membranes were traumatized. Subsequent immunohistochemistry indicated that both immunoglobulin and complement were bound to the tympanic membrane in the area of trauma (Fig 13-1). When these experiments were conducted with serum from nonimmunized rabbits, no antibody or complement deposition was observed. These observations suggest that, under appropriate circumstances, the immune responses proposed by Schiff et al. (1980) will occur. However, they do not provide evidence that the immune response leads to sclerotic disease of the tympanic membrane. In a long-term study, Poliquin et al. (1981) passively sensitized guinea pigs with rabbit anti-guinea pig tympanic membrane antiserum, after which their tympanic membranes were surgically traumatized. The animals were then allowed to survive for 6 months. At the end of this period, white plaques were observed in the traumatized regions of passively sensitized animals, but not in animals that received normal rabbit serum. Histologic examination of the plaques revealed that, while the fibrous layer of the lamina propria and both the mucosal and epidermal epithelia of the membrane were

FIG 13-1. Deposition of rabbit antibody against guinea pig tympanic membrane in the area surrounding a myringotomy (M) is shown by immunofluorescence. Guinea pigs were passively sensitized with the rabbit antiserum, the tympanic membrane was traumatized 1 hr later, and the animals were allowed to survive for 7 days. From Poliquin et al., 1981.

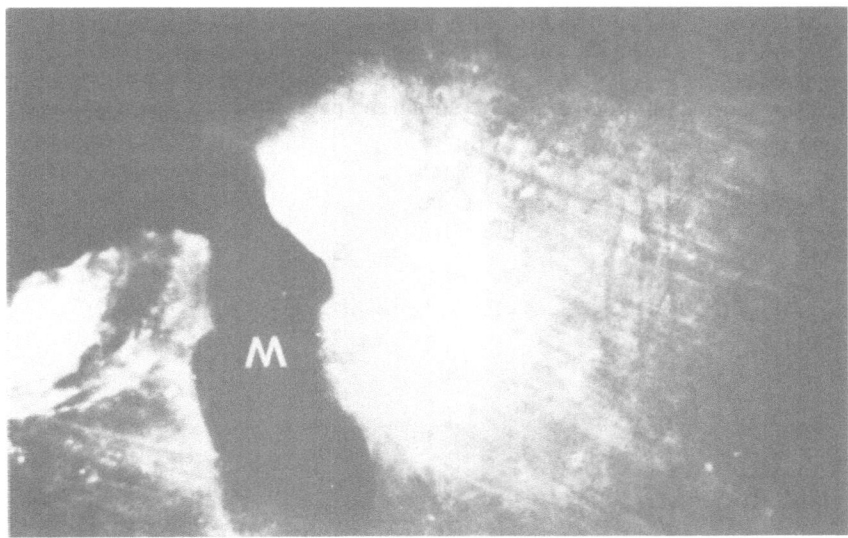

largely unchanged, both subepithelial connective tissue layers were greatly hypertrophied. Calcareous-appearing deposits in the plaque were identified as calcium phosphate (Fig 13-2) by energy-dispersive X-ray analysis (Ryan, Cleveland, Hartman, & Catanzaro, 1982).

The results described above indicate that antibody deposition on tympanic membrane connective tissue, subsequent to injury, can lead to sclerotic changes which in many ways resemble tympanosclerosis. Since animals receiving normal rabbit serum did not show evidence of immunoglobulin or complement binding, or plaques, these responses were clearly related to the specificity of the anti-tympanic membrane antibody. Immediate complement binding also suggests an immunologic origin for the inflammatory changes in the membrane. It should be noted that because rabbit anti-tympanic membrane antiserum was used for the passive sensitization, the resultant immune injury may have included a host response to the rabbit immunoglobulin itself.

Myringitis

Otologists are often frustrated by a condition known as granular myringitis, in which granulation tissue develops over the surface of the tympanic membrane in cases of low-

FIG 13-2. Sclerotic plaque induced by anti-tympanic membrane antibody in the guinea pig. (a). Normal guinea pig tympanic membrane, consisting mostly of a fibrous lamina propria (f). Original magnification, 400×. (b). Tympanosclerotic plaque observed 6 months after passive sensitization with anti-tympanic membrane antiserum and trauma. While the fibrous layer (f) is approximately normal in size, the submucosal connective tissue (SM) on both the epidermal and mucosal sides of the membrane is greatly expanded. (c). Backscattered scanning electron micrograph of a plastic section adjacent to that in (b). Note the dense inclusion material in the submucosa (SM) on the epidermal side of the membrane. (d). Energy dispersive X-ray analysis of the dense inclusion material shown in (c). The spectrum shows high levels of calcium and phosphorus. From Ryan et al., 1984.

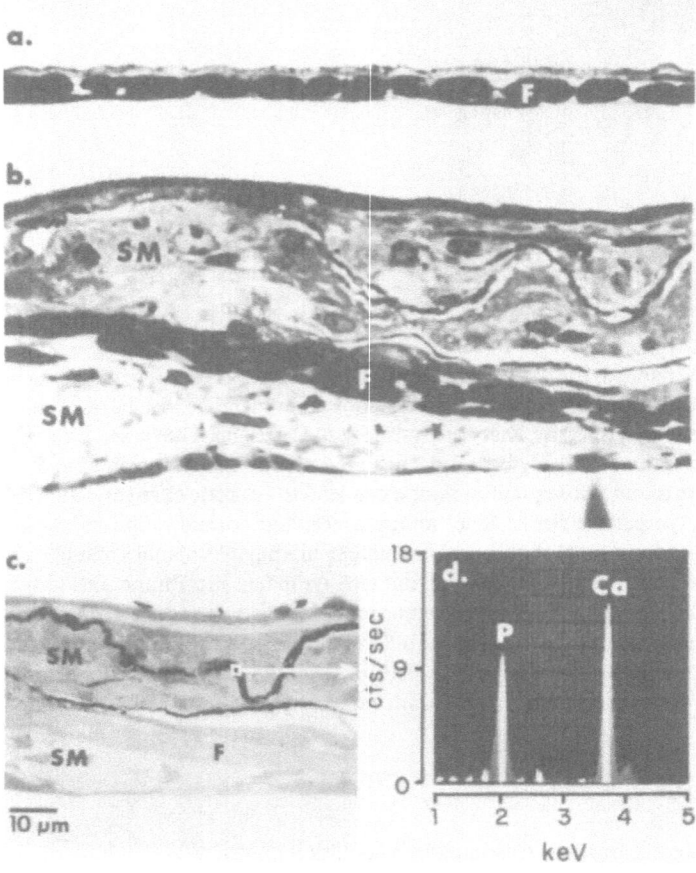

grade chronic otitis externa. This condition is sometimes seen also in the early healing stages following tympanic membrane replacement and if left untreated can result in delayed healing, otorrhea, blunting of the tympanic membrane, and occasional canal stenosis. Histologic examination of this tissue reveals a mixture of inflammatory cells; the condition is often described by pathologists as acute and chronic inflammation. The inciting mechanism for this condition is poorly understood, yet it seems to respond to a variety of local therapeutic regimens that often include corticosteroids and skin grafting when topically applied antibiotic drops fail. While a host response to a bacterium has been assumed to be the etiology of this condition, recent evidence suggests that this may have an immunopathological basis. Frootko (1984) has studied patients who underwent tympanic membrane replacement with dural allograft material and monitored subsequent sensitization of the host to donor transplantation antigens utilizing a cytotoxicity assay against stored donor splenic lymphocytes. Those patients who showed conversion from a negative preoperative donor-specific cytotoxicity assay to a positive postoperative assay had a highly significant association of myringitis ($p < 0.001$). This finding suggests that myringitis may occur solely as the consequence of an immune phenomenon related to graft rejection. Although only a small number of patients was included in this study, it does demonstrate how an immunological event can present as a well-recognized but poorly understood clinical entity. Recently, Veldman (1984) has suggested that Langerhans (interdigitating) cells are present on the surface of the tympanic membrane in myringitis, but not in the normal TM, and that these cells are integrally related to an ongoing immune response involved with this condition. There still appears to be some controversy regarding the uniqueness of the Langerhans cell type in this condition and further research should clarify its role.

IMMUNOBIOLOGY OF THE MIDDLE EAR

Otitis Media

Chronic otitis media with effusion (OME) is a common disease of infants and children. Eustachian tube dysfunction, leading to negative pressure in the middle ear cavity, is a major factor in this condition. However, it has become increasingly apparent in recent years that immune responses are frequently involved in chronic OME. Evidence for this includes the identification of locally produced, specific immunoglobulins directed against upper respiratory pathogens in OME effusions (Juhn, Giebink, Huff, & Mills, 1980; Liu, Lim, Lang, & Birck, 1975). Lymphocytes are frequently observed in effusions (Bryan & Bryan, 1976), as are inflammatory mediators such as components of the complement cascade (Laurell, Nilsson, & Prellner, 1980; Veltri & Sprinkle, 1976) and arachidonic acid metabolites (Juhn et al., 1980). These observations have led to the suggestions that immune responses may play a causative role in this disease. One of the immune mechanisms hypothesized is an acute immediate hypersensitivity response in the eustachian tube leading

FIG 13-3. Middle ear effusion following antigenic challenge of nonimmunized (dashed line) guinea pigs as compared to that seen following challenge of immunized animals (solid line). The antigen used was keyhole limpet hemocyanin (KLH). Middle ear effusion is maximal at 3 days postchallenge in the immunized animals. From Ryan et al., 1984.

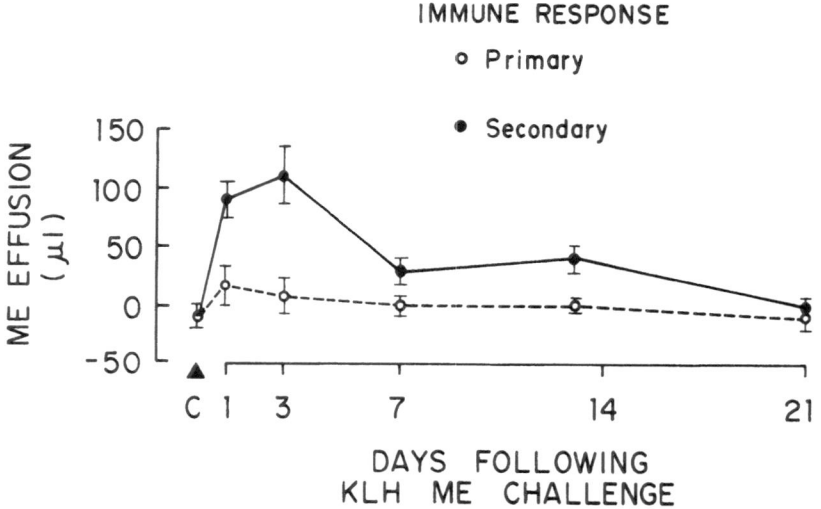

to tubal obstruction, negative pressure in the middle ear cleft, and transudation of serum (Solow, 1958). An alternative hypothesis is that increased vascular permeability occurs in the middle ear mucosa, as a result of immediate hypersensitivity (Ryan & Catanzaro, 1983), complement activation (Veltri & Sprinkle, 1976, chapter 7), or delayed hypersensitivity (Bryan & Bryan, 1976), resulting in the transudation of serum independently of any change in eustachian tube function.

Experimental animal models based upon immunologic responses have been developed to test these hypotheses. Hopp, Elevitch, Pumphrey, Irving, and Hoffman (1965) demonstrated that guinea pigs that were sensitized systemically to an antigen and were later challenged with the same substance in the middle ear developed OME. However, Catanzaro et al. (1982) found that antigen introduced into the middle ear of nonimmunized guinea pigs does not produce OME, even though it elicits a primary immune response both systemically and in the middle ear (Ryan et al., 1982). These investigations further found that OME is a feature only of a secondary immune response in the middle ear (Fig 13-3). The possible contributing role of the eustachian tube was examined in experiments in which antigenic challenge of the pharyngeal mucosa in sensitized animals was performed. This procedure did not result in OME (Yamashita, Okazaki, & Kumazawa, 1980). Ryan et al. (1984) found that OME produced by antigenic challenge of the middle ear of immunized animals was not reduced by tympanostomy tubes, nor did immune-mediated OME have any effect upon eustachian tube function as measured by a forced

FIG 13-4. (a). Middle ear effusion at 3 days after challenge with KLH in actively immunized animals (solid bar) is compared to that observed in animals passively sensitized with various doses of specific IgG (shaded bars). Animals with passively transferred antibody titers of 20 µg/ml or greater showed ME effusion comparable to that seen in actively immunized animals. (b). After passive sensitization with lymphocytes, no effusion is observed upon middle ear challenge. Passive transfer was effective, based upon positive skin test and blastogenesis assay of peripheral blood lymphocytes. From Ryan & Catanzaro, 1983.

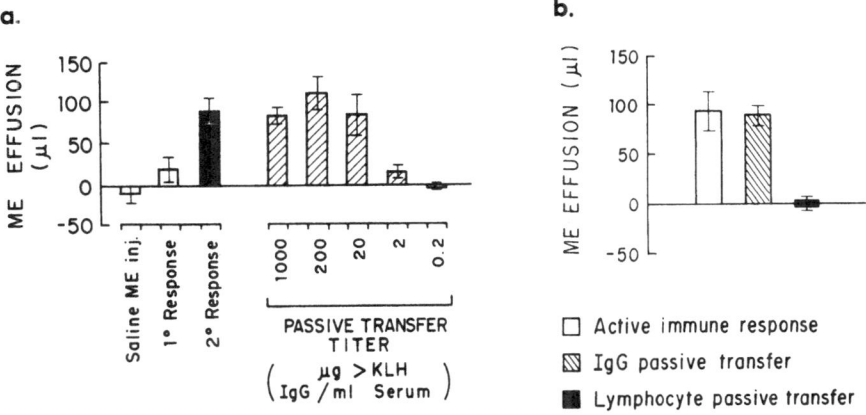

inflation test. These results suggest that immune responses are more likely to produce OME by an increase in vascular permeability in the middle ear mucosa than by edematous closure of the eustachian tube.

Miglets (1973) passively sensitized monkeys with serum from patients allergic to ragweed pollen. When pollen was insufflated into the middle ear through the eustachian tube, the animals developed OME. This result suggests that humoral factors can mediate OME that is produced by immune responses. Ryan and Catanzaro (1983) found that guinea pigs that were passively sensitized only with IgG showed OME upon antigenic challenge of the middle ear. No middle ear response was noted when animals were passively sensitized with lymphocytes (Fig 13-4). These observations indicate that immunologically induced OME is mediated primarily by humoral rather than by cell-mediated immunity. Ryan and Vogel (in press) found that complement depletion with cobra venom factor reduced, but did not eliminate, immune-mediated OME (Fig 13-5). This suggests that complement fixation by immune complexes can be involved in OME. However, since complement depletion does not eliminate immune-mediated OME, it does not appear to be the only mechanism involved. IgG_1 is reagenic in the guinea pig, mast cell degranulation may also play a role. In support of this possibility, Boisvert, Wasserman, Schiff, Catanzaro,

FIG 13-5. Middle ear effusion observed 3 days postchallenge in normal immunized animals, compared with that observed in immunized animals that had been decomplemented with cobra venom factor (CVF). Decomplementation reduced, but did not eliminate, immune-mediated effusion.

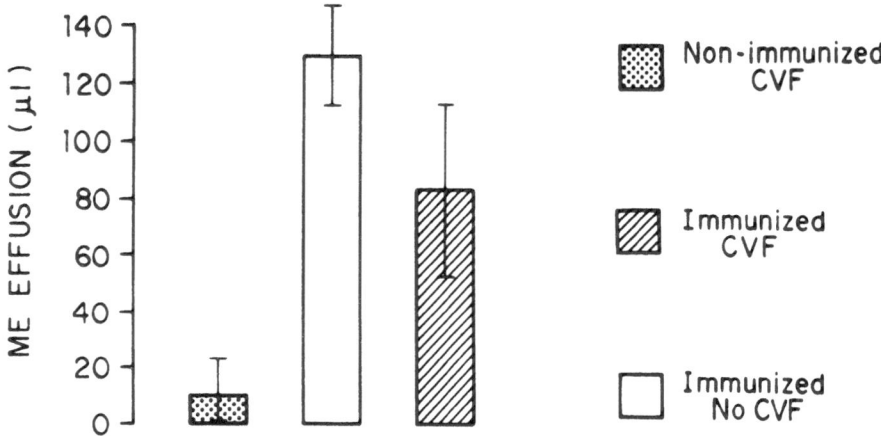

and Ryan (in press) demonstrated that injection of histamine into the middle ear results in effusion, a response that could be partially blocked by antihistamines.

In summary, these experimental models suggest that both immediate hypersensitivity and complement activation have the potential to contribute to OME. There is less experimental evidence to support the role of delayed hypersensitivity. The physical mechanism most likely to mediate OME produced by immune responses is increased vascular permeability in the middle ear mucosa, rather than eustachian tube blockage secondary to edema in the mucosa of the nasopharynx or tube.

Type II Collagen Autoimmunity and Middle Ear Disease

Autoimmunity to Type II collagen, produced by immunization with bovine Type II collagen, has been shown to induce arthritic disease in rats. The effects of this autoimmunity in the ear have been investigated by Yoo and his associates, using primarily rats and guinea pigs. They report that a number of disease states of the middle ear are associated with Type II collagen autoimmunity. These include otospongiotic foci near the tympanic annulus and in the otic capsule (Yoo et al., 1982a), as well as salpingitis (Tomoda and Yoo, 1982). These disease manifestations were frequently associated with mononuclear cell infiltration and vasculitis. An attempt by Harris (1983) to reproduce these findings in a rat model did not result in any manifestations of middle ear disease, even though severe arthritis was produced.

Effect of Middle Ear Immunity on the Inner Ear

Suzuki (1977) previously demonstrated that in the presence of acute middle ear inflammation there was an increase in the protein found within the inner ear. To further investigate the possible passage of immunologic materials across the round window membrane, Harris and Ryan (1984) immunized animals with keyhole limpet hemocyanin (KLH) and bovine serum albumin (BSA) in complete Freund's adjuvant by intradermal injection, and later challenged with KLH in the ME. This resulted in the development of an inflammatory response, which was allowed to continue for 7 days. At the end of this period, the animals were rechallenged in the middle ear with KLH and 3 days later were sacrificed. The resultant ME effusion and perilymph were analyzed for the presence of anti-KLH and anti-BSA antibody by ELISA. Significantly elevated levels of anti-KLH antibody, but not anti-BSA antibody, were present in the inner ear. This result suggests that either antibody or antigen from the ME penetrated the inner ear. Inner ear morphology was normal in these subjects. Injection of KLH into the ME did not result in detectable levels of KLH in perilymph. However, injection of anti-KLH IgG into the ME of unimmunized animals resulted in measurable anti-KLH IgG in perilymph. These results suggest that it was antibody, rather than antigen, which penetrated the round window during immune-mediated otitis media.

The penetration of antibody into the inner ear from a ME immune response is apparently a benign phenomenon in and of itself. However, if antigen, such as bacterial or viral antigen from a middle ear infection, also penetrated the window, this could result in further elaboration of the immune response, with possible damage to the inner ear. This phenomenon could mediate sensorineural hearing loss associated with chronic otitis media.

IMMUNOBIOLOGY OF THE INNER EAR

Experimental Inner Ear Immunology

The inner ear has long been viewed as a delicate neurosensory structure encased in its bony capsule quite isolated from the myriad of organisms which constantly come in contact with our bodies. In considering the natural defenses of the inner ear, one is struck by its lack of apparent lymphatics, regional lymph nodes, or lamina propria rich in macrophages and lymphocytes as seen in other organs of the body. However, upon closer inspection one sees that the perilymph is in communication with the cerebrospinal fluid and is thus a "lymphatic" of sorts and that the connective tissue that encircles the endolymphatic sac does in fact contain immunocompetent cells and may possess lymphatics. Rask-Anderson and Stahle (1980) have shown that the endolymphatic sac is the site of macrophage-lymphocyte interaction. Additionally, Arnold, Morgenstern, and Miyamoto (1981) have demonstrated the presence of immunoglobulin within the endolymphatic sac in humans. Therefore, it is conceivable that this structure plays a role in the defense of the inner ear.

A number of studies have examined the composition of perilymph from humans and animals and have found that it contains immunoglobulins, as well as other blood proteins (Chevance, Galli, & Jeanmarie, 1960; Fritsch & Jolliff, 1966; Mogi, Lim, & Watanabe, 1982; Palva & Raunio, 1967). The predominant immunoglobulin appears to be of the IgG class (Mogi et al., 1982; Palva & Raunio, 1967). The source of inner ear immunoglobulins as well as other proteins appears to be the serum, from which proteins filter across the blood-labyrinthine barrier (Harris, 1983; Juhn & Rybak, 1981; Mogi et al., 1982). Mogi et al. (1982) and Harris (1983) have shown that the higher concentration of immunoglobulin found within the perilymph compared with that found in the CSF is evidence of the independent nature of these fluid compartments with respect to immunoglobulin and may further reflect the independence of their local immune systems.

The appearance of cellular constituents of the immune system as well as immuno-globulin within the inner ear suggests that this organ may have a functioning immune system. To determine whether immune responses occur in the cochlea, or whether the inner ear might be an immunoprivileged site, Harris (1983) performed experiments in which KLH in artificial perilymph was perfused into the perilymphatic compartment of guinea pigs. Two weeks later, animals were found to have low but detectable levels of anti-KLH antibodies. In a second experiment, Harris (1984) immunized animals systemically with both KLH and BSA until high circulating anti-KLH and anti-BSA titers were achieved. These animals were then challenged in the perilymphatic compartment with KLH. All animals developed high anti-KLH titers in perilymph. Moreover, no comparable rise in perilymph anti-BSA titers was observed (Fig 13-6), indicating that the rise in perilymph anti-KLH antibody was locally generated and not derived from serum via increased vascular permeability. Perilymph titers were also independent of CSF titers. These data demonstrate that the inner ear is immunoresponsive, with the capability of generating a primary and a secondary local antibody response. Inner ear immunization was also found to sensitize the host systemically (Harris, 1983), and these observations have recently been confirmed by Mogi (1984).

Kumagami, Nishida, and Dohi (1976) have previously demonstrated the development of a Meniere's-like phenomenon in sensitized rabbits that were challenged within the stylomastoid foramen with the sensitizing antigen. They observed nystagmus and declining cochlear function following this challenge in short-term experiments. Presumably, antigen diffused into the inner ear as a consequence of this injection and resulted in antigen-antibody complexes that produced the observed effects.

To determine the effects of inner ear immune response on cochlear function over a long term, Woolf and Harris performed experiments in which sensitized animals were challenged with KLH in the perilymphatic compartment after baseline electrophysiological recordings. These animals showed a sequential decline in cochlear function, a decline which was not observed in nonsensitized animals that received anti-KLH antibody alone

FIG 13-6. Anti-KLH antibody levels before and 4 weeks after inner ear KLH challenge, in animals previously sensitized to KLH. Note that while serum titers did not change, perilymph titers on the immunized side (Rt.) rose dramatically. Titers in perilymph from the opposite ear (Lt.) and in CSF were much lower: $a > a_3$, $b > b_3$, and $c > c_3$, $p < 0.05$ (Student's t-test). From Harris, 1984.

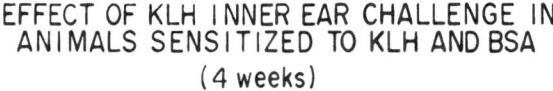

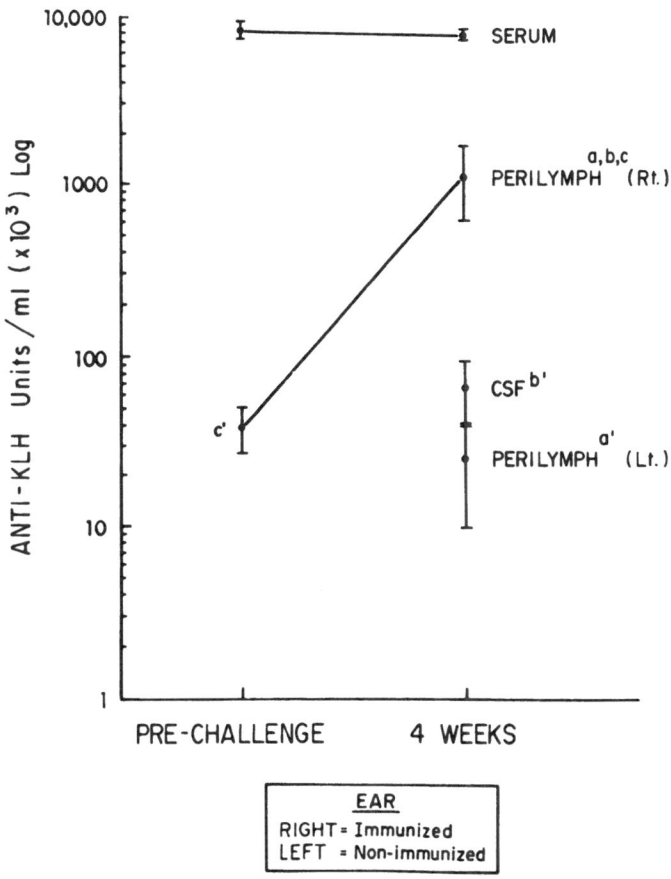

FIG 13-7. Cochlear histology following inner ear inoculation with live guinea pig cytomegalovirus (GPCMV). Arrow demonstrates spiral ganglion cell degeneration. Note the inflammatory infiltrate and hemorrhage within the scala tympani (ST). From Harris et al., 1984a.

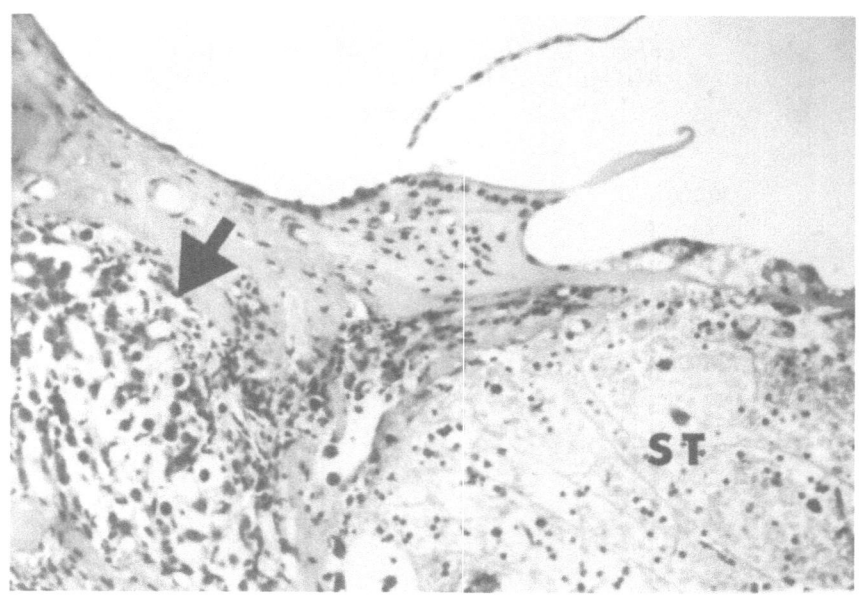

in the inner ear (Woolf & Harris, unpublished observation). These results demonstrate the potentially deleterious effects upon hearing of immune responses in the inner ear.

Recently, Harris, Woolf, Ryan, Butler, and Richman (1984a) developed a model of viral labyrinthitis utilizing guinea pig cytomegalovirus (GPCMV) to assess inner ear immune response to an infectious agent. Animals that were nonimmune to GPCMV showed severe inflammation and hearing loss within 8 days of perilymphatic viral inoculation (Figs 13-7 and 13-8). Animals previously exposed to the virus through systemic inoculation and that developed antibodies to GPCMV showed normal cochlear morphology and hearing preservation when virus was later inoculated into the inner ear (Figs 13-9 and 13-10) (Harris et al., 1984a; Woolf et al., unpublished manuscript). This protection correlated with a rise in specific anti-GPCMV antibody in perilymph (Fig 13-10). These data suggest that inner ear immunity can also serve a protective function in neutralizing this virulent organism. This experiment represents the first demonstration of the protective nature of immunity within the inner ear.

FIG 13-8. Results of a single inner ear inoculation with live GPCMV in nonimmune animals. (a). Note the lack of systemic and inner ear antibody responses to GPCMV by Day 8. (b). Mean eighth nerve action potential recordings demonstrating significantly reduced hearing in the live virus group compared to the group receiving inactivated GPCMV (Psoralen). From Harris et al., 1984a.

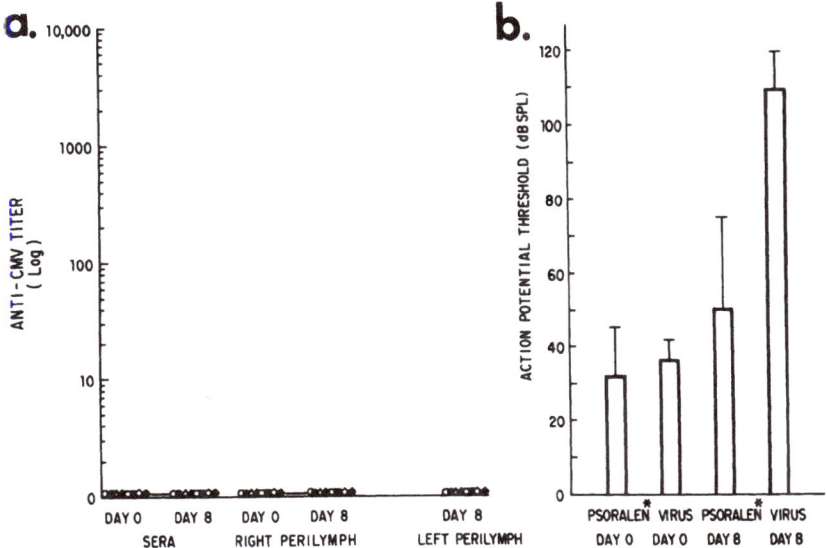

Autoimmune Inner Ear Disease

The role of inner ear immunity in human disease has gained wider acceptance by McCabe's (1979) description of a possibly new clinical entity termed autoimmune sensorineural hearing loss. In this condition, patients suffer from a progressive (over a period of 2 weeks to several months) bilateral sensorineural hearing loss. All patients demonstrate vestibular injury on ENG and 10% of patients have an associated eighth nerve paralysis (McCabe, 1984). They demonstrate increased lymphocyte migration when their peripheral blood lymphocytes are exposed to inner ear antigen in a lymphocyte inhibition assay. However, the nature and specificity of this assay have not been well described. Treatment has involved steroids and cyclophosphamide, often for prolonged periods of time, and plasmaphoresis has been employed for resistant disease. It is of interest that 12 of the currently reported 43 cases have subsequently gone on to develop other autoimmune disorders such as Cogan's syndrome, rheumatoid arthritis, systemic lupus erythematosus, and chronic ulcerative colitis. This is quite important from an etiologic

FIG 13-9. Cochlear histology from an animal with systemic guinea pig cytomegalovirus infection and systemic immunity against GPCMV followed by inner ear challenge with live GPCMV. Note the preservation of sensory structures and the absence of inflammatory cells. From Harris et al., 1984a.

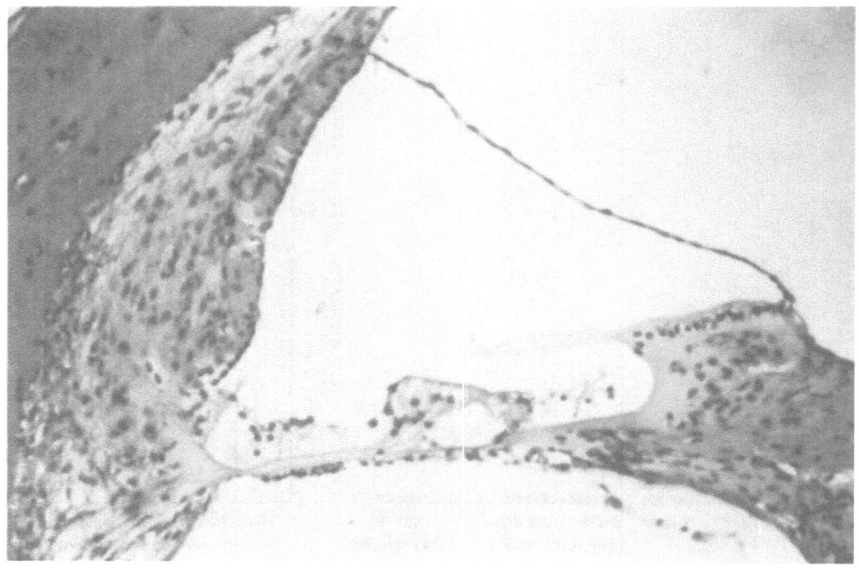

standpoint since inner ear involvement in collagen vascular diseases may be the nonspecific consequence of immune complexes and not the result of specific antibodies and/or cytotoxic T cells directed against inner ear antigens. For instance, the vestibular-auditory symptoms of Cogan's syndrome are believed to be the local manifestation of a generalized periarteritis nodosa (Cody & Williams, 1960; Haynes, Kaiser-Kupfer, Mason et al., 1980; Smith, 1970). Ford and Siekert (1965) reported that 6% of patients with CNS manifestations of periarteritis nodosa had eighth nerve involvement characterized by vertigo and tinnitus. Furthermore, the occurrence of hearing loss, vertigo, and tinnitus in association with Cogan's syndrome following vaccinations for smallpox is further evidence for the role of immune complexes and not specific antibodies to inner ear antigen in this disorder (Cutler, Watters, Hammerstad, & Merlin, 1967; Rosen, 1949). Thus the inner ear is subject to the effects of immune complexes. Hughes, Kinney, Barna, Tomask, and Calabrese (1983) reported the findings of immunological studies performed on two patients with Cogan's syndrome. They found no evidence of humoral immunity toward inner ear antigen or corneal tissue but found one patient who showed lymphocyte transformation on exposure to inner ear antigen. Whether autoimmune sensorineural hearing

FIG 13-10. Results of the development of systemic immunity to GPCMV in guinea pigs, followed by their inner ear challenge with live GPCMV (virus/virus). (a). Note rise of specific anti-GPCMV antibody in the perilymph on the challenged right ear compared to the prechallenged right ear (Day 0) ($p < 0.001$) and nonchallenged left ear ($p < 0.05$). (b). Mean eighth nerve action potential thresholds in these animals compared to a control group that received inactivated GPCMV (Psoralen). Note the protective effect of inner ear antibody on preservation of hearing. From Harris et al., 1984a.

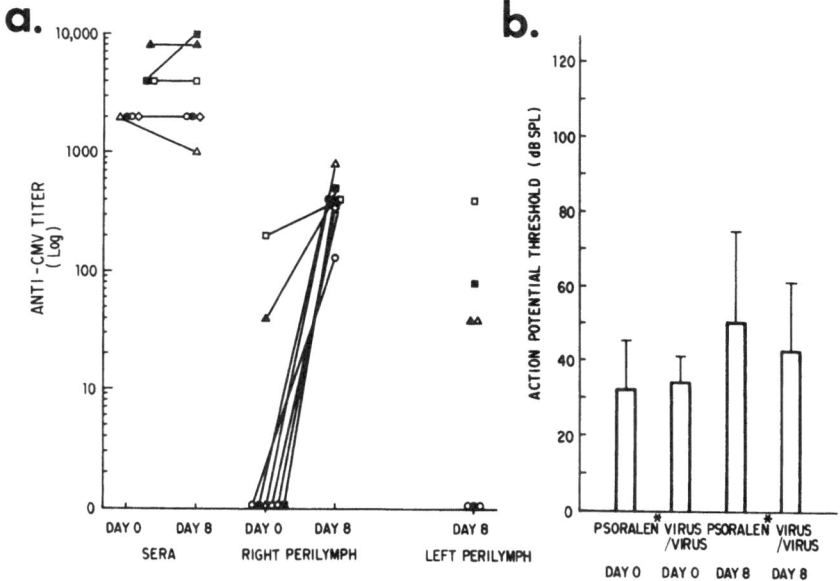

loss is a distinct clinical entity quite apart from a more generalized collagen vascular disease remains to be proven by careful analysis of the inciting antigen and by demonstration of the specificity of the testing procedure.

In an attempt to see if autoimmune inner ear disease might develop as a result of inner ear injury, Harris, Low, and House (1984b) recently undertook a study of the hearing level in the contralateral ear of acoustic tumor patients who underwent unilateral ablative inner ear surgery in the process of tumor removal. It was hypothesized that following this surgery, immunocompetent cells would be exposed and possibly sensitized to hitherto unseen cochlear and vestibular tissue antigens, setting the stage for autoimmunity to the inner ear. Of 380 acoustic tumor patients who successfully underwent removal of their unilateral tumors and had their contralateral hearing assessed audiometrically, 1.3% exhibited unexplained sensorineural hearing losses in the contralateral, uninvolved ear. This incidence was strikingly similar to the reported incidence of sympathetic ophthalmia (0.01%–1%), an autoimmune condition affecting the eye (Liddy & Stuart, 1972; Marak,

1979). Unfortunately, patients were unavailable for immunological investigation; thus, further studies are warranted in order to determine whether an autoimmune event underlies this observation.

Meniere's Disease

The capricious nature of Meniere's disease has defied determination of its etiology. Histopathological studies have demonstrated that there appears to be an overaccumulation of endolymphatic fluid and studies in which the endolymphatic sac is destroyed and the endolymphatic duct is obstructed have resulted in the development of hydrops (Kimura, 1967). Additionally, a number of studies have described histopathological abnormalities of the sac in Meniere's patients, abnormalities which include perisaccular fibrosis, loss of vasculature, degenerating epithelium, and reduction of rugae (Arenberg, Marovitz, & Shaumbaugh, 1970; Schindler, Horn, Jones, & Maglio, 1979; Zechner & Altmann, 1969). Therefore the endolymphatic sac appears to play an important etiological role in this disease. It is also safe to say that Meniere's disease has a number of quite independent causes. Certainly patients who develop delayed endolymphatic hydrops following severe viral inner ear infection, such as mumps, do not have the same etiologic mechanism at play as patients who develop Meniere's disease following a temporal bone fracture which causes physical blockage of the endolymphatic duct. Therefore, in considering an immunological etiology in Meniere's disease, it would be a mistake to assume that every case has an immunological basis. Additionally, even if an immune-mediated disorder originally injured the endolymphatic sac it might be years later that sac dysfunction would result in clinically apparent Meniere's disease, possibly at a time when no further immunological events were occurring. How then might immune mechanisms result in Meniere's disease? A theoretical possibility based upon the apparent lack of other immunological aberrations seen in the vast majority of Meniere's patients would be that host defenses are raised against an inner ear viral infection which, in combination with the cytopathic effects of the virus, nonspecifically causes tissue damage. If the endolymphatic sac were the prime site of this infection, or if the sac were the site where byproducts of the inflammatory process were ultimately cleared from the inner ear, then irreversible injury and dysfunction of the sac might occur. Another mechanism might involve autoimmunity to a specific tissue antigen contained primarily within the inner ear. The origin of autoimmune responses is controversial. However, there are at least two mechanisms by which such responses may be virally induced. In some situations, a virus may contain genetic sequences which are identical to those of the host cell. When an immune response is directed toward this viral epitope, a cross-reacting autoantibody can result (Fujinami, Oldstone, Wroblewski, Frankel, & Koprowski, 1983). Alternatively, antigen might be exposed as the result of an intracellular infection by a virus which may incorporate antigenic determinants of the cell membrane into its capsid, thus provoking an autoantibody when an immune response is directed against the virus. This could ultimately result in both humoral and cell-mediated immunity, causing direct tissue injury in the inner ear. A Gell and Coombs Type II immune response might mediate autoimmune sensorineural hearing loss, as proposed by McCabe (1979) and Yoo (Yoo, Stuart, Kang, Townes, Tomoda, & Dixit, 1982; Yoo, 1984).

Another mechanism may be the development of arteritis within the inner ear from immune complex disease. This might then affect the blood supply and function of the endolymphatic sac and ultimately lead to hydrops. Immune complexes are certainly a well-recognized part of Cogan's syndrome, systemic lupus erythematosus, polyarteritis nodosa, and relapsing polychondritis and may be the cause of the vestibuloauditory symptoms seen on occasion in these disorders. Vasculitis was also the pathological feature seen in the only tissue studied in McCabe's (1979, 1984) series, indicating that immune complex disease was a necessary component of this disorder.

That immediate hypersensitivity reactions mediated through IgE are involved in Meniere's disease seems unlikely since studies of the IgE levels in this disease have uniformly been negative (Stahle, 1976). However, there is some evidence to suggest that immune mechanisms result in endolymphatic hydrops. For instance, in 1961, Fisher and Hellstrom published their findings of temporal bone endolymphatic hydrops in Cogan's syndrome; these findings were subsequently confirmed by Wolff, Bernhard, Tsutsumi et al. (1965). The previously cited animal studies by Kumagami et al. (1976) and Yoo et al. (Yoo, 1984; Yoo et al., 1982) also imply that a Meniere's-like condition can be created by immunological manipulations. Recently, Hughes (1984) presented a preliminary study in which lymphocytes from six patients with Meniere's disease underwent blastogenesis upon exposure to inner ear antigen, suggesting the possibility of an autoimmune event in these individuals. If these results are confirmed and if these patients do not go on to develop other collagen vascular diseases, this would be strong evidence for an immunological basis for Meniere's disease in some patients. It should be cautioned, however, that a necessary requirement for any test of cellular immunity is scrupulous attention to controls of both a positive and a negative nature. For example, when a patient's lymphocytes respond to pooled inner ear tissues it is imperative that a similar pool of "non-inner ear tissue," derived from the same patients from which the inner ear tissues were harvested, be subjected to Meniere's patients' lymphocytes in order to control for nonspecific reactivity of HLA antigens, which are well known stimuli of lymphocyte transformation. Additionally, in tests of immunofluorescence in which patients' sera are incubated with sections of human temporal bone it is absolutely critical that another organ tissue similarly processed be tested in parallel in order to be sure that the fluorescence seen is specific for the inner ear. These tests must be done in conjunction with controls utilizing normal human sera, for in our laboratory we have had many instances of positive fluorescence in the human temporal bone that have proven to be nonspecific when adequate controls have been run simultaneously.

Type II Collagen Autoimmunity and Inner Ear Disease

Recently, Yoo and colleagues have suggested that autoimmunity to Type II collagen may be of etiological importance in otosclerosis and Meniere's disease. This hypothesis is based on their finding that sera of patients with both diseases show increased antibody activity against Type II collagen when compared to sera of normal controls (Yoo et al., 1982). Additionally, animal models of Type II collagen autoimmunity have been produced in rats, guinea pigs, and chinchillas by immunization with homologous Type II collagen (Yoo, 1984; Yoo et al., 1983a, 1983b, 1983c). These animals have been reported to show evidence of otospongiotic changes in the bone of the external meatus and otic capsule (Yoo et al., 1983a), spiral ganglion cell degeneration, arteritis of the cochlear nerve, atrophy of the organ of Corti and stria vascularis (Yoo et al., 1983b), and endolymphatic hydrops with atrophy of the surface epithelium of the endolymphatic duct (Yoo et al., 1983c). Additionally, hearing loss and vestibular dysfunction have been reported in these animals (Yoo et al., 1983b).

Preliminary studies in our laboratory, however, have failed to corroborate these findings in an animal model (Harris, et al., 1983b). Utilizing an identical immunization protocol in Wistar-Furth rats, no short- or long-term (up to 9 months) effects could be found on cochlear microphonic or eighth nerve compound action potential recordings when compared to recordings from control animals. Additionally, no histological lesions could be identified within their temporal bones despite the fact that all of these animals displayed marked arthritis secondary to Type II collagen autoimmunity. The apparent discrepancies between these studies may be the result of the strain differences between our rats and those employed by Yoo and his colleagues. Because this area is one of great interest to many laboratories, additional confirmation should be forthcoming.

CONCLUSION

The ear is an organ that is actively involved in immunologic reactions at several sites. The combination of clinical research and experimental animal models of otoimmunology as described above allows the optimal study of the immune mechanisms involved in human ear disease. As in other organs of the body, many heretofore idiopathic diseases are being recognized as having an immunologic basis. Through immunologic investigation, improved recognition and treatment of these conditions may be realized.

REFERENCES

Arenberg IK, Marovitz W, Shaumbaugh G: The role of the endolymphatic sac in the pathogenesis of endolymphatic hydrops in man. *Acta Otolaryngol (Stockholm)* 1970; Suppl 275.

Arnold W, Morgenstern C, Miyamoto H: Morphology and function of the endolymphatic sac, in Vosteen K-H, Schuknecht H et al (eds): *Meniere's Disease: Pathogenesis, Diagnosis and Treatment.* New York, Thieme-Stratton, 1981, pp 110–114.

Boisvert P, Wasserman SI, Schiff M, Catanzaro A, Ryan AF: Histamine-induced middle ear effusion and mucosal histopathology in the guinea pig. *Ann Otol Rhinol Laryngol* (in press).

Bryan MP, Bryan WTK: Cytologic and immunologic response revealed in middle ear effusions. *Ann Otol Rhinol Laryngol* 1976; 85, Suppl 25: 238–244.

Catanzaro A, Ryan AF, Robb J: Immune-mediated and nonspecific inflammatory events in the middle ear. *Clin Immunol Immunopathol* 1982; 24:361–376.

Chevance LG, Galli A, Jeanmarie J: Immunoelectrophoretic study of human perilymph. *Acta Otolaryngol* 1960; 52: 41–46.

Cody DT, Williams HL: Cogan's syndrome. *Laryngoscope* 1960; 70: 447–478.

Cutler RWP, Watters GU, Hammerstad JP, Merlin E: Origin of cerebrospinal fluid gamma globulin in subacute sclerosing leukoencephalitis. *Arch Neurol* 1967; 17: 620–628.

Fisher ER, Hellstrom HR: Cogan's syndrome and systemic vascular disease. *Arch Pathol* 1961; 72: 96–116.

Ford R, Siekert R: Central nervous system manifestations of periarteritis nodosa. *Neurology* 1965; 15: 114–122.

Fritsch JH, Jolliff CR: Protein components of human perilymph. *Ann Otol* 1966; 75: 1070–1076.

Frootko NJ: Immune responses in allograft tympanoplasty. International Academic Conference in Immunology and Immuno-Pathology as Applied to Otology and Rhinology. Utrecht, The Netherlands. April 12, 1984.

Fujinami R, Oldstone M, Wroblewski Z, Frankel M, Koprowski H: Molecular mimicry in virus infection: Cross reaction of measles virus phosphoprotein or of herpes simplex virus protein with human intermediate filaments. *Proc Natl Acad Sci USA* 1983; 80: 2346–2350.

Harris JP: Immunology of the inner ear: Response of the inner ear to antigen challenge. *Otolaryngol-Head & Neck Surg* 1983; 91: 18–23.

Harris JP: Immunology of the inner ear: Evidence of local antibody production. *Ann Otol Rhinol Laryngol* 1984; 93: 157–162.

Harris JP, Woolf NK, Ryan AF, Butler DM, Richman DD: Immunologic and electrophysiologic response to cytomegalovirus inner ear infection in the guinea pig. *J Infect Dis* 1984a (in press).

Harris JP, Low NC, House WF: Contralateral hearing loss following inner ear injury: Sympathetic cochleolabyrinthitis? *Am J Oto* 1984b (in press).

Harris JP, Woolf NK, Stuart JM: Type II collagen induced autoimmune disease in the inner ear of the rat: Failure to produce pathological effects. Research Forum of the American Academy of Otolaryngology–Head & Neck Surgery and Association for Research in Otolaryngology. Anaheim, CA, October 22, 1983 (manuscript in preparation).

Harris JP, Ryan AF: The effect of a middle ear immune response on inner ear antibody levels. *Ann Otol Rhinol Laryngol* 1984c (in press).

Haynes B, Kaiser-Kupfer MI, Mason P et al: Cogan's syndrome. *Medicine* 1980; 6: 426–441.

Hopp E, Elevitch F, Pumphrey R, Irving T, Hoffman P: Serous otitis media—an "immune" theory. *Laryngoscope* 1965; 74: 1149–1159.

Hughes GB: Immunological Aspects of Meniere's Disease. International Academic Conference in Immunology and Immuno-Pathology as Applied to Otology and Rhinology. Utrecht, The Netherlands. April 11, 1984.

Hughes G, Kinney S, Barna B, Tomask R, Calabrese L: Autoimmune reactivity in Cogan's syndrome. *Otolaryngol-Head & Neck Surg* 1983; 91: 24–32.

Juhn S, Giebink G, Huff J, Mills E: Biochemical and immunochemical characteristics of middle ear effusions in relation to bacteriological findings. *Ann Otol Rhinol Laryngol* 1980; 89, Suppl 68: 161-492.

Juhn SK, Rybak L: Nature of the blood-labyrinth barrier, in Vosteen K-H, Schuknecht H et al (eds): *Meniere's Disease: Pathogenesis, Diagnosis and Treatment.* New York, Thieme-Stratton, 1981, pp 110-114.

Kimura RS: Experimental blockage of the endolymph duct and sac and its effect on the inner ear of the guinea pig. *Ann Otol Rhino Laryngol* 1967; 76: 664-687.

Kumagami H, Nishida H, Dohi K: Experimental labyrinthine lesions through styloid foramen. *ORL* 1976; 38: 334-343.

Laurell A-B, Nilsson N-I, Prellner K: Immune complexes and complement in serous and mucoid otitis media. *Acta Otolaryngol* 1980; 90: 290-296.

Liddy N, Stuart J: Sympathetic ophthalmia in Canada. *Can J Ophthalmol* 1972; 7: 157-159.

Liu Y, Lim D, Lang R, Birck H: Chronic middle ear effusions: Immunochemical and bacteriological investigation. *Arch Otolaryngol* 1975; 101: 278-286.

Marak GE: Recent advances in sympathetic ophthalmia. *Surv Ophthalmol* 1979; 24: 141-156.

McCabe B: Autoimmune sensorineural hearing loss. *Ann Otol Rhinol Laryngol* 1979; 88: 585-589.

McCabe B: Auto-immune Sensorineural Hearing Loss. International Academic Conference in Immunology and Immuno-Pathology as Applied to Otology and Rhinology. Utrecht, The Netherlands. April 11, 1984.

Miglets A: The experimental production of allergic middle ear effusions. *Laryngoscope* 1973; 83:1355-1385.

Mogi G: Inner Ear Immunology. International Academic Conference in Immunology and Immuno-Pathology as Applied to Otology and Rhinology. Utrecht, The Netherlands. April 11, 1984.

Mogi G, Lim D, Watanabe N: Immunologic study on the inner ear. *Arch Otolaryngol* 1982; 108: 270-275.

Palva T, Raunio V: Disc electrophoretic studies of human perilymph. *Ann Otol Rhinol Laryngol* 1967; 76: 23-26.

Poliquin FJ, Catanzaro A, Robb J, Schiff M: Adaptive immunity of the tympanic membrane. *Amer J Otolaryngol* 1981; 2: 94-98.

Rask-Anderson H, Stahle J: Immunodefense of the inner ear? Lymphocyte-macrophage interaction in the endolymphatic sac. *Acta Otolaryngol* 1980; 89: 283-294.

Rosen E: Interstitial keratitis and vestibulo-auditory symptoms following vaccination. *Arch Ophthalmol* 1949; 41: 24-31.

Ryan AF, Catanzaro A: Passive transfer of immune-mediated middle ear effusion and inflammation. *Acta Otolaryngol* 1983; 95: 123-130.

Ryan AF, Cleveland PH, Hartman MT, Catanzaro A: Humoral and cell-mediated immunity in peripheral blood following introduction of antigen into the middle ear. *Ann Otol Rhinol Laryngol* 1982; 91: 70-75.

Ryan AF, Harris JP, Schiff M: Experimental immunology and diseases of the ear. *Ann Otol Rhinol Laryngol* (in press).

Ryan AF, Vogel C-W: Complement depletion by cobra venom factor: Effect on immune-mediated middle ear effusion and inflammation, in Lim D, Bluestone C (eds): *Recent Advances in Otitis Media with Effusion.* Toronto: BC Decker (in press).

Schindler RA, Horn K, Jones P, Maglio M: The ultrastructure of the endolymphatic sac in Meniere's disease. *Laryngoscope* 1979; 89: 95-106.

Schiff M, Catanzaro A, Ryan AF, Poliquin J: Tympanosclerosis: A theory of pathogenesis. *Ann Otol Rhinol Laryngol* 1980; 89, Suppl 70: 1-16.

Smith JL: Cogan's syndrome. *Laryngoscope* 1970; 80: 121–132.

Solow IA: Is serous otitis media due to allergy or infection? *Ann Allerg* 1958; 16: 297–299.

Stahle J: Allergy, immunology, psychosomatic, hypo and hypertonus. *Arch Otol Rhinol Laryngol* 1976; 212: 287–292.

Suzuki Y: Immunological studies on inner ear fluids under the influence of acute middle ear inflammation. *J Otolaryngol Jpn* 1977; 6: 618–626.

Tomoda K, Yoo TJ: Type II collagen induced autoimmune salpingitis. Research Forum of the American Academy of Otolaryngology-Head & Neck Surgery and Association for Research in Otolaryngology. New Orleans, October 15–17, 1982.

Veldman JE: Immunopathology of cholesteatoma. International Academic Conference in Immunology and Immuno-Pathology as Applied to Otology and Rhinology. Utrecht, The Netherlands. April 11, 1984.

Veltri R, Sprinkle P: Secretory otitis media: An immune complex disease. *Ann Otol Rhinol Laryngol* 1976; 85 Suppl 25: 135–139.

Wolff D, Bernhard WG, Tsutsumi S et al: The pathology of Cogan's syndrome causing profound deafness. *Ann Otol Rhinol Laryngol* 1965; 74: 507–519.

Woolf NK, Harris JP: Unpublished observation.

Woolf NK, Harris JP, Ryan AF, Butler B, Richman D: Experimental cytomegalovirus infection of the inner ear of the guinea pig: Systemic immunity prevents hearing loss (unpublished manuscript).

Yamashita T, Okazaki N, Kumazawa T: Relation between nasal and middle ear allergy: Experimental study. *Ann Otol Rhinol Laryngol* 1980; 89 (Suppl 68): 147–152.

Yoo TJ: Etiopathogenesis of Meniere's disease. *Abstracts, ARO.* St. Petersburg Beach, FL, Feb, 1984.

Yoo TJ, Stuart JM, Kang AH, Townes AS, Tomoda K, Dixit S: Type II collagen autoimmunity in otosclerosis and Meniere's disease. *Science* 1982, 217: 1153–1155.

Yoo TJ, Tomoda K, Kang AH, Stuart JM, Townes AS: Type II collagen-induced autoimmune otospongiosis: A preliminary report. *Ann Otol Rhinol Laryngol* 1983a; 92: 103–108.

Yoo TJ, Tomoda K, Stuart JM, Cremer MA, Townes AS, Kang AH: Type II collagen-induced autoimmune sensorineural hearing loss and vestibular dysfunction in rats. *Ann Otol Rhinol Laryngol* 1983b; 92: 267–271.

Yoo TJ, Yazawa Y, Tomoda K, Floyd R: Type II collagen-induced autoimmune endolymphatic hydrops in the guinea pig. *Science* 1983c; 222: 65–67.

Zechner G, Altmann F: Histological studies of the human endolymph duct and sac. *Pract Oto-rhino-laryngol* 1969; 31: 64–83.

Author Index

A

Aalberse, R. C., 163, 164
Aaron, T. H., 178
Aas, K., 160, 183, 190
Abdou, N. I., 269
Ada, G. L., 294
Adamson, I. Y. R., 108
Ades, E. W., 107
Adkinson, N. F., Jr., 184, 191, 197
Adorini, L., 31
Ahlstedt, S., 123
Albini, B., 147, 148, 152
Albrite, J. P., 279
Alderson, M., 268
Alexander, H. L., 160
Alexander, J. C., 261, 267
Alexander, S., 260
Ali, M., 130
Allegra, J., 268
Alling, D. W., 252
Alper, Ch. A., 106
Alroy, J., 224
Alspaugh, M. A., 224
Altenau, M. M., 283
Altman, A., 69, 72, 74
Altmann, F., 338
Amadio, F. J., 191
Ammann, A. J., 240, 258, 265
Anderson, B., 123
Anderson, C. L., 162
Anderson, M. C., 190
Anderson, V., 131, 219
Andre, C., 125
Araneo, B. A., 31
Arbesman, C. E., 117, 195
Arenberg, I. K., 338
Arnason, B. G., 294
Arnaud, P., 107

Arnold, W., 331
Arrendal, H., 268
Arroyave, C. M., 219
Askenase, P. W., 94, 109, 238, 240
Astaldi, G., 266
Atassi, M. Z., 27
Atkinson, J. P., 252
Atrache, V., 166
Augustin, R., 194
Aune, T. M., 91
Austen, K. F., 64, 67, 69, 161, 164, 165, 166, 167, 168, 170, 219, 252
Austen, W. G., 168
Austin, D. F., 279

B

Babb, J. L., 123
Bach, F. H., 248
Bach, M. K., 162
Back, N., 143, 148, 150, 152
Backman, R. Z., 133
Baer, H., 190
Baggiolini, M., 8
Bainton, D. F., 2
Baklien, K., 121, 122
Baldwin, R. W., 263
Balestra, S. T., 268
Ballantyne, J. C., 297
Balner, H., 295
Banas, J. M., 199
Bansal, S. C., 263
Barker, C. F., 298
Barna, B., 336
Barnard, J. H., 160
Basham, C., 263
Baskies, A. M., 267
Bass, D. A., 169, 170

T

U

Y

Z

Subject Index

Page numbers in *italics* refer to illustrations; (t) indicates tables.

A

Adenoid(s), cellular immunity and, 131–132
  humoral immunity and, 130
  immunology of, 129–132
  microbiology of, 132
Adenoiditis, 129–133
Adenotonsillectomy, guidelines for, 132–133
Adjuvant(s), 31–32
  definition of, ix
Agammaglobulinemia, acquired, 238
  X-linked infantile, 234–238, *239*
Aging, and cancer, 270
Alcoholism, and head and neck cancer, 269
Allergen(s), bridging of IgE Fab portions
      by, 161, *161*
  nature of, 173
  standardization of, 190–191, 190(t)
Allergic diseases, controversial diagnostic
      and treatment procedures for,
      196–197
Allergic hypersensitivity reactions, types of,
      x
Allergy, nasal, 159–202. See also *Rhinitis*.
  and genetics of atopic disease, 172–173
  basic mechanisms of, 160–164, *161*
  chemical mediators in, 164–168, 165(t)
  complications of immunotherapy or
      skin testing, 192–194, 193(t)
  controversial diagnostic and treatment
      procedures for, 196–197
  diagnostic procedures for, 179–184
  immunoglobulins in, 160–163, *161*
  immunopharmacology of, 168–169
  skin testing in, 179–181
  treatment of, 184–192
  by tolerogens, 200–201
  immunotherapy of, 189–202

Allograft(s), in tympanoplasty, immuno-
      histophysiology of, 291–311
  middle ear, cell biological considerations,
      311–312
    immunological considerations, 312–317,
      318, 319
    reaction by, and X-irradiation, 296–297,
      297
Alum-precipitated extracts, for treatment of
      allergy, 198
Autoinjection, of urine, as allergy
      treatment, 196
Amyloidoses, 226
Anaphylatoxin(s), 60
  C5a, biological properties of, 60, 62(t)
  role of in nasal allergy, 165(t), 168
Angioedema-urticaria, 219
Angioneurotic edema, hereditary, 252, *253,*
      254
Antibody(ies), blocking, in nasal allergy,
      163
  conformational changes in antigen-
      antibody reactions, 48
  definition of, ix
  production of, regulation of, 71–72
Antigen(s), 24–32
  and antigenic determinants, 25–32
  complex, antigenic determinants of,
      28–29
  definition of, ix
  excess of, serum blocking activity and,
      263–264, *265*
  immunogenicity of, physical and chemical
      requirements for, 24–25
  low levels of, serum blocking activity
      and, *266*
  recall, 259–260
  T independent, 31

O

Opsonization, C3b, 60
Organisms, specific classes of, and special
    susceptibility to infection, 233(t)
Ossiculoplasty, 280–291
Otitis media, 327–330
    acute, cellular immune response in, with
        effusion, 140–141
    experimental, animal models in,
        141–142
    humoral, immune response in, 139–140
    immunology of, 139–143
    specific immunotherapy for prevention
        of, 142–143
    immunology of, 137–152
    middle ear effusion in, 138, 328–330,
        328, 329, 330
    nonacute, nonpurulent with effusion,
        immunopathogenesis of, 143–152
Otolaryngology, transplantation in, 278–317

P

PAF. See *Platelet activating factor.*
Peptidase, role of in nonspecific host
    defense, 105
Peptidase inhibitors, role of in nonspecific
    host defense, 105
Peyer's patches, 112–113
Phagocytes, mononuclear, 11–13, *12*
Phagocytosis, disorders of, 251
Plasma cells, 6, *7*
Plasmocytes, in lamina propria of colon,
    121
Platelet activating factor, 78
    role of in nasal allergy, 165(t), 167
Pollinex, 200
Polymorphonuclear leukocytes, 7–11, *8*
Polyps, nasal, and rhinitis, 177–178

Precipitin curve, between antigen and
    antibody, *47*
Prostaglandins, role of in nasal allergy,
    165(t), 167
Proteoglycans, structural, 80
Pseudoepinephrine, combined with
    antihistamines, in treating nasal
    allergy, 187
Pyridine-treated extracts, for treating
    allergy, 198

R

Radioallergosorbent test, for nasal allergy,
    183–184
Radioimmunosorbent test, for IgE, in nasal
    allergy, 183
RAST. See *Radioallergosorbent test.*
Reactions, late phase IgE-mediated, 181
Reactivity, lymphocyte, in cancer, 262–263
Recall antigens, 259–260
Reticuloendothelial system, 7–13
Rhinitis, allergic, 175–176. See also *Allergy,*
        nasal.
    intranasal immunotherapy for, 194
    treatment of, 185–189. See also
        Immunotherapy, for nasal allergy.
    classification of, 174–175
    clinical diagnosis and management of,
        174–184
    diagnostic procedures for, 179–184
    eosinophilic nonallergic, 174–175
    hormonal, 177
    IgE-mediated versus non-IgE-mediated,
        216–218
    nasal polyps and, 177–178
    nonallergic, 176–179
    vasomotor, 174–175
Rhinitis medicamentosa, 177
Rinkel method, 196–197
RIST. See *Radioimmunosorbent test.*

X